Fine Needle Aspiration Biopsy of the Head and Neck

Austin,

Congrats on a great year.

We are delighted you are joining our family.

May all your aspirations come true

Colette
2016

Fine Needle Aspiration Biopsy of the Head and Neck

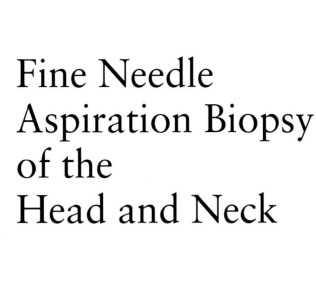

Celeste N. Powers, M.D., Ph.D.

Associate Professor of Pathology and Otolaryngology,
Director of Cytopathology, State University of New York
Health Science Center, Syracuse, New York

William J. Frable, M.D.

Professor of Pathology and Director of Surgical and
Cytopathology, Medical College of Virginia,
Richmond, Virginia

Butterworth-Heinemann

Boston Oxford Johannesburg Melbourne New Delhi Singapore

Every effort has been made to ensure that the drug dosage schedules within this text are accurate and conform to standards accepted at time of publication. However, as treatment recommendations vary in the light of continuing research and clinical experience, the reader is advised to verify drug dosage schedules herein with information found on product information sheets. This is especially true in cases of new or infrequently used drugs.

Recognizing the importance of preserving what has been written, Butterworth–Heinemann prints its books on acid-free paper whenever possible.

Library of Congress Cataloging-in-Publication Data
Powers, Celeste N.
Fine-needle aspiration biopsy of the head and neck / Celeste N. Powers, William J. Frable
p. cm.
Includes bibliographical references and index.
ISBN 0-7506-9503-X
1. Head—Biopsy, Needle. 2. Neck—Biopsy, Needle. I. Frable, William J. II. Title.
[DNLM: 1. Biopsy, Needle—methods. 2. Head and Neck Neoplasms—pathology. 3. Salivary Gland Diseases—pathology. 4. Thyroid Diseases—pathology. 5. Lymphatic Diseases—pathology. WE 707 P888f 1996]
RC936.P69 1996
617.5′107582—dc20
DNLM/DLC
for Library of Congress 96-5026
CIP

British Library Cataloguing-in-Publication Data
A catalogue record for this book is available from the British Library.

The publisher offers special discounts on bulk orders of this book.

For information, please write:
Manager of Special Sales
Butterworth–Heinemann
313 Washington Street
Newton, MA 02158-1626
Tel: 617-928-2500
Fax: 617-928-2620

For information on all medical publications available, contact our World Wide Web home page at: http://www.bh.com/bh/

10 9 8 7 6 5 4 3 2 1

Printed in the United States of America

To my mentors at Virginia Commonwealth University, the Medical College of Virginia, Richmond, Virginia, and Dr. Paula R. Larson, my first fellow.

CNP

To the fellows and residents, graduates of the Department of Pathology, Virginia Commonwealth University, Medical College of Virginia. Your success has made it all worthwhile.

WJF

Contents

Preface

Fine needle aspiration biopsy continues to evolve as a rapid, safe, and cost-effective procedure for the diagnosis of palpable masses from a variety of both superficial and deep sites. This book, representing another example of site- or area-specific monographs on fine needle aspiration biopsy, focuses on lesions of the head and neck. It is intended for clinicians, pathologists, and fellows and residents who are interested in the techniques of fine needle aspiration biopsy, cytopathologic criteria, and clinical correlations that are necessary to diagnose the large variety of lesions occurring in the head and neck.

This book represents the accumulated experience of interventional cytopathologists and includes detailed descriptions of the various techniques used to obtain suitable material for diagnosis with minimal clinical impact on the patient. In addition to highlighted diagnostic criteria, the major sections of this work also present problems, pitfalls, and complications that can occur and ways to avoid them. Because of the development of rapid staining methods, aspiration biopsy is available for immediate, on-site interpretation as an important aid in patient diagnosis and management. As a result, the reader will find many color illustrations of both Romanowsky- and Papanicolaou-stained aspiration smears.

CNP and WJF

Acknowledgments

The authors wish to thank the following individuals for their support in this project: Dr. Robert M. Kellman, Professor and Chair, Department of Otolaryngology, State University of New York, Health Science Center, at Syracuse, New York; Dr. Patricia J. Numann, Professor of Surgery, State University of New York, Health Science Center, at Syracuse, New York; Dr. Paul E. Wakely Jr., Director of Cytopathology, Virginia Commonwealth University, Medical College of Virginia, Richmond, Virginia; and many former faculty members of the Division of Surgical and Cytopathology, Virginia Commonwealth University, Medical College of Virginia, Richmond, Virginia—fellows, residents, and referring pathologists who have contributed interesting fine needle aspiration cases.

We would also like to thank the following individuals for administrative and technical support: Cindy T. Steele, SCT (ASCP), Senior Cytotechnologist, State University of New York, Health Science Center, at Syracuse, New York; Diane Street, Administrative Secretary, Cytopathology, State University of New York, Health Science Center, at Syracuse, New York; and Kit L. Hefner, MS, CMI, Medical Illustrator, State University of New York, Health Science Center, at Syracuse, New York.

Chapter

1 Introduction and Techniques

Fine needle aspiration biopsy (FNAB) is a simple, quick, and inexpensive method that is used to sample superficial masses and usually is performed in the office or clinic setting. It causes minimal trauma to the patient and carries virtually no risk of complications. Masses located within the region of the head and neck, including salivary gland and thyroid lesions, can be readily diagnosed using this technique. The intent of this book is to provide a concise, practical approach to the performance and diagnosis of FNAB of the head and neck.

HISTORY OF FINE NEEDLE ASPIRATION BIOPSY

In 1930, Dr. Hayes Martin, an American surgeon and radiotherapist, first published a paper on the needle aspiration method, using an 18-gauge needle.[1] Sixty cases from a variety of body sites, including breast, lung, and head and neck organs (lymph nodes, thyroid and salivary glands), were described in his original series. Martin worked in close collaboration with Dr. Fred Stewart, attending pathologist and successor to James Ewing as Director of Pathology at Memorial Sloan Kettering Cancer Center in New York. Dr. Stewart became proficient in interpreting both aspiration smears and histologic sections of the very small core fragments of tissue that were procured with the 18-gauge needle. Stewart's 1933 publication on diagnosis by the aspiration method is still one of the largest personal series ever reported.[2]

The development of the fine needle method, using yet smaller diameter needles, occurred in Europe after World War II in The Netherlands at Leiden, at the Karolinska Institute in Stockholm, Sweden, and in Lund, also in Sweden.[3–6] The physicians at these centers, with one exception, were not pathologists but hematologists. Like Martin, they wished to have a quick bedside diagnostic method for palpable tumors, and they were capable of both obtaining and interpreting their own aspiration smears. They adapted the Romanowsky staining methods (May-Grunwald-Giemsa, Giemsa alone, and Wright's stain) for the interpretation of epithelial lesions, as well as hematologic processes. They found that the use of fine needles, rather than the larger 18-gauge needles, allowed rapid, good cytologic sampling, with little or no discomfort to the patient. This method was also virtually free of complications. In the late 1960s and early 1970s, a few pathologists and some clinicians in the United States were exposed to the work of the group at the Karolinska Institute in Stockholm.[7,8] This kindled a revival of aspiration biopsy using fine needle techniques in the United States; interest was subsequently fueled by radiologists when diagnostic imaging became available.[9,10] The practice of FNAB continues to evolve.[11–16]

DEFINITION OF FINE NEEDLE ASPIRATION BIOPSY

While the original concept used an 18-gauge needle and local anesthesia to sample relatively large masses thought to be neoplastic, the current *fine needle* aspiration method employs 22, 23, and 25 or higher gauge needles. The use of these thin needles causes very few problems; by contrast, it can be demonstrated that the larger the external diameter of the needle, the greater the likelihood of complications. A recent comprehensive review by one of the authors (CNP) found that complications from superficial FNAB of the head and neck are exceedingly rare and result from poor technique, an inappropriate number of passes, and the use of large gauge (larger than 22-gauge) needles.[17] Currently, most physicians

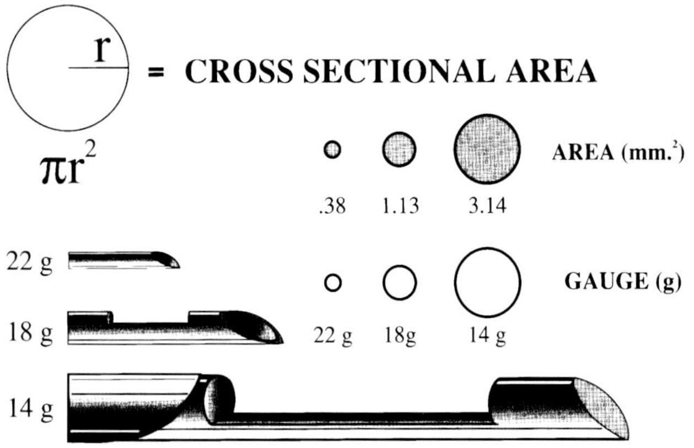

FIGURE 1.1 Comparison of needle size with cross-sectional area. (Reprinted with permission from Powers CN. *1995 Cytopathology Annual.* ASCP Press, Chicago, Illinois: 1996.)

experienced with aspiration biopsy agree that needles with an outside diameter greater than 1.4 millimeters (larger than 22-gauge) should not be categorized as *fine needles* (Figure 1.1). The selection of the appropriate needle gauge will depend on the location and consistency of the mass to be aspirated. Aspiration biopsy performed in the area of the head and neck as well as all other body sites, by the authors, involves the use of 22- to 25-gauge needles.

The concept of fine needle *aspiration* biopsy implies the use of negative pressure to facilitate the withdrawal of cells and/or fluid from masses. During FNAB, attempts to manipulate a 10- or 20-milliliter syringe attached to the fine needle to create some suction is very cumbersome and often results in an inadequate sample and/or excessive bleeding. A variety of syringe holders have been developed that allow application of negative pressure with one hand, while the other hand maintains a firm grasp of and isolates the target lesion.[18]

Fine needle biopsy *without aspiration* is a technique that can be useful in a variety of situations, particularly aspiration of the thyroid, the so-called needle-only method.[19,20] A fine needle without attached syringe is used to penetrate the mass. Cells are drawn up into the needle hub by a combination of rapid back-and-forth movements within the mass and the effects of capillary pressure. If fluid is encountered, a syringe can be attached to the needle to collect the material for specimen processing. A surprisingly large sample can be obtained using the needle-only technique. Because the aspirator has more direct control over the needle, this procedure is quite valuable for very small, superficial masses such as skin lesions and small lymph nodes and for lesions of the thyroid where it tends to reduce the amount of blood that is obtained. This technique is also useful in children who are often nervous and uncooperative during the biopsy.

PRECAUTIONS IN PERFORMING FINE NEEDLE ASPIRATION BIOPSY

Obviously, fine needle aspiration biopsy is a procedure in which the physician works directly with uncapped needles. Any insecurity with the aspiration biopsy procedure can result in trauma to the patient and potential endangerment to the person performing the FNAB. The potential for needle sticks is greater when the patient is extremely nervous or agitated. Proceeding with FNAB in this situation is questionable. It is not wise to attempt aspiration with an uncooperative patient. If FNAB is the modality of choice, then mild to moderate sedation with or without restraint is recommended. Restraint may be necessary in the pediatric population, in which even slight movement of the head can result in not sampling a small head or neck mass.

WHO PERFORMS THE ASPIRATION BIOPSY?

The question, "Who should perform FNAB?" has been debated in the literature as well as in many clinics and hospitals across the United States.[3,7,11,12,15,21–24] To achieve success with aspiration biopsy, a close working relationship needs to be established between the clinician and the cytopathologist, regardless of who performs the biopsy. However, the general consensus is that only individuals who have been trained or have acquired the necessary experience—be they surgeons, clinicians, or pathologists—should perform FNAB. Interventional cytopathologists are pathologists with added qualifications in cytopathology who perform as well as interpret aspirations. Stewart's admonition of 60 years ago still holds today:

> "Aspiration biopsy is as good as the combined intelligence of the clinician and [the] pathologist [who] makes it."[2]

EQUIPMENT

The ease and affordability of FNAB are major reasons for its popularity. A syringe holder (*aspiration gun*) is perhaps the only piece of "capital" equipment required; the remaining items, such as syringes, needles, and slides, are all disposable and can be found in clinics and hospitals as routinely stocked supplies. Special needles with a side slot, *side-port needles,* have been designed for FNAB to increase the yield of sample, but the authors have found them to be more traumatic than conventional needles of 22 gauge and higher. However, this type of needle may sometimes be useful in breast aspiration but is not recommended for masses in the head and neck. Table 1.1 lists the ancillary supplies needed for superficial FNAB.

A small plastic tray conveniently holds all the equipment and can be taken to clinics, to the bedside,

TABLE 1.1 Basic Equipment Required for Fine Needle Aspiration Biopsy

1. Syringe holder or *aspiration gun.*
   a. Cameco Syringe Pistol, 20.0 and 10.0 mL. Available from Precision Dynamics Corporation, 13,880 Del Sur St., San Fernando, CA 91340-3490. 1-800-847-0670.
   b. Aspir-Gun. Available from Everst Company, 5 Sherman Street, Linden, New Jersey 07036.
   c. Inrad Aspiration Biopsy Syringe Gun. Available from INRAD Inc., 620 Watson S.W., Grand Rapids, Michigan 49504. 1-800-253-1540.
2. 10.0 or 20.0 mL disposable plastic syringe with Luer Lok® Tip (Becton Dickinson & Company, Rutherford, NJ), depending on aspiration gun handle size. Available from Becton Dickinson, Division of Becton Dickinson & Company, Rutherford, NJ 07070.
3. 22–25 gauge 0.6–1.0 mm external diameter disposable needles, 3.8 cm and 8.8 cm, 15.0 and 20.0 cm long, with or without stylus (used for most aspirations of palpable lumps and deep masses). Available from Becton Dickinson, Division of Becton Dickinson & Company, Rutherford, NJ 07070.
4. Alcohol prep sponges. Antiseptic sponges for deeper aspirations, transabdominal, transthoracic, bone, or deep soft tissue.
5. Sterile gauze pads.
6. Microscopic glass slides with frosted ends.
7. Small vial of balanced salt solution and/or RPMI® (Bio Whittaker, Walkersville, MD) tissue culture transport media.
8. Suitable alcohol spray fixatives for immediate fixation of wet smears.
9. Vial of local anesthetic, 1–2% lidocaine, is optional. Topical spray anesthesia for aspirates in children or intraoral aspirates is useful.
10. Small vial of buffered glutaraldehyde for fixing aspirate for electron microscopy if required.

and into the operating room.[25] Local anesthetic is recommended for FNAB of oral mucosal masses but is rarely necessary for other clinically palpable lumps. The authors use a few milliliters of 1 percent lidocaine after checking with the patient for any history of an allergic reaction to anesthetics. It is important not to use too much local anesthesia, because the mass may get lost within a large area infiltrated with the anesthetic. There are also topical spray and "gun injection" types of anesthesia that can be useful to numb the skin surface or the oral mucosa. Deeper anesthesia in the oral cavity can be administered in the same manner as a dentist using a 30-gauge needle attached to a special gun that contains a small vial of lidocaine.[15] FNAB may be repeated during one procedure as many times as necessary to procure sufficient amounts of cellular material for conventional diagnostic purposes and for special stains, immunohistochemistry, flow cytometry, molecular diagnostic techniques, and electron microscopy.

INFORMED CONSENT

As with any biopsy procedure, the patient should be informed about what to expect. The authors have used the analogy of drawing blood. That is, the procedure will take no longer to perform nor be more uncomfortable than a successful venipuncture. An explanatory brochure that reviews the FNAB procedure can be provided to the patient for the initial visit. This should include the general indications for FNAB, what the biopsy is intended to accomplish, and a brief discussion of the few potential complications. The brochure can be sent ahead with an appointment letter in the case of referrals to the cytopathologist, or it can be made available at the time the patient registers, to be read in the waiting room.

Obtaining written consent for FNAB is a matter of personal choice and clinic and/or hospital policy, depending upon the potential exposure to medical liability. Some may choose to have the patient sign a standard procedure consent form or a specific consent form developed for the FNAB Service.[15] The former tends to have unrelated and often serious complications listed that may needlessly worry patients. A simple and concise form designed for FNAB can save time and energy (see Appendix 1.1). While written consent for the aspiration of superficial masses may be optional in some hospitals, most interventional cytopathologists will recommend that written consent be obtained from one or both parents in the case of a child's FNAB. The initial meeting between patient and the cytopathologist or clinician who will perform the aspiration is an appropriate time to explain the procedure, obtain a brief history, answer any of the patient's questions, and obtain verbal or written consent.

HISTORY AND PHYSICAL EXAM

Knowledge of the clinical problem of any patient undergoing FNAB is important. Prior to the aspiration biopsy, the cytopathologist or clinician should carefully review the patient's history and determine the clinical problem in relation to the lesion to be biopsied. This will first enable the physician to decide whether the biopsy is appropriate. A specific and detailed description of the location of the mass for biopsy, its consistency upon aspiration, the clinical history of the patient, and the clinician's differential diagnosis need to be clearly communicated on the requisition and report forms by the aspirator or personally provided to the cytopathologist. A requisition form designed specifically for FNAB enables rapid documentation of appropriate data (see Appendix 1.2).

To successfully perform FNAB, it is very important to correctly position the patient and locate and stabilize the mass. Take the time to examine patients thoroughly and reassure them while they wait for the actual FNAB. The region containing the mass should be palpated not only to determine the exact location of the lesion to be sampled but to determine its relationship to surrounding structures. The aspirator should determine the depth of the target for biopsy as well as the optimal direction to approach the lesion to accomplish the aspiration biopsy. Subcutaneous or deep-seated masses are usually best approached directly and perpendicular to the skin surface. Superficial and very small tumors are best sampled by penetrating the skin in a nearly horizontal plane, subsequently probing for the mass with the tip of the needle.

While techniques specific for the various organs or regions of the head and neck are discussed in the appropriate chapters, the main concern is that the patient is placed in a comfortable position for the aspiration biopsy with the mass readily palpable and easily stabilized during the procedure (Figure 1.2).

Positioning is extremely important for head and neck masses, where the prominence of an enlarged lymph node or lump may depend on whether the patient is lying down or sitting up. Most patients instinctively want to be supine for the FNAB, but this may not always be the best position for masses in the head and neck region. If an adjustable examination chair with head rest is not available, it is useful to begin the examination with the patient sitting on the edge of the examination table facing you.

The sternocleidomastoid muscle and its relationship to the cervical lymph nodes mandates positioning the patient so that a minimum of soft tissue is traversed before reaching the target. Aspirating through any large muscle mass should be avoided because muscle tissue may fill the needle and grossly simulate a good sample.

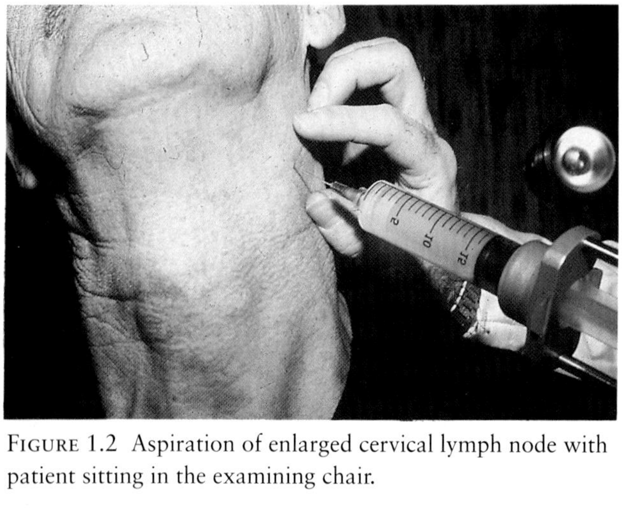

FIGURE 1.2 Aspiration of enlarged cervical lymph node with patient sitting in the examining chair.

The sternocleidomastoid muscle is also an important landmark with respect to thyroid aspirations. This muscle forms the lateral border of a groove bounded medially by the trachea. Within this groove, nodules of the thyroid can be isolated and immobilized. Aspirating in a perpendicular plane along this groove can be done with no fear of puncturing the carotid artery or plugging up the needle with muscle tissue. A reference point for deep-lying thyroid nodules is the transverse vertebral process.[16] Hitting this process with the tip of the needle indicates that the entire substance of the thyroid has been traversed.

THE ASPIRATION BIOPSY PROCEDURE

Once FNAB is determined to be justified, several sequential steps should be followed (Table 1.2). The mass should be firmly grasped with one hand, usually with two fingers. For a very small mass, it may be better to push the lesion into a position where it seems fixed and stable, keeping the skin taut over the mass. Prepare the skin with an alcohol sponge as for a venipuncture. The tip of the needle with syringe pistol attached is laid against the skin at the predetermined puncture site. With a quick and smooth motion, the needle is inserted through the skin and advanced into the mass. Puncture of the target lesion may be tested by differences in resistance, sensing that a capsule is penetrated. Slight lateral motion of the syringe may also indicate that the mass has been penetrated because it will move under the palpating fingers. When the mass has been penetrated, about one-third suction should be applied to the aspirating syringe. The amount of suction is modified in accordance with the type of target. For example, in the thyroid, which is quite vascular, minimal or no suction is often sufficient to obtain a biopsy. Exceptions to that observation may occur with some tumors and chronic forms of thyroiditis where there is significant fibrous tissue. Cases of chronic sialoadenitis and reactive lymph nodes may also produce excessive blood if too much suction is applied.

The needle should be moved back and forth within the target mass with quick and short strokes and in very slightly different directions. The aspiration needle should describe a small cone within the mass to be most effective.[16] The apex of the cone is at the point where the needle penetrates the skin. If the target is large, multiple separate aspirates are indicated describing overlapping cones.[16] For obtaining aspirates of high quality, it is critical to keep the sample within the needle, avoiding aspirating excessive blood or fluid that dilutes the cellular composition of the specimen. The first appearance of any sample at the junction of the syringe and the needle (needle hub) is the appropriate time to release the trigger of the syringe pistol and let the vacuum in the syringe equate to normal. For most cases, the aspiration itself is of very short duration.

TABLE 1.2 Performance of the Aspiration Biopsy

1. By palpation, attempt to determine the location of the lesion to be biopsied in relation to surrounding structures. Estimate its depth. Assess the optimal direction for approach to accomplish the aspiration biopsy.
2. Place the patient in a comfortable position for the procedure but with the mass readily palpable and easily grasped during the aspiration biopsy.
3. Grasp the lesion with one hand, usually between two fingers, or push it into a position where it seems fixed and stable.
4. Prepare the skin with an alcohol sponge as for venipuncture.
5. Lay the syringe pistol with attached needle against the skin at the determined puncture site and angle.
6. With a quick motion, insert the needle through the skin.
7. Advance the needle into the mass.
8. Puncture of the target may be tested by differences in resistance, feeling that a capsule was penetrated, or by moving the syringe pistol very slightly laterally to detect a corresponding movement of the mass beneath the fingers.
9. Apply suction to the aspirating syringe, usually about one-third the length of the syringe barrel.
10. Move the needle back and forth within the tumor with short, quick strokes and in slightly different directions.
11. Note at all times the junction of the needle and the hub of the syringe for the appearance of any specimen.
12. At the first appearance of any sample at the junction of the syringe and the needle, release the trigger of the syringe pistol and let the vacuum in the syringe equate to normal.
13. With air pressure in the syringe equalized, withdraw the needle from the mass.
14. Apply gentle pressure to the puncture site with a sterile gauze pad. The patient, a nurse, or an assistant may apply pressure to the puncture site while the aspirator turns to smear preparation and appropriate fixation.

The needle is withdrawn from the mass with air pressure equalized in the syringe, and pressure is applied to the puncture site with a sterile gauze pad. Never withdraw the needle from the mass with any vacuum in the syringe pistol because the small aspirate biopsy will be pulled into the syringe. The sample becomes quite difficult to recover from the barrel of the syringe and it begins to dry immediately. The specimen can be irretrievably lost and may be of poor quality if recovered. When a cyst is encountered, it is evacuated as completely as possible. Following the aspiration of any cyst, it is essential to reexamine the area for any residual lesion. If detected, that residual mass should be reaspirated. Remember that inclusion of additional blood or fluid is not better for aspiration biopsy, but rather it dilutes what tissue fragments and cells are present. When aspirating masses in and around the thyroid, a cyst with water clear fluid may be encountered. The finding of this clear fluid is essentially diagnostic of a parathyroid cyst. This fluid is usually acellular. A portion may be submitted for determination of parathormone levels, which are often quite elevated.

No aspirate may appear in the needle hub/syringe interface with 10 to 12 passes in the lesion, but this does not necessarily indicate an unsuccessful aspiration. After this number of excursions within the mass, if no sample is seen, the aspiration is stopped by allowing the air pressure in the syringe to return to normal.

It takes practice to become adept at FNAB. Both cadavers and surgical specimens may be used to learn and to improve one's technical skills with FNAB. Smears from these practice sessions, using normal tissues as well as tumors, may be prepared and are a useful microscopic reference to compare to actual cases.[8] Excellent instructional videos are now available that emphasize the points above, and others, for successful application of aspiration biopsy to clinical problems.[26,27] The technical aspects of handling needles and the syringe gun for FNAB can also be practiced using an apple or orange.

DIAGNOSIS

To render an accurate and appropriate diagnosis, the cytopathologist needs to have all the pertinent clinical information, the clinician's differential diagnosis and the patient's physical findings clearly recorded in the requisition and/or report form or preferably obtained by the cytopathologist at the time he or she performs the FNAB. This is crucial if the clinician or surgeon is the one performing the aspiration biopsy and if the cytopathologist does not have an opportunity to examine the patient or to review the clinical problem first hand. As the algorithm in Table 1.3 illustrates, the initial process of the FNAB begins with adequate *clinical information*. A variety of stains and procedures can and should be applied to the FNAB material to ensure the maximum yield of *cytologic information*. The blending of both sets of data results in an extremely accurate diagnosis. Conversely, should either set be ignored, incomplete, or absent, a diagnostic error is likely.

The cytopathologist must render a report meaningful to the clinician, a report that makes sense within the framework of the clinical presentation.[16,24] The diagnosis should include the site as well as the morphology; for example, "squamous cell carcinoma, keratinizing,

TABLE 1.3 FNA Algorithm

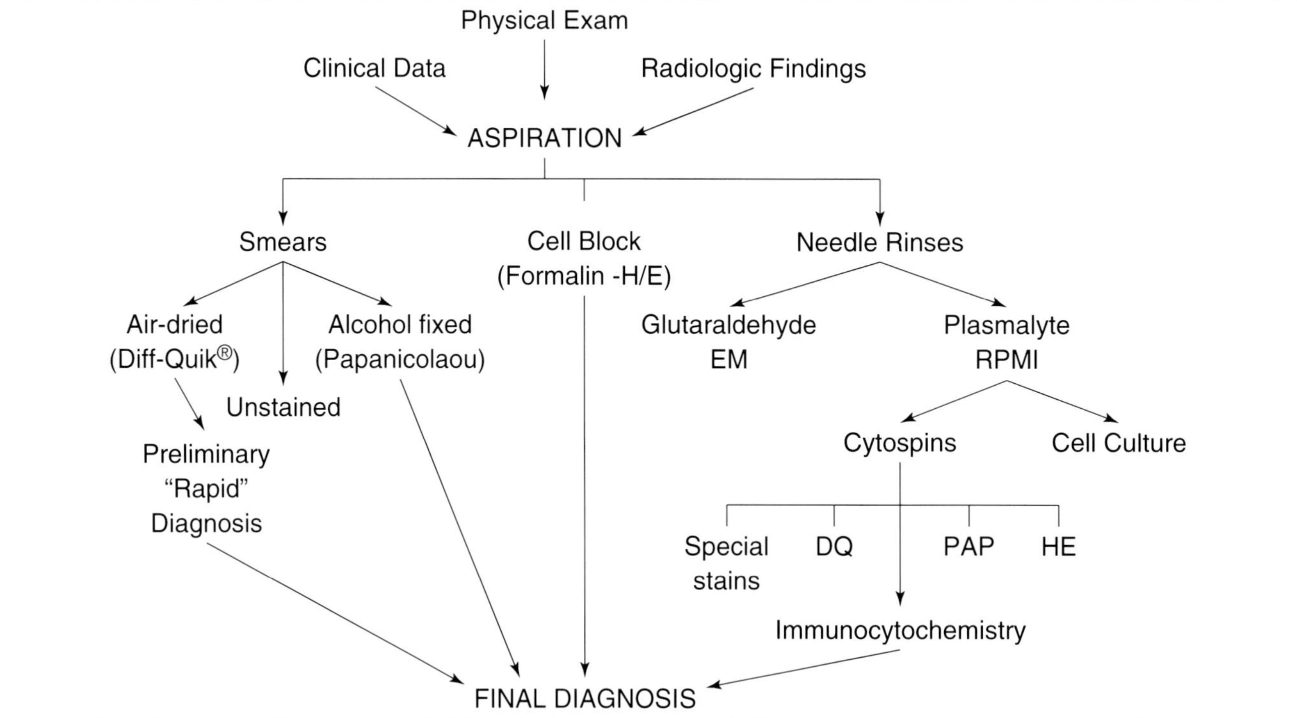

metastatic to right cervical lymph node following same from tongue." These cytologic diagnoses are rendered in the same manner as standard surgical pathology diagnoses. They are complete diagnoses. If the cytopathologist is unsure or feels a definitive diagnosis cannot be made, this need to be stated. These are much less specific diagnoses. Examples are "atypical cells of undetermined type or significance, from aspirate of right cervical lymph node." The quality of the aspirate obtained needs to be reported as well.

No attempt should be made to develop a definitive interpretation on inadequate material or even on a good aspirate with incomplete clinical information.[11,14] Also, when the initial cytologic diagnosis does not fit the clinical situation, caution is advised in terms of making major therapeutic decisions on the basis of cytologic findings alone.

Recommendations

Recommendations for appropriate additional studies are indicated, including a possible request for repeat aspiration biopsy. A recommendation for an open biopsy may be made in some cases, depending on the degree of certainty of the cytopathologist in the reporting of the aspiration biopsy. An intraoperative frozen section should be specifically suggested in some cases after aspiration biopsy if the cytopathologist cannot make a definitive diagnosis of malignant, and major surgery would be indicated for such a neoplasm. In view of the current legal climate in the United States, it may be advisable to confirm a malignant aspiration biopsy diagnosis by intraoperative frozen section, particularly if the contemplated surgery is extensive. Even with this caveat, the aspiration biopsy is still quite useful, because among patients with suspected malignant tumors, it distinguishes between those definitely requiring immediate surgery and those that do not.

Complications and Liability

Most "lumps and bumps" considered for FNAB are superficially located or at least located in such a position that they are not directly in relation to anatomic structures that are hazardous for biopsy. Complications from fine needle aspiration biopsy of superficial masses are few and of little consequence.[17] These include some minor discomfort in the area of the aspiration (usually lasting no more than a few hours), some bruising and discoloration of the aspiration site, and rarely, small hematomas. Complications are directly related to needle size and have been less than 0.03 percent in a review of published series when needles of finer gauge than 20 gauge have been used.[17] Needle tract seeding of tumors has been reported only rarely with this size needle; most such cases are poorly documented.[17] One of the authors (WJF) has observed no cases of needle tract seeding in either superficial or deep aspiration biopsies while performing or assisting in this procedure since 1972. With superficial aspiration biopsy, particularly in the area of the head and neck, some patients may experience lightheadedness or actual syncope.[17] Most of these patients have had similar vasovagal responses to needle puncture (venipuncture) in the past. A history of such tendency can be elicited prior to biopsy allowing suitable precautions to be taken.

There are three areas of vulnerability to legal action following FNAB. These are false-negative diagnosis of malignancy, a false-positive diagnosis of malignancy, and complications of the needle aspiration procedure itself.[16]

A false-negative diagnosis may arise in diverse ways: failure to find or recognize malignant cells that are present; inadequate or poorly prepared samples; missing the actual tumor by aspiration; and characteristics such as sclerosis, which are intrinsic to some tumors and render them poorly suited to the FNAB approach. Avoiding the first problem, that of failure to recognize malignant cells, is fully the responsibility of the cytopathologist, while most of the remaining problems are the responsibility of the aspirator.[16] They reflect the importance of attention to details in all aspects of the aspiration biopsy method. As Stewart concluded, the surgeon and the pathologist must function as an intelligent team.[2] Ultimately, the surgeon or clinician must decide in each case, on the basis of its clinical features, the likelihood of a representative FNAB and the confidence in its interpretation, whether to accept a diagnosis of negative for malignancy as a final step in the patient's evaluation.

False-positives are invariably the result of overreading atypical-appearing cells, usually few in number.[8] If a malignant diagnosis from FNAB does not fit the clinical picture, the patient's physician is wise to ask for a review of the slides specifically with this information in mind. Good sampling is important to accurate diagnosis because masses that consistently yield few cells despite the performance of a technically good aspiration biopsy, regardless of suspicion of abnormality, are nearly always benign.[16]

Problems for the Surgeon/Clinician

The most common problem for both surgeons and clinicians is failure to procure a good specimen from aspiration biopsy. This should not be judged on the total volume of sample but rather on the numbers of cells obtained and their distribution upon the slide. More sample is not necessarily better if most of it is only blood or cyst fluid. *There is no substitute for proper technique.*

The target of aspirate must be clearly and completely identified and there should be a clinical differential diagnosis transmitted to the pathologist. The clinician must have clear indications for the aspiration biopsy and know how that information will influence patient management after the biopsy.[8,16]

Problems for the Pathologist

The pathologist's most obvious problem is trying to read too much into limited material, particularly with inadequate clinical information. Listed below are the seven golden rules of FNAB; they are worth remembering at all times:[28]

1. Be aware of the limitations of FNAB for the body site being sampled.
2. Obtain cellular samples that are adequate and well prepared.
3. Be aware of the diagnostic pitfalls for each body site sampled.
4. Correlate cytologic impressions with the patient's history and physical findings.
5. Live within your experience and limitations.
6. Compare the cytology of FNAB with tissue samples whenever they are available.
7. Maintain good lines of communication among clinician, cytopathologist, and patient.

SPECIMEN PREPARATION

The utility of FNAB rests not only on the interpretive skills of the cytopathologist but also on the technical competence of the aspirator. Technical expertise does not end with the aspiration itself but includes the ability to handle the specimen. Although the sample obtained from FNAB can be rinsed directly into saline for cytospin preparations or into formalin to prepare as a cell block, the vast majority of cytopathologists rely on smears made directly from material expressed from the needle onto glass slides. Well-prepared smears, with the preservation of microfragments of tissue, can provide an architectural framework, upon which to base a diagnosis as well as to evaluate individual cells. This is the primary reason for the term fine needle aspiration *biopsy.* Tables 1.4 and 1.5 as well as Figures 1.3 and 1.4 list the steps that are necessary for making high-quality smears.

It is very important to place the bevel of the needle against the slide while expressing the biopsy from the syringe so that there is no intervening air gap. In this way, splattering of the sample or excessive air-drying prior to fixation is lessened. With enough practice, it is possible to place all the aspirated material, normally 4 or 5 drops within a 3.8-centimeter needle, on a series of three or four slides and then to begin actual smear preparation without encountering significant drying artifacts in those smears that are then wet-fixed. However, the maneuvers described must be done quickly to obtain high-quality smears. With the recent introduction of a rapid Papanicolaou stain that allows all smears to be air-dried, speed in smear preparation has become less critical.[29]

A critically important point in making smears is that they should occupy only a small area of the slide. The objective is to create a tissuelike pattern to the smears and reduce the area of the smears that must be screened for diagnostic features.

Pulling the slides apart vertically, what the author (WJF) has labeled "compression smears," will also be consistently accomplished by confining the smear to a

TABLE 1.4 Smear Preparation and Fixation (refer to Figure 1.3)

1. Immediately following completion of the aspiration, detach the needle from the syringe and fill the syringe with air.
2. Reattach the needle and place the needle in the center and on the surface of a plain glass slide.
3. Advance the plunger of the syringe to express a small drop of aspirate, 2–3 mm in diameter, onto the slide.
4. Carry out this procedure over a series of slides as quickly as possible.
5. Invert a second plain glass slide over the drop and, as it spreads, gently pull the two slides apart horizontally.
6. Alternatively, as the drop spreads, pull the two slides apart vertically.
7. Repeat this procedure for all slides, immediately fixing those to be stained by other than Romanowsky methods (Diff-Quik® (Biochemical Sciences, Inc., Swedesboro, NJ), May-Grunwald-Giemsa, etc.) with 95% alcohol. Simply drop the slide into a suitable container of alcohol as for a conventional cervicovaginal (Pap) smear or use a pump sprayer with alcohol (several are commercially available, see Appendix 1.2) to spray the material on the slides.
8. Allow unfixed smears to air-dry.

TABLE 1.5 Smear Preparation: Bloody or Other Fluid Aspirates (refer to Figure 1.4)

1. Place the drop of biopsy material on the slide (A) as above, usually 5–10 mm in diameter.
2. Hold slide A with the drop of biopsy in the left hand.
3. Hold a second slide (B) with the right hand and bring the edge of slide B up to the drop.
4. The drop will spread along the edge of slide B. As it does, push the edge of slide B toward the end farthest from the drop of bloody aspirate in the manner of making a blood smear and about halfway down slide A.
5. At that point, lift slide B straight up.
6. Immediately tilt slide A away from the leading edge of the smear so that the blood runs back toward the original point of the placement of the biopsy sample.
7. Continue smear preparation by rotating slide B 90 degrees so that there is a clean edge. Use this edge of slide B to make a smear from the leading edge of slide A.

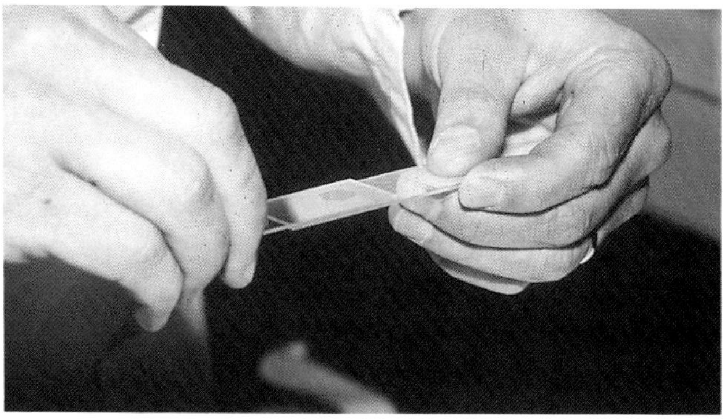

FIGURE 1.3 Smear preparation. A drop of aspirate is placed in the center of a plain glass slide. A second slide is inverted over the drop, and the slides are gently pulled apart vertically or horizontally *once*.

small area of the slide. When pulling the slides apart horizontally to make a smear, do it only once. Do not scrub the specimen back and forth as this tears the cytoplasm from the nucleus, destroying any tissuelike pattern and cell detail. Optimal smears are very difficult to prepare from aspiration biopsy specimens diluted by blood or excessive fluid.

These smears inevitably cover large areas of the slide, and the cells are separated and diluted by the blood and fluid that is present. There is the mistaken belief by many clinicians that aspiration of large bloody samples is of value, the philosophy that "more is better." This is not true. All of the blood pulled into the syringe may be placed entirely into a small tube of 10 percent buffered formalin and processed as a cell block. The majority of cells in this situation will still remain in the needle. Smears should be made only from that part of the sample. Both large volumes of blood or even a few milliliters may result in quick clotting. Clotting of blood greatly interferes with good smear preparation. The fibrin in clotting blood entraps cells and distorts the picture of the smear, often resulting in heavy and uneven staining. In summary, it is important to learn the mechanics of FNAB and smear preparation and to be quick and sure with all aspects of this procedure.[8,13]

Frustration may occur with aspirate material that clots and remains in the hub of the needle or the tip of the syringe. A solution to the problem of aspirate in the needle hub is to first insert the needle firmly into a rubber stopper, Figure 1.5, or into the rubber top of a vacutainer tube. As illustrated in Figure 1.5, snap the needle hub against a glass slide to dislodge the material. Be careful to anchor the needle firmly and to wear protective eye covering; do not perform this maneuver near the patient or other personnel to avoid any accidental needle stick.[16] Figure 1.6 demonstrates the method of removing residual material from the syringe tip. Hold the syringe over a glass slide with the plunger withdrawn a short distance. Aim the tip of the syringe at the center of the slide and slightly above its surface. Strike the plunger of the syringe sharply while firmly holding the barrel.[16]

When a specimen that is largely fluid is encountered, for example, thyroid cysts, place the sample into a clean container with an equal volume of 50 percent alcohol for initial fixation, and transport the sample to the

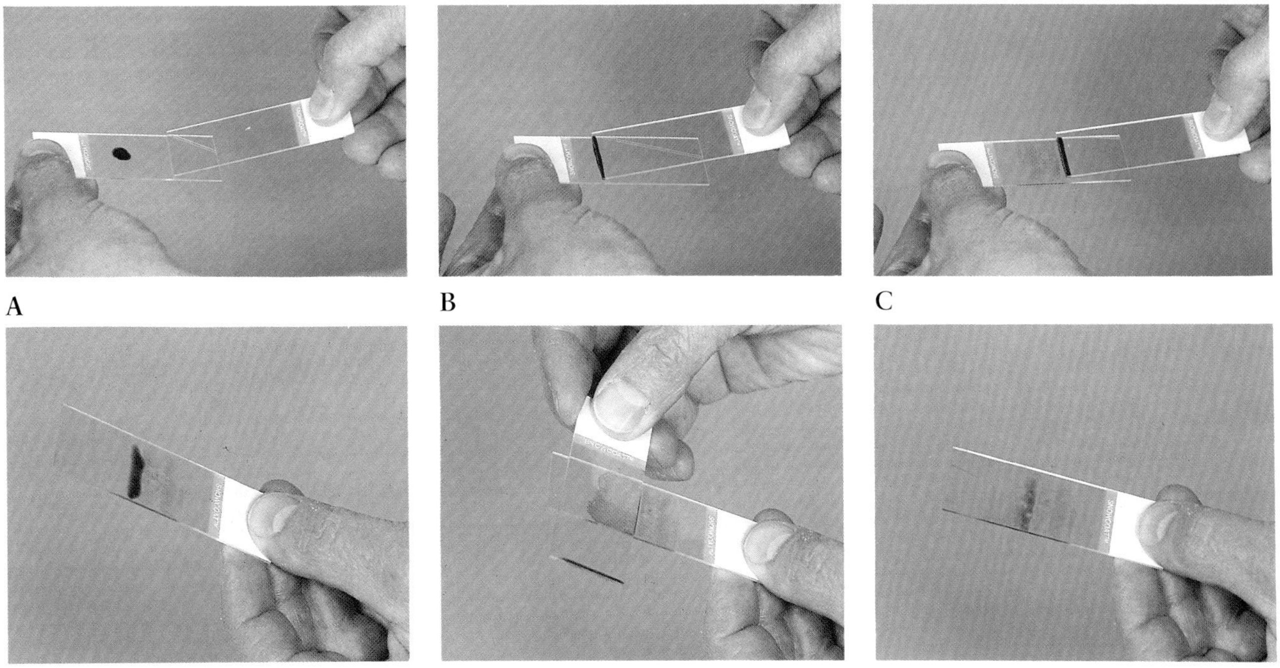

FIGURE 1.4 Multiple steps in preparing smears from bloody or fluid specimens. (A) Drop placed near the frosted end of slide held in the left hand. A second slide is advanced toward the drop. (B) Bloody material spreads along the edge of slide held in right hand. (C) Material is pulled gently down the slide in the manner of making a blood smear, then it is lifted off the slide. (D) Slide in the left hand (slide with the partially made smear) is tilted toward the frosted end so that the blood runs back toward that end. (E) The long edge of the slide in the right hand is then used to continue making the smear from the leading edge of the original smear (slide in the left hand). (F) Finished smear will have any cell fragments present concentrated between the thick area of the smear and the edge farthest away from the frosted end.

pathology laboratory. For fluid specimens *do not* use concentrations of alcohol higher than 50 percent. The laboratory's preferred method for examining cyst fluids cytologically may require that they be submitted fresh and unfixed. That can be best accomplished by placing the fluid into a clean container with an equal volume of balanced salt solution. Refrigerate (but do not freeze) the sample until it can be transported to the laboratory. Fluids placed in balanced salt solution will retain good cell preservation, if refrigerated, up to 48 hours and even longer. Where clinicians are performing the FNAB, they should work closely with the cytopathologist regarding how to best preserve aspiration biopsies and fluids to ensure optimum samples for interpretation.

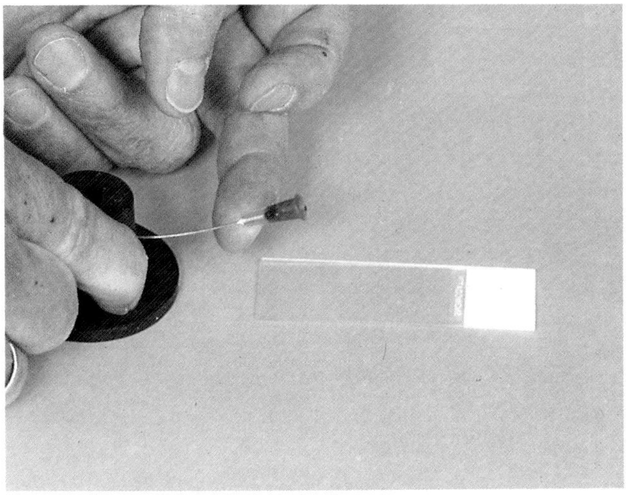

FIGURE 1.5 Method of dislodging aspirate that is stuck in the hub of the needle. Perform this maneuver out of range of the patient or other personnel. Wear a protective eye shield.

The Cell Block

Cell blocks can be quite valuable in some aspiration biopsies. They reinforce tissue patterns that may be seen on smears, thus aiding in making a more specific diagnosis. They also provide more consistency with immunoperoxidase staining, with the exception of aspirates of lymph nodes where lymphoproliferative disease is suspected. Cell blocks may be handled by either the plasma thrombin clot method or with the new cytoblock system (see Appendix 1.3).[30,31] The author (WJF) has found the cytoblock method excellent for preserving the maximum amount of material submitted for cell block preparation.[31]

Small tissue fragments or microcores can sometimes be found in material expressed from the needle or lodged within the needle tip. This is particularly true

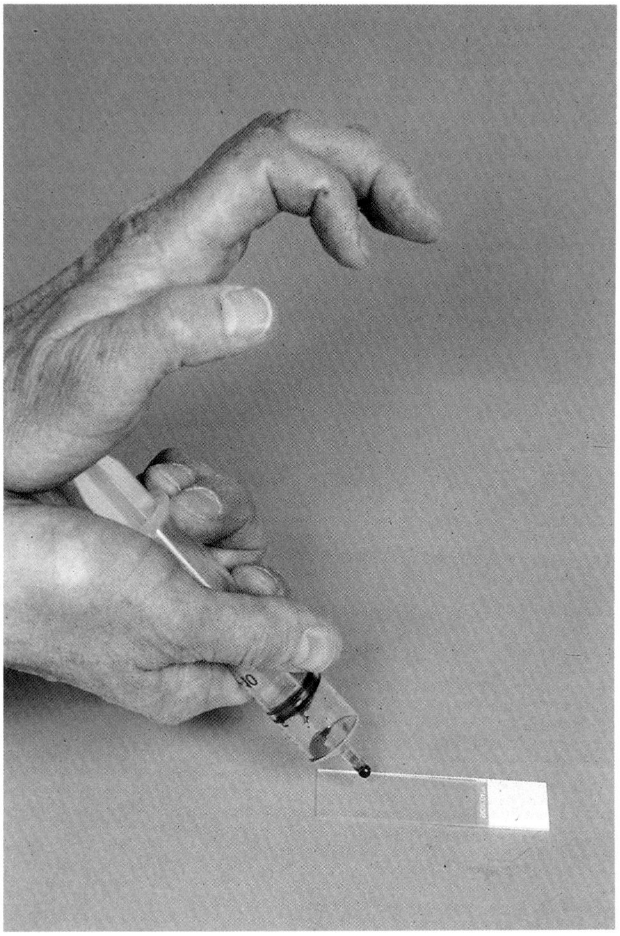

FIGURE 1.6 Method of dislodging aspirate from the tip of the syringe. Hold the barrel firmly when striking the plunger. Aim the tip of the syringe at the surface of a glass slide.

with Franseen-style needles, which have a tendency to obtain microcores. It is important to keep the stylus close at hand to dislodge these very small pieces of tissue from the needle, expressing them onto a plain glass slide. Do not attempt to smear these small cores because they will tear and become distorted. They should not be crushed, but they can be gently rolled over a small area of the slide to make a smear that is like a touch preparation. This is done quickly because it is most important to place these small fragments in fixative for small biopsy tissue processing. For both cell blocks and these microcores, the histology laboratory personnel should be trained to trim the final paraffin block carefully and to retain as many levels from these samples as possible, even if they are not stained immediately. With care, there is often plenty of FNAB specimen for special stains if required for diagnosis.

Following initial evaluation of rapid stains from an FNAB, a lymphoproliferative process may be suspected. A separate aspirate should then be taken and preserved in balanced salt solution for flow cytometry or the preparation of cytospins (see Appendix 1.4). A large number of these cytospins can usually be made from a single FNAB for typing of lymphomas and/or determining monoclonality. Material can be preserved in a similar fashion for molecular diagnostic methods including fluorescent *in situ* hybridization (FISH).

Fixatives and Stains

Personal preference and experience will dictate what stains are used on aspiration biopsy smears. Surgical pathologists with limited experience in cytopathology may feel more comfortable with hematoxylin and eosin because that stain on FNAB smears simulates what they see every day in histologic sections. Experience in cytopathology usually results in a preference for the Papanicolaou stain because of its transparency for viewing the nucleus. Following the influence of those individuals trained in hematology, the authors like the Romanowsky stains, Diff-Quik®, May-Grunwald-Giemsa, straight Giemsa, or Wright's stain.[3,4,6,7,13] Azure A, which is oxidized to Azure B, forms the basis of the Romanowsky effect, that is, contrasting metachromasia of various elements, cytoplasm, nucleus, and background stroma or cell substances such as mucin. Use of rapid versions of these stains, which are applied to either air-dried or alcohol-fixed smears, have the added advantage of leading to an immediate diagnosis following the FNAB. The quality of the aspirate and the smears is also routinely checked. Repeat FNAB, if necessary, can be performed for both diagnosis and special studies.

Air-dried smears are stained by the Romanowsky methods. There are three steps to the Diff-Quik® stain: fixation in methyl alcohol, staining in eosin Y, and staining in Azure A. The authors wash the slides in water, a few dips between the eosin Y and Azure A. The procedure takes less than 20 seconds to perform. It is important *not* to follow the manufacturer's directions slavishly, because this stain was developed for blood smears that, unlike FNAB smears, are of uniform thickness. The final color of the stained aspirate should be a blue-purple, not a red or orange-blue. If the smear is not stained to satisfaction when viewed microscopically, it usually needs only to be stained for an additional few seconds in the Azure A (solution II). It is very difficult to overstain smears with Diff-Quik®, but it is easy to understain them. Over time, the Azure A deteriorates and requires a longer staining time to accomplish the same result. Like any stains and fixative solutions, these need to be filtered, and additional stain should be added periodically.

The authors keep a Diff-Quik® stain setup near the frozen section area and gross rooms for staining both the aspirates and touch smears from frozen sections—an invaluable addition to that procedure that not only assists in diagnosis but aids in teaching cytopathology to residents. This rapid stain technique will also occasionally pick up metastatic carcinomas in lymph nodes that will not be recognizable on conventional frozen sections.[25] Tables 1.6 and 1.7 compare the general and some spe-

TABLE 1.6 Comparison of General and Some Specific Properties of Romanowsky Stains and the Papanicolaou Stain[13]

	Air-Dried Smear Romanowsky Stain	*Wet-Fixed Smear Papanicolaou Stain*
Dependence on smear technique	Strong	Moderate
Dry smear	Fixation good	Drying artifacts often
Wet smear	Artifacts common	Fixation good
Tissue fragments	Cells poorly visualized, heavy staining of ground	Individual cells seen clearly
Cell and nuclear area	Differences exaggerated and enhanced	Similar to tissue sections
Cytoplasmic detail	Demonstrated very well	Demonstrated poorly
Nuclear detail	Chromatin pattern different from Pap stain	Excellently demonstrated
Nucleoli	Not always visible	Demonstrated well
Stromal components	Differentially stained and well demonstrated	Poorly demonstrated
Partially necrotic tissue	Poor cell definition and detail	Good definition of single and intact cells

cific properties of air-dried versus wet-fixed smears and the features emphasized by Romanowsky stains and the Papanicolaou stain. These comparisons are discussed in more detail by Orell.[13]

Smears designated for staining with the conventional Papanicolaou method are spray-fixed with 95 percent ethyl, methyl, or isopropyl alcohol or submerged directly in these fixatives. Smears should be fixed *immediately* following preparation, before the surface dries. Spray-fixed smears should dry at least 1 hour prior to staining. Be careful when using aerosol-spray fixatives, and do not hold the spray can closer than about 30.5 centimeters (1 foot) from the slide to prevent freezing artifacts that result from the propellant.[32]

There have been a number of reports detailing the use of rapid Papanicolaou stains developed for FNAB smears. Most of these have reduced staining times and the number of alcohol and clearing solutions and have increased stain concentrations. They require prior fixation, which is difficult to shorten significantly, and they still result in the same cell loss that has plagued the staining of aspiration biopsy smears with conventional Papanicolaou staining. The authors have recently been provided with a 90-second rapid Papanicolaou that seems to overcome these problems. This method has the added advantage of being performed on air-dried smears, so that rapid preparation and fixations are no longer important. The smears are rehydrated briefly in normal saline, which has the added effect of lyzing most or all of the red blood cells present, considerably reducing the effect of bloody smears on staining. The immediacy of this rapid Papanicolaou stain makes both Romanowsky stained smears and Papanicolaou stained smears available at the same time for complete signout. The authors have found good nuclear detail with this method, excellent preservation of cell structure, and greatly enhanced cellularity of the smears.[29]

For those laboratories that prefer staining by rapid hematoxylin and eosin, FNAB smears will benefit from immersion for a few seconds in equal parts of 50 percent ethyl alcohol and 10 percent neutral buffered formalin. This fixation is identical to that used for conventional frozen sections in surgical pathology. Use of any of the rapid stains at least allows the quality of the aspirate and the smears to be checked. In many cases, an immediate diagnosis can be made following the aspiration biopsy. If necessary, repeat aspirates can be obtained for both conventional preparations and ancillary studies that will aid in the diagnosis.

TABLE 1.7 Features Highlighted by Romanowsky and Papanicolaou Stains[13]

Features Emphasized by Romanowsky Stain
Epithelial
Mucin, extracellular or intracellular, colloid (thyroid); basement membrane globules (adenoid cystic carcinoma); amyloid; secretory granules (prostate); fire flares (thyroid); lipofuscin granules (seminal vesicles); lipid vacuoles; bare bipolar nuclei (benign breast); bile plugs.
Lymphoid
Lymphoglandular bodies; hematopoietic cells; cytoplasmic basophilia; lipid vacuoles.
Features Emphasized by Papanicolaou Stain
Epithelial
Squamous differentiation with keratinization; oncocytes (salivary gland tumors and thyroid); psammoma bodies.
Lymphoid
Nuclear chromatin pattern; nucleoli nuclear outline.

Special Preparation Methods for Ancillary Studies

Immunocytochemistry, electron microscopy, and most recently, molecular diagnostic methods may be of value in selected cases to precisely define a diagnosis. Common differential problems include large cell lymphomas versus anaplastic carcinoma versus sarcoma, the differential diagnosis of small round-cell tumors in children, and identification of small numbers of tumor cells in necrotic metastatic tumor in lymph nodes. Evaluation of the initial rapidly stained smears may establish the necessity for these types of ancillary studies. For immunocytochemistry, cell block material is the most valuable. A separate aspiration should be taken for these studies. Material for cell block can be placed directly into buffered 10 percent formaldehyde or other suitable fixative. Cytospin preparations for immunohistochemistry should be prepared from a rinse of the aspirate in balanced salt solution. Cytospins may be air-dried or fixed in 95 percent ethyl alcohol. We prefer air-drying. Air-dried or fixed slides for immunocytochemistry may be stored in a freezer for up to 4 weeks.

APPENDICES

Appendix 1.1. Sample of Fine Needle Aspiration Biopsy Consent Form

(see pg. 13)

Appendix 1.2. Sample of Fine Needle Aspiration Biopsy Requisition/Report Form

(see pg. 14)

Appendix 1.3: Cell Block Preparation

CYTOBLOCK Cell Block Preparation System. Available from Shandon Inc., 171 Industry Drive, Pittsburgh, PA 15275. 1-800-245-6212. Kit includes: Cytoblock Cassettes, Cytoblock Reagent 1 (clear fluid), Cytoblock Reagent 2 (colored fluid)

Directions

1. Record patient information on the Cytoblock.
2. Use samples previously fixed in neutral buffered formalin.
3. Concentrate the fixed cells by centrifuging the sample for several minutes. Pour off the excess fluid and drain the tube on a paper towel.
4. Estimate the amount of sample present. If the total amount of sample is 2 drops or less, add 4 drops of Reagent 2 to the specimen pellet and mix by vortexing.
5. If the sample is more than 2 drops, divide into several cell blocks based on 2 drops per block. For example, if there is 4 drops of sample (enough for two cytoblocks), add 8 drops of Reagent 2 and vortex.
6. Assemble Cytoblock cassettes into Cytoclip (Cytospin standard equipment) and keep it horizontal. The locating peg on the back of the Cytoblock cassette fits into the hole in the Cytoclip to be properly oriented.
7. Add 3 drops of Reagent 1 into the center of the well in the board insert. Reagent 1 should coat the entire circumference of the well in the board insert. Use care and avoid any Reagent 1 on the top surface of the board insert.
8. With the backing paper projecting toward the top of the Cytoclip, place a Cytofunnel (Cytospin equipment) disposable chamber over the prepared Cytoblock and secure the metal clip holder in the usual manner (see Cytospin operating instructions).
9. Place the assembled Cytoclip into the Cytospin rotor.
10. Place the mixed cell suspension in each Cytofunnel.
11. Close the Cytospin and set for 5 minutes at 1500 rpm. Use the LOW acceleration setting. Start the Cytospin.
12. When the Cytospin stops, remove the Cytofunnel assemblies and place in a horizontal position. Release the clip and remove the funnels. Removal may require rocking the funnel to the side to separate the funnel assembly from the underlying board insert. Be certain the cell button is in the well and has not adhered to the funnel. Then discard the funnel.
13. Place 1 drop of Reagent 1 in the center of the insert board well, on top of the cell button. Close the Cytoblock cassette and place it in fixative to await tissue processing.
14. After processing in the standard tissue processor, open the Cytoblock cassette. Fold back paper and remove the board insert. Use fine forceps inserted through holes under the board insert.
15. Dislodge the cell button into the base mold and embed flat. Discard the board insert and backing paper.
16. Reclose the Cytoblock cassette and place FLAT SIDE UP (round peg side down) on top of base mold. Fill with paraffin.
17. Handle as any paraffin block but trim carefully because cell buttons may be quite thin.

UNIVERSITY HOSPITAL
SUNY Health Science Center
at Syracuse

CONSENT FOR FINE NEEDLE ASPIRATION

1. I authorize C. N. Powers, M. D. (Attending Physician) and such physicians as may be selected by her to perform upon ________________ (State "myself" or name of patient) the following diagnostic or therapeutic procedure:
   Fine needle aspiration - withdrawal of cells from tissue (State nature of procedure in layman's terms)
   for microscopic evaluation
   Body site: ________________

2. If any condition arises during the course of the procedures calling, in the judgement of the physician, for procedures in addition to or different from those described, I further authorize the physician to alter the procedures as deemed advisable.

3. The benefits and purpose of the procedure and the risks and discomforts involved have been fully explained to me. No guarantees have been made with respect to the results that may be obtained.

4. I understand that in addition to the risks explained to me, the possibility of other risks and consequences may arise. I have been advised that if I ask for any further information, it will be given to me.

5. I have been advised of possible alternative procedures and they have been explained to me.

6. I have read this entire document and understand its contents. In addition, I have been told that I am free to withdraw any portion of my consent.

7. I have either completed or crossed off any unacceptable statements prior to my signing.

Date ________ Time ________ Signature of Patient ________

If consenting party is other than patient:

Date ________ Time ________ Signature of Parent or Guardian ________

Witnesses:

Date ________ Time ________ Signature of Witness ________

Date ________ Time ________ Signature of Witness ________

Physician:
I have discussed the treatment described above with the patient or relative whose signature appears on this document.

Date ________ Time ________ Physician's Signature ________

CROSS OUT ANY OF THE ABOVE PARAGRAPHS WHICH DO NOT APPLY AND INITIAL

Rev. 2/93 CNP/CTS M-1

Appendix 1.1 Sample of Fine Needle Aspiration Biopsy Consent Form

REQUEST FOR FINE NEEDLE ASPIRATION

Name ____________________
Address ____________________
____________________ Zip ________
Birthdate ____________________ Sex ☐ M ☐ F
Chart # ____________________
Social Security No. ____________________

Requesting MD ____________________
Address ____________________
Phone/Beeper ____________________
Date: ______ /______ /______
Body Site: ____________________

VIRGINIA COMMONWEALTH UNIVERSITY
MEDICAL COLLEGE OF VIRGINIA HOSPITAL
DEPARTMENT OF PATHOLOGY
CYTOLOGY LABORATORY
RICHMOND, VIRGINIA 23298
MAS 232

Patient Location: ☐ Consult ________
☐ InPt ________ CT OR
☐ OutPt ________

Dx of Malignant Neoplasm	199.1	☐
Dx of Benign Neoplasm	229.9	☐
Dx of Unspecified Neoplasm	239.9	☐
Dx of Infectious Disease	686.9	☐

Insurance Co. ____________________
Policy # ____________________

diagram

Hx:
____
____
____
____

Rinse: **Plasmalyte RPMI Formalin Alcohol**
Cyst Fluid ______cc
Spec Studies: **Flow Cell Block Cytospins______**
IP: *ER/PR*
Spec Stains:

Preliminary Diagnosis:
____
____________________ ____________________ M.D.

MEDICAL RECORDS COPY

Interpretation:
☐ **NEGATIVE** — Malignant Tumor Cells Are Not Seen
☐ **Unsat** — Entirely Unsatisfactory
☐ **NES** — Not Entirely Satisfactory

Limited Cells
Drying Artifact
Exudate

Excess Blood
Degeneration
____

Final Diagnosis:
____
____
____
____

Recommendation: NONE BIOPSY EXCISION REPEAT F/S CONFIRM

CT__________ Date __________ Signed ____________________ M.D.

57-048 (Rev. 2/94)
H-MR 386

DQ/Pap____/____

APPENDIX 1.2 Sample of Fine Needle Aspiration Biopsy Requisition/Report Form

Appendix 1.4: Cytospin Preparation

Preparation of Cytospins for Tumor Markers

1. Aspirates for cytospin preparation and tumor markers are received as a needle rinse into balanced salt solution. Enough sample should be present so that the fluid is slightly cloudy. If the sample is grossly bloody, saponization should be performed (see below). If the sample is grossly cloudy, it should be diluted with balanced salt solution until it becomes slightly cloudy before being used for cytospin preparations.
2. Follow the manufacturer's directions to set up the Shannon Cytospin.
3. Samples that are blood tinged or have required saponization should be washed in balanced salt solution and centrifuged for 15 minutes at 1500 rpm. Restore the original volume.
4. Break the Cytospin filter seal by scraping your fingernail around the edge of the circle on the filter a couple of times. This allows for better absorption of fluid.
5. Load the Cytospin with sample chamber, filter, and slides so the chamber is balanced.
6. Using a disposable pipette, add specimen dropwise to the specimen chamber. Usually 2 to 5 drops, depending on cellularity of the sample.
7. Cellularity can be checked initially by using 1 drop of sample on a slide and 1 drop of supravital stain. Mix thoroughly with an applicator stick and coverslip. Examine under the microscope with high power field (400X). If every other field has 5 to 10 cells, then 1 drop of sample will provide an adequate Cytospin sample. If the cell estimate is higher than this, dilute with balanced salt solution to at least this distribution of cells or lower.
8. Follow the addition of sample drops to the Cytospin chamber with 2 drops of 20% fetal calf serum in RPMI® (tissue culture transport media).
9. Spin for approximately 5 minutes at a speed of 500 rpm.
10. When Cytospin stops, remove slides and filters. Discard filters.
11. Allow slides to air-dry.
12. Determine again the Cytospin quality by using a representative slide and staining it with Diff-Quik®. Examine the slide for adequate cellularity under the microscope.
13. If necessary, add or decrease the number of sample drops used. Cells should not overlap as this produces confusing staining patterns and edge effects.
14. Prepare an adequate number of quality slides to process the immunohistochemistry tests ordered.
15. Wash sample chambers in bleach, rinse with water, and allow to dry after use.

Saponization

This procedure may be applied to visibly bloody fluids and may be used in small amounts on samples that exhibit traces of blood.

Materials

1% saponin (w./v.)
1.0 g saponin
0.2 g sodium *p*-hydroxybenzoate (preservative)
99.0 mL distilled water
3% calcium gluconate (w./v.)
3.0 g calcium gluconate
0.2 g sodium *p*-hydroxybenzoate (preservative)
97.0 mL distilled water

Prepare solutions above in beakers. Mix thoroughly. Filter into clear brown bottles, date, and label. Expiration for these solutions is 2 weeks.

Methods

1. Pour sample into designated centrifuge tube, leaving sufficient space for addition of saponization solutions (see steps 2 to 4).
2. If specimen is grossly bloody, add 2 disposable pipettes full of 1% saponin and vortex for 30 seconds. Let sit for an additional 30 seconds. Coloration and/or transparency of the sample should change noticeably.
3. Add 3 disposable pipettes full of 3% calcium gluconate and vortex for 30 seconds.
4. The saponin and calcium gluconate must always be used in a 2:3 ratio. The actual amounts may be varied according to the amount of blood present in each specimen. It is feasible to use only 2 drops:3 drops if blood is present only in minute amounts.
5. Proceed to centrifugation and Cytospin preparation.
6. If the presence of blood is detected only after initial centrifugation, saponin may still be used. Decant supernatant, vortex suspension, and add the solutions in a ratio of 2 drops: 3 drops, respectively. Proceed with preparation of Cytospins.

Appendix 1.5: FNAB Staining Procedures

1. Papanicolaou
2. Rapid Papanicolaou
3. Diff-Quik®
4. May-Grunwald-Giemsa
5. Modified Wright's
6. Hematoxylin and Eosin
7. Vital Stain

Staining Techniques

1. Papanicolaou Stain. Any of the modifications available in most laboratories are satisfactory. The authors prefer Gills Hematoxylin®, available from Polysciences, Inc., Paul Valley Industrial Park, Warrington, PA 18976. (215) 343-6484. Staining times may need to be adjusted for variations in thickness of smears. We also use Gill's modified Orange G-6 (OG-6) and Eosin (EA) for our Papanicolaou stain. These are also available from Polyscience, Inc., Bayshore, NY.[31]
2. Papanicolaou Stain, Rapid Method.[29] This is a 90-second staining protocol that has proven quite effective in producing a high-quality Papanicolaou stained slide and at the same time has reduced or eliminated blood in the background of aspiration smears. Smears are made in the usual fashion and allowed to air-dry.

Staining protocol

Normal saline	30 seconds
Alcoholic formalin*	10 seconds
Water	6 slow dips (at speed of 1 dip/second)
Richard-Allen Hematoxylin 2	2 slow dips
Water	6 slow dips
95% ethanol	6 slow dips
Richard-Allen Cyto-Stain†	4 slow dips
95% ethanol	6 slow dips
100% ethanol	6 slow dips
Xylene	10 slow dips

Mount in mounting media and add coverslip.

3. Diff-Quik® Stain Set. This commercial stain kit, a modified Wright stain, is a three-solution, three-step method that is both fast and practical. It provides good cell detail and identifies stromal fragments by metachromasia. This stain is comparable to the May-Grunwald-Giemsa and the Wright-Giemsa, but it is much quicker. Fixation is with methanol containing 1.8 mg/L Triarylmethane Dye, 100% pure dye content. Solution I is buffered Eosin Y. Solution II is a buffered solution of thiazine dyes, methylene blue, and Azure A. Azure A undergoes slow constant oxidation to Azure B, which is the actual staining solution of the original Romanowsky method. This is available from American Scientific Products, Div. of American Hospital Supply Corp., McGaw Park, Illinois 60085.

Staining procedure

The air-dried smears are dipped for 5 seconds (five dips) in solutions I, II, and III, respectively. The excess stain is drained from the slides between solutions. Following the last staining solution, the slide is rinsed with water and either allowed to dry or examined wet. When the smear completely dries, it may be made permanent by immersing it in xylene for several seconds and mounting it with Permount (Fischer Chemical/Fischer Scientific, Fairlawn, NJ) and a coverslip. Staining times may need modification depending on the thickness of the smear and the age of the stain. Examination of the finished stain should have a gross purple-blue color, not brown or orange. If the latter color is seen, the slide is understained. It is quite difficult to overstain with Diff-Quik®. We prefer to rinse the slide briefly in water following immersion in Solution I before dipping the slide in Solution II.

4. Modified May-Grunwald-Giemsa Stain

May-Grunwald stock stain	1.0 g eosin-methyl blue 1000 mL methyl alcohol
Giemsa stock stain	Add 1.0 g Giemsa powder to 66.0 mL glycerin. Incubate at 37 degrees for 3 hours, mixing occasionally. Add 66.0 mL methyl alcohol to the incubated stain. Store in the refrigerator.
May-Grunwald working stain	To 40.0 mL of stock stain add 20.0 mL methyl alcohol in a Coplin jar.
Giemsa working stain	Add 45.0 mL of Giemsa stock stain to 45.0 mL of distilled water in a Coplin jar.

Staining procedure

Immerse the air-dried aspiration smears in May-Grunwald working stain for 15 minutes. Rinse gently in tap water. Immerse the smears in Giemsa working stain for 15 minutes. Rinse gently with tap water. Allow to air-dry. Dip in xylene for 10 seconds and mount in Permount.

Prepare May-Grunwald working stain fresh weekly. Prepare Giemsa stain fresh daily. The stock Geimsa stain

---

*Three liters of alcoholic formalin is conveniently prepared by combining 300.0 mL of 38–40% formaldehyde, 2053.0 mL of 95% ethanol, and 647.0 mL of distilled water. This makes a mixture that is 65% ethanol and 4% formaldehyde. This is a potent fixative, and smears should not be transported in it. Prolonged immersion in this fixative will adversely effect the cytomorphology.

† Richard-Allen Cyto-Stain® is an alcoholic mixture of Orange G, Eosin-Y, light green, and aniline blue. Both this stain and Richard-Allen Hematoxylin 2® are available from Richard Allen, Richland, Michigan. There are small volume portable staining rackets that will easily accommodate this number of solutions and can be transported to any site (radiology). The Richard-Allen dyes are quite stable but should be filtered at least weekly. All other solutions need to be changed daily.

is good for 6 months if refrigerated. The stock May-Grunwald stain is good indefinitely and does not require refrigeration.

5. Modified Wright-Giemsa Stain

Wright	Any formula in standard laboratory use is satisfactory.
Giemsa	See Giemsa stock stain
Buffer solutions	pH 6.4 and pH 6.8
Giemsa working stain	Dilute 1 part Giemsa stock stain with 9 parts of buffer pH 6.8. Prepare fresh daily.

Staining procedure

Flood the air-dried aspiration smears with methyl alcohol and allow the alcohol to evaporate completely. Then flood the smears with Wright's stain for 3 minutes. Add buffer solution of pH 6.4 drop by drop to the Wright's stain, blowing on the slide to mix stain and buffer. The stain develops a green sheen when enough buffer has been added. Allow to stand for 4 minutes. Wash in tap water and dry completely. Stain in working Giemsa 3 minutes. Wash with tap water and dry completely. Dip in xylene for 10 seconds and mount in Permount and coverslip.

6. Hematoxylin-eosin stain

Eosin Y

Harris Hematoxylin

Dilute ammonium hydroxide

Add 1 drop of concentrated ammonium hydroxide to 100.0 mL of distilled water.

Staining procedure

Use on air-dried aspiration smears.

1. Absolute ethyl alcohol	1 minute
2. 95% ethyl alcohol	1 minute
3. Tap water	several dips
4. Harris Hematoxylin	2 minutes
5. Tap water	several dips
6. Dilute ammonium hydroxide	1 to 2 dips
7. Eosin Y	30 seconds
8. Tap water	several dips
9. Tap water	several dips
10. 95% ethyl alcohol	several dips
11. 95% ethyl alcohol	several dips
12. Absolute ethyl alcohol	several dips
13. Acetone	several dips
14. Xylene	1 minute
15. Mount with Permount and coverslip	

Supravital stain

Toluidine Blue

0.5 g Toluidine Blue

20.0 mL 95% ethyl alcohol

80.0 mL distilled water

Dissolve Toluidine Blue in alcohol, add distilled water, filter and store in dark bottle in the refrigerator.

Appendix 1.6: Immunocytochemistry Procedures

Immunostaining of Cytospins: DAKO® LSAB Kit (DAKO, Santa Barbara, CA), Peroxidase

1. Etch a circle around the Cytospin area with a diamond-tipped etching pencil. Brush lightly to remove glass particles. Also label the slide with patient identification.
2. Fix in cold acetone (4°C) for 10 minutes.
3. Allow to air-dry for 5 minutes or more on a flat surface.
4. Rehydrate by placing in modified phosphate buffered saline (PBS) for 10 minutes.
5. Wipe off excess PBS. Cytospins must be kept wet at all times.
6. Place the slide in humidified chamber and apply primary antibody (mouse monoclonal in preference to rabbit polyclonal). Incubate for 15 minutes at room temperature.
7. Rinse gently with PBS. Wash by placing in PBS (fresh) for 5 minutes.
8. Wipe off excess PBS. Cytospins must be kept wet at all times.
9. Place in humidified chamber and apply Link Antibody (Biotinylated/Anti-Mouse Immunoglobulins, Biotinylated Anti-Rabbit Immunoglobulins). Incubate for 10 minutes.
10. Rinse gently with PBS. Wash by placing in PBS (fresh) for 5 minutes.
11. If quenching of endogenous peroxidase activity is desired, apply enough 3% hydrogen peroxide to cover specimen in a Coplin jar. Incubate 5 min. Note: To prepare 3% hydrogen peroxide, dissolve 3 tablets of Urea-H_2O_2 in 100 mL of deionized water immediately before use.
12. Wash slides in PBS for 5 minutes.
13. Wipe off excess PBS. Cytospins must be kept wet at all times.
14. Place in humidified chamber and apply Streptavidin (peroxidase conjugated) to cover specimen. Incubate for 10 minutes.
15. Rinse gently with PBS. Wash by placing in PBS (fresh) for 5 minutes.
16. Wipe off excess PBS. Cytospins must be kept wet at all times.
17. Place in humidified chamber and apply DAB solution (*d,d*-Diaminobenzidine). Incubate for 5 minutes. Note: DAB solution must be prepared immediately before use.
    a. Add 10.0 mL of Tris buffer (0.05M, pH 7.6) to a 10 mg bottle of DAB (Polysciences, Bayshore, NY), (Cat #04008); mix.

b. Add 0.16 mL 0.3% H_2O_2, prepared by dissolving 1 tablet of Urea-H_2O_2 in 100.0 mL of deionized water immediately before use.

18. Rinse gently with PBS. Wash by placing in PBS (fresh) for 5 minutes.
19. Slides are now ready to counterstain. Rack slides and dip in each solution approximately 10 times with the exception of hematoxylin:

    PBS
    Distilled water
    Hematoxylin (3–4 minutes)
    Distilled water
    PBS
    Distilled water
    80% ethyl alcohol
    95% ethyl alcohol
    100% ethyl alcohol
    Xylene
    Xylene
    Xylene

20. Coverslip slides with Permount or other suitable mounting media.

Estrogen Receptor (ER) and Progesterone Receptor (PR) on FNA Aspirates from Breast Tumors

1. Use Silane-coated slides (Columbia Diagnostics, Inc., Springfield, VA, Cat.# G740C) Procedure: Same as for Cytospins using DAKO® LSAB Kit. Using Anti-Estrogen Receptor (Coulter-Immunotech, Miami, FL, Cat.# 1344) Progesterone Receptor (Novacastra-Vector Laboratories Ltd. Claremont Place, Newcastle Upon Tyne, UK, Cat.# NCL-PGR)
   ER dilution 1/100ER-/PR-labeled slides
   PR dilution 5/100ER test labeled slides
   PR test 5/100 ER test labeled slides
   Note: 1. Do not peroxide block slides
2. After washing slides after DAB, counterstain using ethyl green (CAS®), Cell Analysis Systems, Inc., Elmhurst, IL) for image analysis.

Staining Procedure for the CAS® using Ethyl Green[33]

The ethyl green staining procedure has been developed as a nuclear counterstain for nuclear immunological staining procedures. The staining has been optimized for measurement on the CAS® image analyzer. The staining can be combined with immunocytochemical staining for estrogen receptor, progesterone receptor, and antigens in proliferating cells.

Packaging. Each bottle of stain contains 10 grams. The recommended staining concentration is 0.4 g per 100 mL of solution. This is sufficient for about 15 slides. In 100-mL batches, 50 stainings can be accomplished, or approximately 750 slides.

Precautions. For investigational use only. Not for *in vitro* diagnostic use. Standard laboratory precautions should be taken in handling this dye.

Reagent Storage and Stability. The ethyl green dye should be stored in a dry place at room temperature (18°–28°C). Do not expose to bright light.

Materials Required

Deionized water
Sodium acetate ($CH_3COONa \cdot 3H_2O$; analytical grade or ACS certified)
Glacial acetic acid (98% or greater, analytical grade or ACS certified)
1-butanol (analytical grade or ACS certified)

Specimen Preparation. The ethyl green methodology has been developed as a nuclear counterstain for a variety of (nuclear) immunocytochemical procedures for measurement on the CAS® image analyzer. The ethyl green staining is used as a poststaining procedure. Therefore, cytologic specimens (e.g., Cytospins, touch preparations, fine needle aspirates, smear preparations) and histologic specimens (frozen and paraffin sections) that are immunocytochemically stained can be counterstained with ethyl green. The ethyl green staining should be conducted immediately upon conclusion of the immunocytochemical staining procedure.

Limitations. The use of other reagent dilutions, incubation times, and rinse procedures can alter stain intensity and affect quantitation results. The ethyl green solution should be freshly made each day prior to use. (The properties of the stain solution may change upon storage resulting in erroneous CAS® measurements.) Having applied the stain solution, deionized water rinsing and butanol dehydration times should not be exceeded, otherwise the ethyl green staining intensity will be too low.

Preparation of 0.1M Sodium Acetate Buffer pH 4.0 and Ethyl Green Solution. 0.1*M* sodium acetate buffer, pH 4.0, is made from 0.2*M* acetic acid and 0.2*M* sodium acetate stock solutions according to the following scheme:

0.2*M* acetic acid (12 mL acetic acid made up to 1000 mL with deionized water 82.0 mL
0.2*M* sodium acetate (27.2 g of $CH_3COONa \cdot 3H_2O$ made up to 1000 mL with deionized water) 18.0 mL
Deionized water 100.0 mL
Total volume 200.0 mL

Ethyl Green Solution

Dissolve 0.4 g ethyl green in 100 mL of 0.1M sodium acetate buffer, pH 4.0.

Stir with a magnetic stirrer until dissolved (a few minutes).

Staining Procedure

The ethyl green counterstain is performed at room temperature (18° to 28°C) and follows the last water rinse after the chromogen incubation in the immunocytochemical staining procedure.

1. 0.1M sodium acetate buffer pH 4.0	10 minutes
2. Ethyl Green	10 minutes
3. Deionized water	10 dips
4. Deionized water	10 dips
5. Deionized water	10 dips*
6. 1-butanol	10 dips
7. 1-butanol	10 dips
8. 1-butanol	10 dips†
9. Xylene	2 minutes
10. Xylene	2 minutes
11. Mount in a synthetic resin (e.g., Coverbond mounting Media‡, Permount§)	

Results. The staining results in green stained nuclei that contrast well with the brown DAB staining. The cytoplasm should not stain.

Specimen Collection Procedure

1. Collect fresh fine needle aspirates and prepare smears on Silane-coated slides immediately. Place smears, while still wet, in a Coplin jar of 3.7% formaldehyde in PBS for 10–15 minutes. Make a minimum of six smears that contain tumor cells. DO NOT ALLOW CYTOSPIN SLIDES TO DRY AT ANY TIME. Aspirates are preferable to cytospins from FNA of tumors, which have given inconsistent results and are usually low in cellularity. Touch preparations or scrapes from small tumors prepared as smears can also be used.
2. After fixation, place slides in PBS for 4–6 minutes.
3. Transfer slides to cold methanol at −10° to −25°C for 3–5 minutes, then transfer to cold acetone at −10° to −25°C for 1–3 minutes. Rinse in PBS at room temperature for 4–6 minutes.
4. Transfer slides to a container of fresh PBS and rinse for an additional 4–6 minutes.
5. Using a diamond-tipped pen, make a circle around the sample area on the slide.
6. Return slides to PBS.
7. Proceed to the staining procedure within 2 hours of completing fixation, OR immediately after preparation, remove specimen from PBS and place in −10° to −25°C Specimen Storage Medium (see below). Store at −10° to −25°C for up to 4 weeks.

Materials Required but not Provided

3.7% formaldehyde-PBS Solution‖
1 volume formaldehyde (37%)
9 volumes PBS

Specimen Storage Medium

To make 500 mL of Specimen Storage Medium, dissolve 42.8 g sucrose and 0.33 g magnesium chloride (anhydrous) in PBS.
Adjust final volume to 250 mL
Add 250 mL glycerol and mix by stirring
Store at −10° to −20°C

Prior to Performing the Assay

1. Refer to Specimen Collection and Preparation for Analysis.
2. If fixed specimens have been stored at −10° to −20°C, place them in PBS bath for 5 minutes. Repeat, using fresh PBS bath.
3. Prepare a humidified chamber by placing moistened paper towels in a container with a lid. The chamber should contain a rack on which slides can be positioned horizontally.
4. Bring all reagents except Control Slides to room temperature for use.

Procedural Notes

1. Apply kit reagents dropwise in sufficient quantity to cover the circled aspirate smear; usually 2 drops are sufficient.
2. Perform all incubation steps in the humidified chamber at room temperature.
3. Drain excess buffer or reagent from a slide onto a paper towel and then wipe the area around the etched circle of the smear with an absorbent wipe or equivalent. Note: Do not touch the smear or the estrogen test (ET) positive cells (control slide) within the circle. Touching will destroy the smear or the cells.
4. When adding ER antibody and PR antibody to the control slide, do not allow reagents to mix. Use Abbott (Abbott Park, IL) ER Control Slides.

Assay Procedure

Note: Note under Immunocytochemical Staining Procedure

1. Remove excess PBS from fixed smear and control slide.

*Stay in third water wash, step #5, until 30 seconds is up. For Cytospins and touch preparations, differentiate fast with a few dips through water washes.
†Stain in third butanol until a total of the 3 minutes is up; for Cytospins and touch preparations, differentiate fast with a few dips through the butanol washes.
‡Trademark of EM Industries (distributed by American Scientific Products, Columbia, MD)
§Trademark of Fischer Scientific, Fairlawn, NJ

‖This fixative solution should be prepared fresh daily.

2. Place in humidified chamber and apply primary antibody (mouse monoclonal in preference to rabbit polyclonal). Incubate for 15 minutes at room temperature.
3. Rinse gently with PBS. Wash by placing in PBS (fresh) for 5 minutes.
4. Wipe off excess PBS. Cytospins must be kept wet at all times.
5. Place in humidified chamber and apply Link Antibody (Biotinylated Anti-Mouse Immunoglobulins, Biotinylated Anti-Rabbit Immunoglobulins). Incubate for 10 minutes.
6. Rinse gently with PBS. Wash by placing in PBS (fresh) for 5 minutes.
7. Wipe off excess PBS. Cytospins must be kept wet at all times.
8. Place in humidified chamber and apply Streptavidin (peroxidase conjugated) to cover specimen. Incubate 10 minutes.
9. Rinse gently with PBS. Wash by placing in PBS (fresh) for 5 minutes.
10. Remove excess PBS.
11. Place in humidified chamber and apply DAB solution (*d,d*-Diaminobenzidine). Incubate 5 minutes.

Note: DAB solution must be prepared immediately before use:
   a. Add 10.0 mL of Tris buffer (0.05*M*, pH 7.6) to a 10-mg bottle of DAB from Polysciences, Cat.# 04008. Mix.
   b. Add 0.16 mL 0.3% H_2O_2 prepared by dissolving 1 tablet of urea-H_2O_2 in 100.0 mL deionized water immediately before use.

12. Rinse gently with PBS. Wash by placing in PBS (fresh) for 5 minutes.
13. Remove excess PBS.
14. Slides are now ready to counterstain with ethyl green for quantitation on the CAS® image system or for observation using the staining procedure that follows. For the staining method below, rack the slides and dip in each solution approximately 10 times with the exception of hematoxylin:

    PBS
    Distilled water
    Hematoxylin (1 minute)
    Distilled water
    PBS
    Distilled water
    80% ethyl alcohol
    95% ethyl alcohol
    100% ethyl alcohol
    Xylene
    Xylene
    Xylene
15. Coverslip slides with Permount or other suitable mounting media.

Specimen Results

If estrogen receptor is detected in the specimen, the immunocytochemical staining will be located in the nuclei of the cells treated with the Primary Antibody and will appear reddish brown. The nuclei of the cells that do not contain significant amounts of estrogen receptor will be blue. Other brown staining that might occur in the cytoplasm, in leukocytes, erythrocytes, or necrotic cells will also be apparent in the specimen treated with control antibody and should be considered nonspecific.

REFERENCES

1. Martin HE, Ellis EB. Biopsy by needle puncture and aspiration. *Ann Surg* 1930;92:169–181.
2. Stewart FW. The diagnosis of tumors by aspiration biopsy. *Am J Pathol* 1933;9:801–812.
3. Lopes Cardozo P. *Clinical cytology.* Leiden: Stafleu, 1954.
4. Soderstrom N. *Fine needle aspiration biopsy.* Stockholm: Almqvist & Wiksell, 1966, pp. 13–18.
5. Dahlgren SE, Nordenstrom B. *Transthoracic needle biopsy.* Stockholm: Almqvist & Wiksell, 1966, pp. 13–18.
6. Zajicek J. Aspiration biopsy cytology, Part I. Cytology of supradiaphragmatic organs. *Monographs in clinical cytology,* Vol. 4. New York: S. Karger, 1974, pp. 1–15, 20–26.
7. Linsk JA, Franzen S. *Clinical aspiration cytology.* 2nd ed. New York: J.B. Lippincott Co., 1989, pp. 1–15.
8. Frable WJ. Thin needle aspiration biopsy. In Bennington J (ed.), *Major problems in pathology,* Vol. 14. Philadelphia: W.B. Saunders Co., 1983.
9. Salzman, AJ. Imaging techniques in aspiration biopsy. In Linsk JA, Franzen S (eds.), *Clinical aspiration cytology,* 2nd ed. Philadelphia: J.B. Lippincott Co., 1989, pp. 17–38.
10. Moulton JS, Moore TP. Coaxial percutaneous biopsy technique with automated biopsy devices: Value in improving accuracy and negative predictive values. *Radiology* 1993;186:515–522.
11. Hadju SI. The value and limitations of aspiration cytology in the diagnosis of primary tumors. *Acta Cytologica* 1989;33:741–790.
12. Cohen MB, Miller TR, Gonzales JM, Sacks ST, Bottles K. Fine-needle aspiration biopsy: Perceptions of physicians at an academic medical center. *Arch Pathol Lab Med* 1986;110:813–817.
13. Orell SR, Sterrett GF, Walters Max N-I, Whitaker D. *Manual and atlas of fine needle aspiration cytology,* 2nd ed. New York: Churchill Livingstone, 1992.
14. Koss LG, Woyke S, Olszewski W. *Aspiration biopsy. Cytologic interpretation and histologic bases,*

2nd ed. New York: Igaku-Shoin, 1993, pp. 12–53, 55–108.

15. Abele JS, Miller TR. Implementation of an outpatient needle aspiration biopsy service and clinic: A personal perspective. In Schmidt WA (ed.), *Cytopathology annual.* Baltimore: Williams & Wilkins, 1993, pp. 43–71.

16. Stanley MW, Lowhagen T. *Fine needle aspiration of palpable masses.* Boston: Butterworth-Heinemann, 1993.

17. Powers CN. FNAB complications: The reality behind the myths. *1995 Cytopathology Annual.* Chicago, IL: ASCP Press, 1996.

18. Hopper KD, Abendroth CS, Sturtz KW, Matthews YL, Shirk SJ. Fine-needle aspiration biopsy for cytopathologic analysis: Utility for syringe handles, automated guns, and the nonsuction method. *Radiology* 1992;185:819–824.

19. Zajdela A, Zillhardt P, Voillemot N. Cytological diagnosis by fine needle sampling without aspiration. *Cancer* 1987;59:1201–1205.

20. Kinney TB, Lee MJ, Filomena CA, Krebs TL, Dawson SL, Smith PL, Raafat N, Mueller PR. Fine-needle biopsy: Prospective comparison of aspiration versus non-aspiration techniques in the abdomen. *Radiology* 1993;186:549–552.

21. Frable WJ. The role of the clinician in cytology and the society: Non-gynecologic cytology. *Acta Cytologica* 1977;21:659–660.

22. Frable WJ. Fine-needle aspiration biopsy: A review. *Hum Pathol* 1983;14:9–28.

23. Stanley MW. Who should perform fine-needle aspiration biopsies? *Diagn Cytopathol* 1990;6:215–217.

24. Orell SR. The two faces of fine-needle biopsy: Its role in the teaching hospital and in the community. *Diagn Cytopathol* 1992;8:557–558.

25. Bloustein PA, Silverberg SG. Rapid cytologic examination of surgical specimens. *Pathol Ann* 1977; 12(2):251–278.

26. Ljung B. *Thin needle aspiration biopsy: An instructional video.* San Francisco: Department of Cytopathology, University of California, 1991.

27. Grohs HK. *Fine needle aspiration and smear making techniques: An instructional video.* Manchester MA: International Institute for Applied Cyto Science, 1991.

28. Kardos TF. Personal communication.

29. Yang GCH, Alvarez II. Ultra-fast Papanicolaou stain: An alternative preparation for fine-needle aspiration cytology. *Diagnostic Cytopathology* (In Press).

30. Harris MJ. Cell block preparation. Three-percent bacterial agar and plasma-thrombin clot methods. *Cytotech Bull* 1974;11:6–7.

31. Gill GW. The Shandon Cytospin 2 in diagnostic cytology: Techniques, tips, and troubleshooting. *Cytospin 2 Handbook.* Sewickley, PA: Shandon Southern Instruments, Inc., 1982, pp. 1–73.

32. Holmquist MD. The effect of distance in aerosol fixative of cytologic specimens. *Cytotech Bull* 1979;15:25–27.

33. *Technical manual. Ethyl Green.* Elmhurst, IL: Cell Analysis Systems, Inc. 1992.

Chapter 2

Salivary Glands

INTRODUCTION

Fine needle aspiration may be utilized in the evaluation of both the major salivary glands, the parotid and submaxillary, and the minor salivary glands, either extraoral or intraoral, when a palpable lesion is present. Aspiration biopsy of the salivary glands was used at Memorial Sloan Kettering Cancer Center some 50 years ago but was abandoned despite good results.[1] It was reestablished as a viable biopsy method at the Karolinska Institute in Stockholm, Sweden, albeit with less than optimal results in early reported series.[2,3] After some experience and a more precisely applied classification of salivary gland tumors from histologic material, the results of aspiration biopsy of this organ have become quite accurate.[4–8]

Indications for Fine Needle Aspiration

Aspiration biopsy of an enlarged salivary gland or one containing a definitive mass will accomplish at least one of three objectives in most cases:

1. Distinguish inflammatory from neoplastic lesions.
2. Aid in planning therapy when a tumor is identified.
3. Establish that there has been recurrence of a neoplastic lesion.

Problems in Diagnosis

Cytologic interpretation of fine needle aspirates from salivary glands, to be most effective, requires considerable experience. There are a variety of neoplastic and nonneoplastic lesions that may involve the salivary glands, making interpretation of aspiration biopsy smears one of the more difficult tasks.[9,10] This is particularly true if the lesions are cystic.[11] There is an overlap of cytologic patterns from salivary gland neoplasms. For example, benign mixed tumors and low-grade mucoepidermoid carcinomas both may have a myxoid appearing stroma and bland epithelial cells (Figures 2.1 and 2.2). Warthin's tumor, benign lymphoepithelial lesion, and cysts of the salivary gland, particularly those seen in patients with AIDS, may have quite similar cytologic features (Figures 2.3 and 2.4). Monomorphic adenoma, acinic cell carcinoma, and adenoid cystic carcinomas may also look quite similar on aspiration biopsy smears (Figures 2.5, 2.6, and 2.7).

There may be a variability of pattern in any one type of lesion, as seen with benign mixed tumor and low-grade mucoepidermoid carcinoma, depending on the volume of myxoid stroma and mucinous material versus the epithelial elements. Patterns may vary from area to area, for example, in Warthin's tumor with squamous metaplasia (Figure 2.8). Finally, as noted, cyst formation in the benign mixed tumor, monomorphic adenoma, Warthin's tumor, and low-grade carcinomas of adenoid cystic and acinic cell type may merge the apparent cytologic patterns causing diagnostic problems.[12]

In spite of these difficulties, by keeping in mind the limitations and pitfalls of the procedure, FNA of the salivary glands can be utilized effectively. In some instances, surgery can be avoided while in other situations the preoperative diagnosis by aspiration biopsy can direct the best surgical approach.[13,14]

Method

Standard aspiration techniques, as utilized in other percutaneous aspirations, are employed and are described

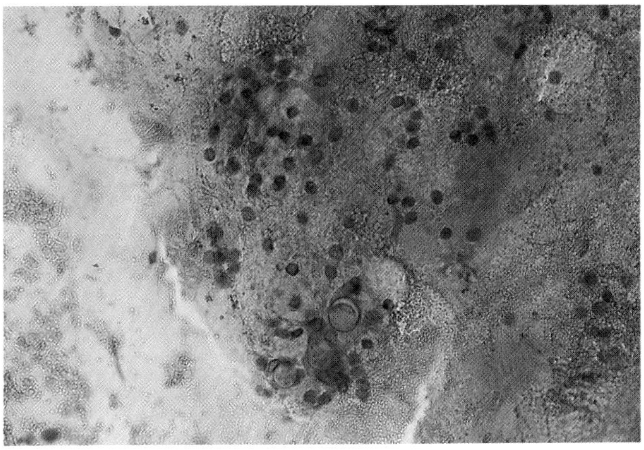

FIGURE 2.1 Low-grade mucoepidermoid carcinoma of parotid gland. Small sheets of bland epithelial cells embedded in myxoid appearing stroma. Papanicolaou stain 400×.

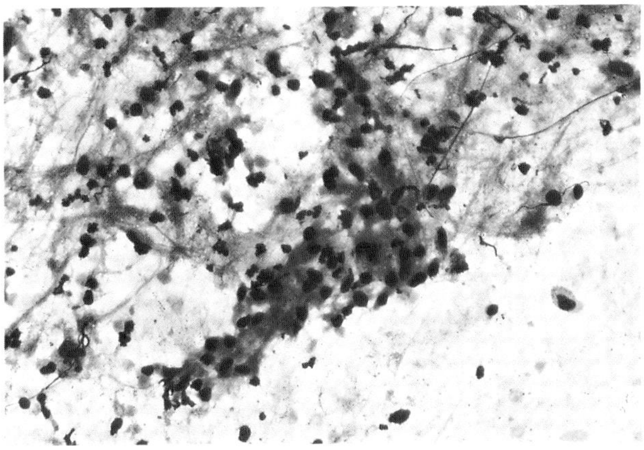

FIGURE 2.2 Benign mixed tumor of parotid gland. Sheet of degenerated epithelial cells in metachromatic myxoid background. Cystic degeneration has caused cytologic atypia that, coupled with the myxoid appearing background, simulates low-grade mucoepidermoid carcinoma. Compare to Figure 2.1. Diff-Quik® 400×.

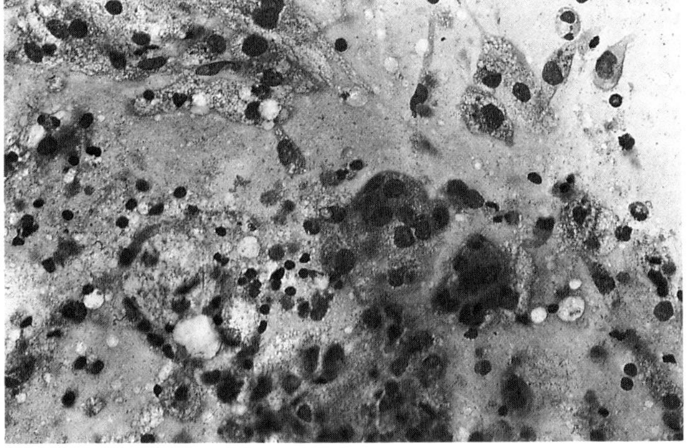

FIGURE 2.3 Warthin's tumor of parotid with cystic degeneration. Loose sheets of degenerated cells without specific features for Warthin's tumor. Many of the cells are finely vacuolated and do not have any features of the oncocytic cells of typical Warthin's tumor. Diff-Quik® 400×.

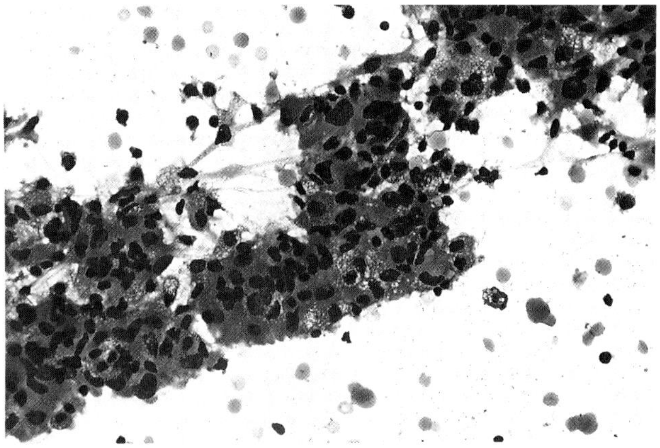

FIGURE 2.4 Benign lymphoepithelial lesion of parotid with cystic degeneration. Large sheet of oncocytic appearing cells that suggests Warthin's tumor instead of the correct diagnosis of benign lymphoepithelial lesion. Diff-Quik® 400×.

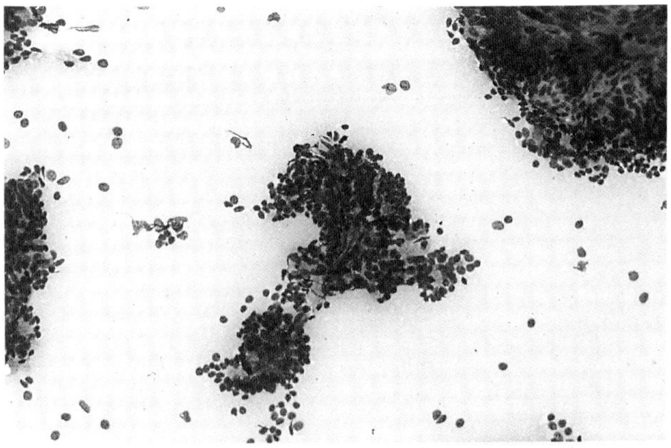

FIGURE 2.5 Monomorphic adenoma of the parotid. Sheets and clusters of small monotonous epithelial cells in some foci surrounding small mass of metachromatic stroma simulate adenoid cystic carcinoma. Diff-Quik® 250×.

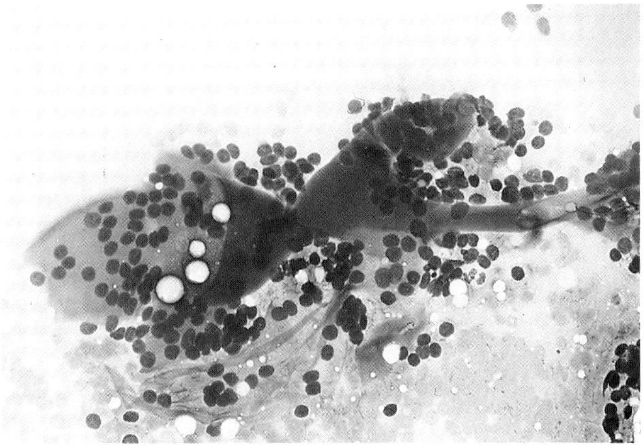

FIGURE 2.6 Adenoid cystic carcinoma of submaxillary gland. Similar monotonous cells as in Figure 2.5 with intervening metachromatic dense stroma but no recognizable pattern of adenoid cystic carcinoma in this field. Diff-Quik® 400×.

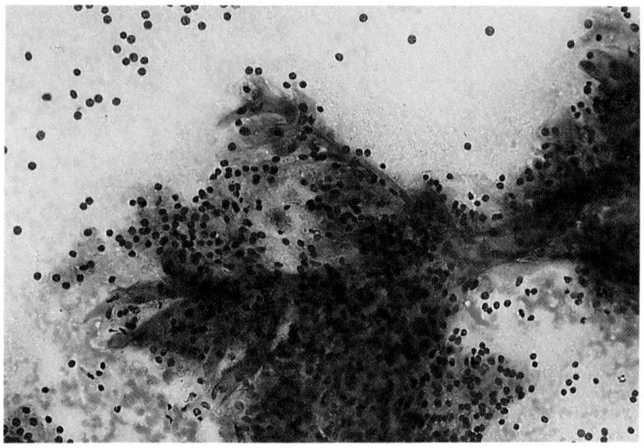

FIGURE 2.7 Acinic cell carcinoma of parotid gland. Small monotonous cells but with more abundant cytoplasm. Note the close approximation of metachromatic stroma and the resemblance in this field to the adenoid cystic carcinoma illustrated in Figure 2.6. Diff-Quik® 250×.

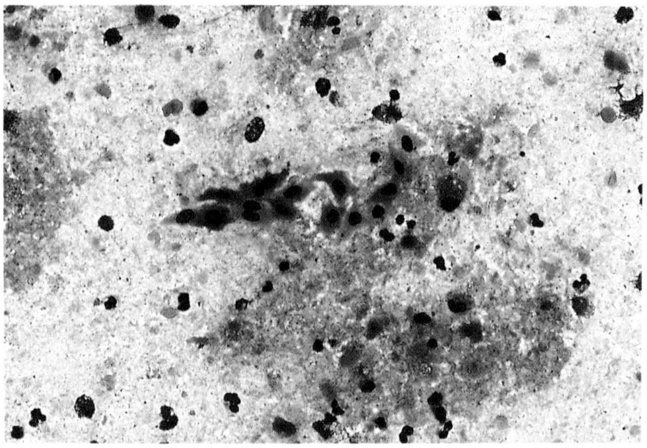

FIGURE 2.8 Warthin's tumor of parotid gland. Cystic mass with sheet of squamous appearing cells, some lymphocytes in the background with proteinaceous debris. This is a typical appearance of Warthin's tumor that has undergone cystic degeneration with squamous metaplasia. This pattern may mimic metastatic squamous cell carcinoma with necrosis. Diff-Quik® 400×.

in Chapter 1. Because of the heterogeneous patterns encountered in many salivary gland neoplasms, it is often useful to perform several aspirations of a single mass. One variation of the aspiration technique that is often used in the thyroid and is also of value with some intraoral masses is to insert the needle directly into the mass (needle-only technique) without an attached syringe or gun.[15] The capillary pressure may be sufficient to extract a sample. After making 15 to 20 passes of the needle alone, withdraw the needle, attach it to the syringe and expel the material onto a plain glass slide. Then prepare the smears in the conventional manner.

NORMAL SALIVARY GLAND

Salivary glands—both major and minor—are composed of multiple lobular acinar units, each suspended in a fatty matrix and joined by ductular structures. The parotid gland is triangular in shape and is situated with one base along the anterior border of the ear and another immediately beneath the zygomatic arch. The tail of the parotid extends inferiorly to a point between the ear lobe and the angle of the jaw. The gland partially overlies the temporomandibular joint superiorly and the carotid artery inferiorly.[16]

The submandibular gland is located beneath the mandible and immediately anterior to the emergence of the neurovascular complex over the ridge of the mandible.

Many people have prominent salivary glands.[17] Salivary glands are also often enlarged in association with liver cirrhosis, diabetes, endocrine insufficiencies, and nervous system disorders. Occasionally one of these enlarged glands will be mistakenly identified as an enlarged lymph node or some other type of potential tumor, clinically requiring aspiration biopsy.[18]

Normal Structures—Cytologic Characteristics

Acinar cells occur in flat sheets interspersed with fat in aspirates from normal salivary glands. The serous cells have a granular cytoplasm while the mucinous cells have a clear cytoplasm. Small sheets of these two cells in aspirates from the parotid may show serous cells wrapping around groups of mucinous cells, recapitulating the histologic pattern of demilunes as seen predominantly in the parotid salivary gland (Figure 2.9). A third type of

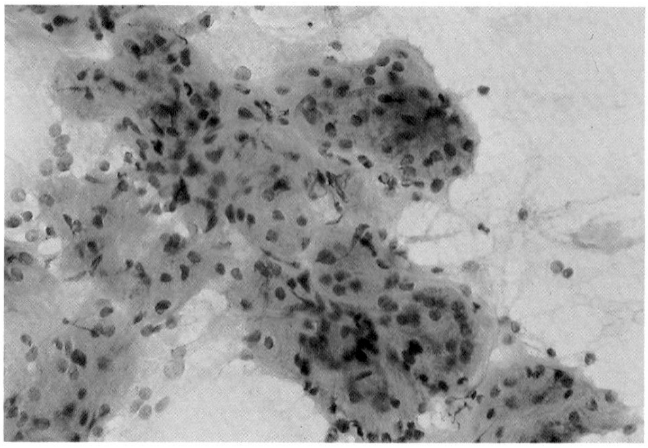

FIGURE 2.9 Normal salivary gland acini. Scattered clear cells represent the mucus cells surrounded by larger numbers of serous cells in an aspirate from normal parotid. Arrow indicates small flattened myoepithelial cell. These cells are difficult to detect in aspiration biopsies. Papanicolaou 400×.

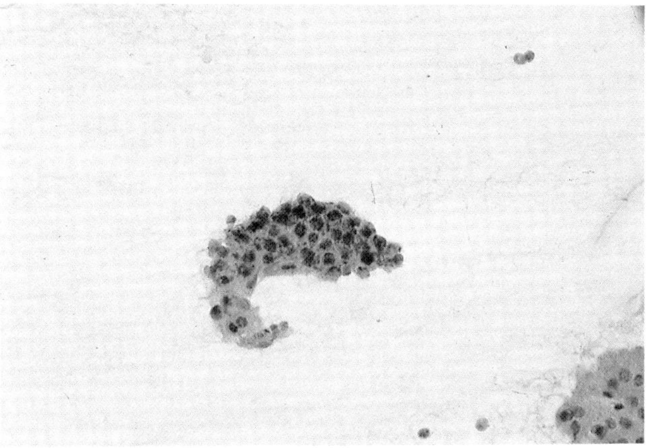

FIGURE 2.10 Small sheet of intercalated ducts. Aspirate from enlarged, chronically inflamed parotid gland. Fine red granularity of the cytoplasm indicates their somewhat oncocytic appearance as seen histologically. Papanicolaou 400×.

cell, the myoepithelial cell, is not prominent in normal glands but may be seen as a small flattened cell at the periphery of intact salivary gland acini that are aspirated. This cell may also be identified in aspiration smears by positive staining for smooth muscle actin and S-100 protein. The S-100 protein staining is less specific. With aging, the acinar cells become progressively more oncocytic. As a result, the aspiration smear may be dominated by oncocytes in the older patient with nonspecific salivary gland enlargement.

The duct cells in normal aspirates are chiefly of intercalated duct type. They are found in flat and usually small sheets with round oval and hyperchromatic nuclei (Figure 2.10). Small nucleoli may be present in these cells. The overall cellularity of salivary gland aspirates from normal glands or those enlarged by cirrhosis, diabetes, or endocrine dysfunction is usually low. Rarely are cells from excretory ducts present. When seen, they have a nonspecific squamous appearance and are larger than intercalated duct cells.

INFLAMMATORY DISEASE

As listed below, four entities may be seen on aspiration biopsy of salivary glands in the presence of inflammation:

1. Acute suppurative sialadenitis.
2. Subacute and chronic sialadenitis.
3. Intra- or paraglandular lymph node enlargement.
4. Granulomatous sialadenitis.

Acute inflammation of the salivary glands seldom produces a discrete mass but is often unilateral and without demonstrated duct obstruction. Acute sialadenitis is painful and the gland is tender. It is also quite painful for patients to undergo aspiration of an inflamed salivary gland, particularly one in which the inflammation is acute. If the clinical history is sufficient to substantiate acute sialadenitis, the author believes aspiration biopsy is not indicated. A history of episodic swelling of the gland is usually encountered only with sialadenitis and most often with a chronic inflammatory process. Chronic inflammation can sometimes result in a hard, partially fixed salivary gland that cannot be clinically distinguished from a malignant tumor. Even though the aspiration is sometimes painful in this situation, the technique can quite reliably rule out the presence of a salivary gland neoplasm.

Acute Suppurative Inflammation—Clinical and Cytologic Characteristics

Clinically, the patient experiences acute swelling and pain of one or more salivary glands with acute suppurative inflammation. On palpation, the gland is quite tender but there is no discrete mass. If the clinical picture is obviously that of acute inflammation, such as in the case of mumps, there is nothing to be gained from the aspiration biopsy.

If there is a compelling reason to perform the biopsy, then the smears will be composed mostly of neutrophils and a background of edema and blood. A few enlarged duct cells and some degenerated acinar cells may also be present, with the duct cells showing the cytologic features of tissue repair (Figure 2.11). Necrosis is present and occasionally fragments of crystalline material suggesting that a stone blocking the main excretory duct may have been the initiating cause. As the process begins to resolve, lymphocytes and plasma cells increase in number, and loosely textured granulomas (granulation tissue) may also be present.

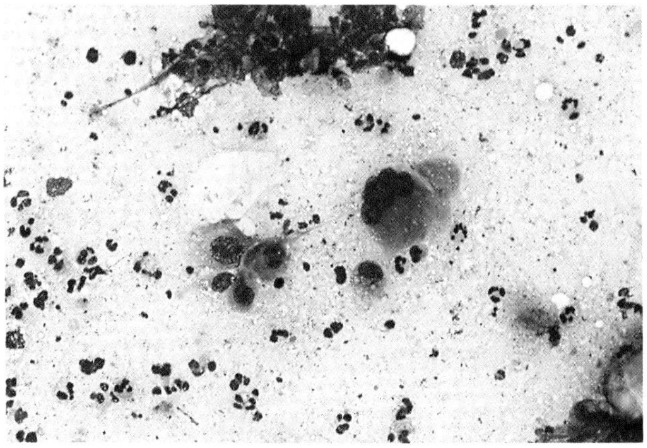

FIGURE 2.11 Aspirate from acutely inflamed parotid gland. Scattered atypical duct cells in a background of neutrophils. Degenerating acinar cells at the top of the photomicrograph. Diff-Quik® 400×.

ACUTE SUPPURATIVE SIALADENITIS

Background of
- **–Acute inflammatory cells**
- **–Blood and necrosis**

Enlarged, atypical duct cells

Degenerated acinar cells

Fragments of crystalline material (stone)

****Resolving phase: granulation tissue/repair**

Subacute and Chronic Inflammation—Clinical and Cytologic Characteristics

Subacute and chronic inflammation of the salivary glands is more likely to clinically present as a mass although careful palpation usually reveals that, while the gland is enlarged and firm, there is really no separate lesion distinguished from the gland itself. The aspirates in subacute and chronic sialadenitis are of low cellularity with scattered lymphocytes and plasma cells, blood, and some small sheets of squamouslike cells that have relatively small dark nuclei. There are usually no acinar elements because they are destroyed first by the inflammatory process. Because of their hyperchromatic nuclei, the intercalated duct cells may appear atypical and even suggest metastatic or primary malignancy, but they are really quite homogeneous in appearance and do not have nuclear chromatin abnormalities or nucleoli. They are few in number—an observation that is very much against any kind of malignant diagnosis. Because obstruction plays a part in subacute and chronic sialadenitis, there may be some cyst formation resulting in a mucinous-like fluid as a background to the smear.[13] Psammoma bodies have also been seen in aspirates from chronic sialadenitis. Their presence can lead to a mistaken diagnosis of adenocarcinoma[19] (Figure 2.12).

SUBACUTE AND CHRONIC SIALADENITIS

Low cellularity specimen

Background of
- **–Lymphocytes and plasma cells**
- **–Blood and occasional mucinous material (cyst)**

Sheets of atypical ductal epithelium (intercalated ducts)
- **–Hyperchromatic nuclei**
- **–Uniform chromatin**
- **–Inconspicuous nucleoli**

Psammoma bodies (rarely)

****Acinar cells absent**

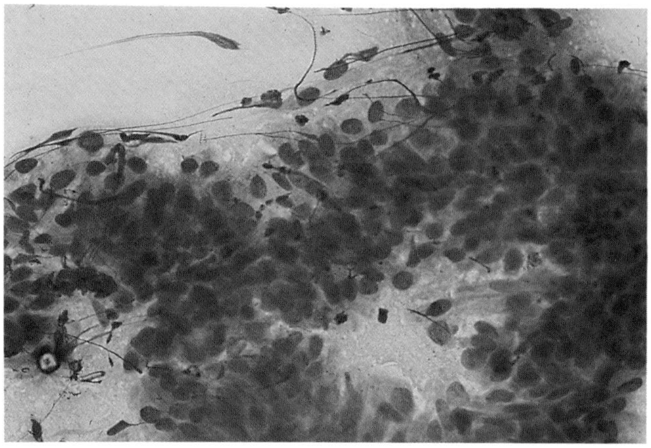

FIGURE 2.12 Aspirate of enlarged parotid gland. Sheet of intercalated ducts with uniform but hyperchromatic nuclei. At first glance, sheets of intercalated ducts seem worrisome because of their hyperchromatic cells. Nuclei have a uniform chromatin pattern and nucleoli are very inconspicuous. Diff-Quik® 400×.

Intra- or Paraglandular Lymph Nodes—Cytologic Characteristics

The parotid gland usually contains a lymph node within its substance. There are also lymph nodes in close proximity to the submaxillary glands as well as lymph nodes in the upper cervical area that may often contain salivary gland inclusions.[20] These lymph nodes may respond by hyperplasia and proliferative activity in the presence of sialadenitis. Distinguishing an enlarged lymph node from the salivary gland itself may be difficult and on aspiration there is often a mixture of lymphoid elements and salivary gland cells that come from one of these nodes. If there is a dominant pattern of lymphoid cells with a reactive pattern of small, intermediate, and large cells, then it is quite likely that a lymph node has been aspirated, particularly in the area of the parotid gland. The duct epithelium and, occasionally, acinar cells that may be found in the smear look quite bland and normal; they are present in small numbers and indicate only that these are inclusions that may be normally found in these nodes.

Granulomatous Sialadenitis—Cytologic Characteristics

The most common type of granulomatous sialadenitis is that secondary to sarcoidosis. The clinical picture is usually quite obvious but sarcoid may present initially as a mass in the major salivary glands, usually the parotid.[13] Cytologic characteristics of sarcoid are cohesive or "hard" granulomas with many spindle-shaped epithelioid cells (Figure 2.13). These are very cohesive and well-formed granulomas that incorporate multinucleated giant cells that are quite obvious on the usual aspiration biopsy. The background contains a few

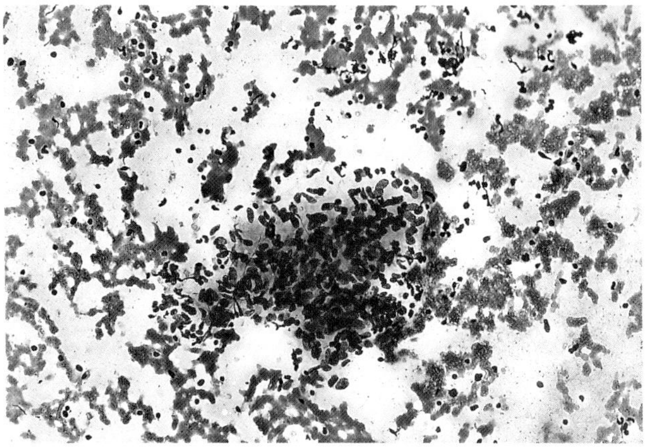

FIGURE 2.13 Aspirate of nodular parotid gland. Discrete cohesive collection of epithelioid cells with a few scattered lymphocytes in the background. A few multinucleated giant cells are present at the periphery of this granuloma and intimately incorporated within it to the right. Diff-Quik® 400×.

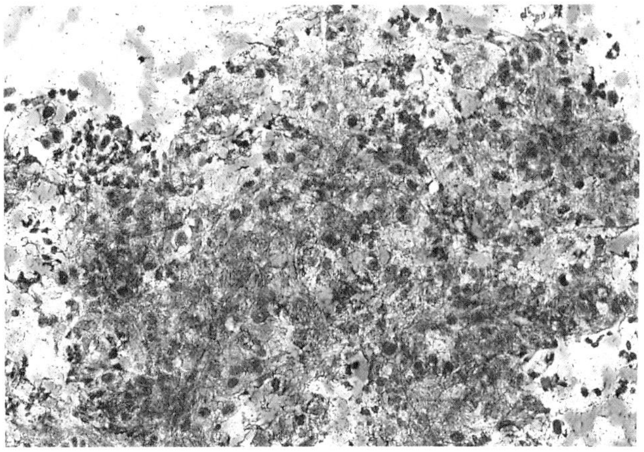

FIGURE 2.14 Aspirate of parotid gland. Very loosely textured granuloma dominated by necrosis and including only vague epithelioid cells. Neutrophils are also present. Presence of poorly formed granulomas dominated by necrosis should initiate a search for acid-fast organisms. Diff-Quik® 400×.

lymphocytes but is often quite clean so that the granulomas appear naked within the few background inflammatory cells as they do in histologic sections of sarcoid.

GRANULOMATOUS SIALADENITIS

Epithelioid histiocytes—cohesive "hard" granulomas

Few multinucleated giant cells

Scattered lymphocytes in clean background

Infrequently, granulomatous processes secondary to organisms such as *Mycobacterium tuberculosis* or actinomycosis involve the salivary gland. With the epidemic of HIV infection and AIDS, mycobacterial infections, particularly from the atypical organisms, have become much more prevalent, while drug therapy used in conventional tuberculosis in AIDS patients is resulting in the production of drug-resistant strains capable of infecting individuals who have normal immune systems.[21] We have seen several examples in aspiration biopsy, more often of lymph nodes in the head and neck, but also involving salivary glands. The granulomas in tuberculosis are not well formed and present in a background of necrosis with scant multinucleated giant cells (Figure 2.14).

Aspirates of salivary glands, but more often lymph nodes, infected with atypical mycobacteria may have few lymphocytes and a rather amorphous background containing enlarged histiocytic cells (see Chapter 4). Both within the cytoplasm of these cells and often in the background there are clear thin and curved lines representing the organism. The cytoplasm of the cells may be filled with these clear lines giving the cells an appearance similar to Gaucher cells.[22] This feature is only seen in air-dried smears, presumably because the waxy capsule of the organisms does not allow penetration of stains, thus creating an artifact referred to as a "negative image."

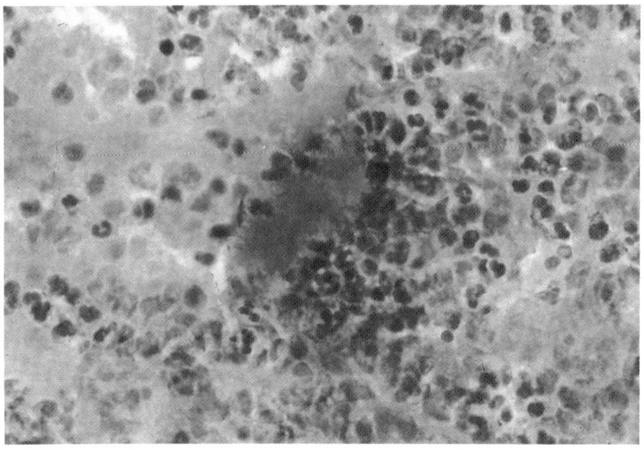

FIGURE 2.15 Aspirate of parotid gland. Organisms of actinomycosis in the center of the field surrounded by acute inflammatory exudate. Papanicolaou 400×.

With infection by *Actinomyces*, the background is both necrotic and acutely inflamed. The organisms are visible in both Romanowsky-stained and Papanicolaou-stained smears (Figure 2.15). The Papanicolaou stain demonstrates the filaments at the periphery of a deeply hematoxylin-stained, homogeneous, amorphous mass, while the filaments appear dark purple to blue with Romanowsky stains.[23]

CYSTS

Cysts are of the simple retention type due to a blocked duct or the so-called "branchial cleft cyst" found within the upper cervical or intraparotid lymph nodes. In most cases, these latter cysts represent degeneration of epithelial inclusions in the upper cervical and/or the parotid lymph node and are not true congenital epithelial cysts from embryonal branchial cleft arches.[24] Tense salivary gland cysts can simulate tumors. Once a cyst has been evacuated, it is necessary to carefully palpate and reaspirate any residual mass.

SIMPLE (RETENTION) CYST

Clear, yellow fluid

Essentially free of cells or few scattered inflammatory cells

Branchial Cleft (Branchiogenic) Cyst—Cytologic Characteristics

These cysts have fluid that is often turbid and variably dark colored. They contain benign squamous cells and keratin debris. Inflammation may be present. Degeneration can occur within these cysts leading to squamous atypia (Figure 2.16). The background is seldom extensively necrotic and the number of atypical cells is few, unlike a cystic metastasis from a squamous cell carcinoma, which would be the major differential diagnosis (Figure 2.17). Other diagnostic problems that occur with cysts of the upper cervical and salivary gland area are cystic degeneration in Warthin's tumor; low-grade mucoepidermoid carcinoma that has undergone cystic degeneration; cystic changes in a benign lymphoepithelial lesion; and the cystic changes that may occur in the salivary glands in some patients with AIDS.[12,25–27] This cystic change may bring all of the aspiration smear patterns closer together so that in some cases only a list of the differential diagnosis can be offered in the report of the aspiration biopsy.

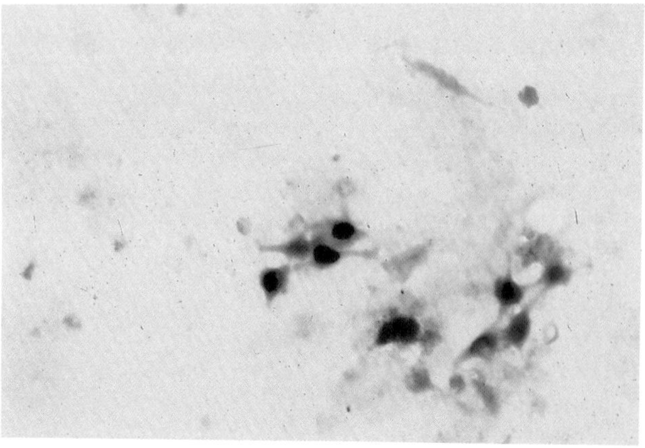

FIGURE 2.16 Aspirate of upper cervical-parotid mass. A few atypical squamous cells with small dark irregular nuclei are found in a background of inflammation with some necrosis in the aspirate from this cystic mass. Such cells raise the possibility of metastatic necrotic squamous cell carcinoma. A careful search is needed to find some well-preserved and clearly malignant cells before an unequivocal diagnosis of carcinoma is made. Diff-Quik® 600×.

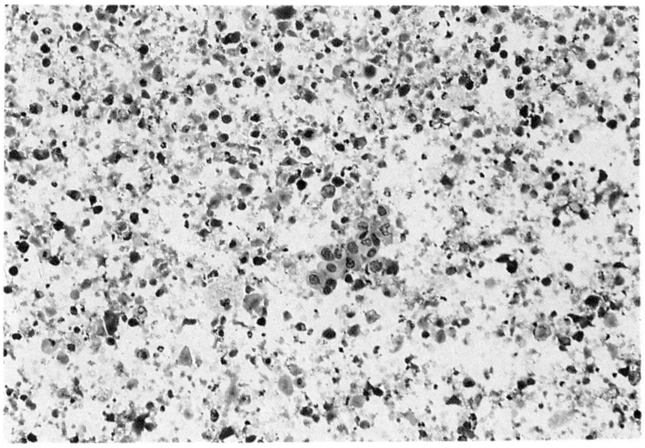

FIGURE 2.17 Aspirate of upper cervical-parotid mass. Note the very necrotic background with scattered degenerated atypical cells. The necrosis is out of proportion to what would be expected with an inflamed branchial cleft cyst. Careful search is necessary to find a few clearly malignant squamous cells. Occult primary tumors producing this type of necrotic metastasis are found commonly in the tonsil. Diff-Quik® 250×.

BRANCHIAL CLEFT CYST

Fluid is dark and turbid

Keratin debris and inflammatory cells

Benign squamous cells

****Degeneration causes atypia**

AUTOIMMUNE DISORDERS

Autoimmune disorders that produce salivary gland enlargement include benign lymphoepithelial lesion, Sjogren's disease, Sjogren's syndrome, and Mikulicz's disease. These entities are interrelated. Benign lymphoepithelial lesions are usually localized, presenting as a distinctive tumor mass, but the salivary gland may be diffusely involved. When the lesion is present as part of Sjogren's syndrome the patient can have a constellation of symptoms including keratoconjunctivitis sica, xerostomia, and evidence of connective tissue disease, usually rheumatoid arthritis.[28]

The histopathologic appearance of the salivary glands varies with the stage of the process. The sequence of changes includes infiltration by chronic inflammatory cells, chiefly lymphocytes and plasma cells, progressive atrophy of acinar parenchyma, and ductal proliferation resulting in the formation of "epimyoepithelial islands" (Figure 2.18). Cytologic features depend upon the stage at which the gland is aspirated. The

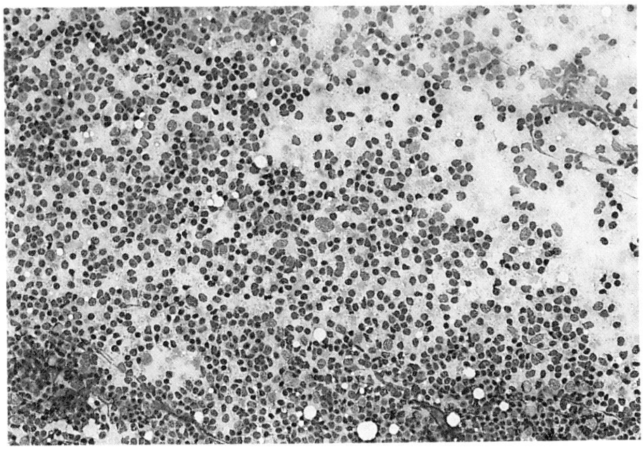

FIGURE 2.18 Parotid gland aspiration. Cellular aspirate with mixed lymphoid infiltrate dominated by small lymphocytes. The center of the photomicrograph shows a loosely textured mixture of lymphoid cells, including some follicular center cells representing the cytologic picture of a lymphoid follicle. No epimyoepithelial elements are present in this smear. Diff-Quik® 250×.

commonly encountered aspiration biopsy findings are summarized below.

BENIGN LYMPHOEPITHELIAL LESION

Cyst fluid (occasionally) with degenerative changes in the duct cells and lymphoid elements

A proteinaceous background more prevalent if there is cystic degeneration

Numerous lymphocytes

Fragments of ductal cells in cohesive sheets

The differential diagnostic problems most often found to be confusing are cystic degeneration in epidermoid or mucoepidermoid carcinomas; Warthin's tumor; and nonspecific chronic obstructive sialadenitis.[12,29] A primary lymphoma presenting as a totally or partially infarcted lymph node may also result in diagnostic problems as the exact identification of the cells may be impossible. Infarction and inflammation may also alter the appearance of salivary gland duct cells that may be contained in lymph nodes in the upper cervical, parotid area.[30]

NEOPLASMS

Tumors of the salivary glands comprise less than 3 percent of all neoplasms in the head and neck. Between 75% and 85% are found in the parotid glands. Approximately 10% to 20% of all salivary gland tumors arise outside of the major salivary glands, occurring in lacrimal glands, mucous glands of the palate, lips, tongue, nasopharynx, accessory sinuses, and larynx. The palate is the most common site of minor salivary gland tumors.[31]

Benign tumors are much more common than malignant ones; they account for over four-fifths of parotid tumors but for less than half of the tumors of other major salivary glands or the minor salivary glands.[31] According to Enroth, one of six tumors in the parotid gland, one of three in the submandibular gland, and almost half of the tumors of the palate will be malignant.[32]

Clinically, rapid growth and fixation are features suggesting a malignant salivary gland tumor, but sometimes these same findings can be encountered in benign neoplasms as well as inflammatory conditions of the salivary glands. Facial nerve paralysis is an ominous sign for malignancy with salivary gland tumors and usually occurs late in the clinical course. Lymphadenopathy may reflect metastatic disease but also can be encountered just as often with inflammatory conditions.

BENIGN NEOPLASMS

Listed below are the benign neoplasms of salivary glands that include the morphologic variants of adenoma and the most common major salivary gland tumor, pleomorphic adenoma (mixed tumor):

1. Pleomorphic adenoma (benign mixed tumor)
2. Monomorphic adenoma (basal cell adenoma)
3. Adenolymphoma (Warthin's tumor)
4. Oncocytoma
5. Hemangioma-hemangioendothelioma

Pleomorphic Adenoma (Benign Mixed Tumor)—Clinical and Cytologic Characteristics

This tumor is slow growing and usually well demarcated. It occurs most commonly in the parotid, accounting for more than 70 percent of all parotid tumors. It is particularly found in the tail of the parotid, but is also encountered in the other major as well as minor salivary glands. Usually this neoplasm is painless and has been present for a long time with very slow increase in size. On examination the tumor is usually firm or hard, smooth and mobile. Size is quite variable and related to duration.[33]

The aspiration smears reveal a fibrillary metachromatic chondromyxoid ground substance with blunt-ended spindle mesenchymal cells lying free, adjacent to and embedded within this stromal matrix. Epithelial cells occur both singly and in clusters and are intimately mixed with the fibrillary and chondroid stromal matrix (Figure 2.19). Even examination of the freshly smeared aspirate may reveal the white granular matrix found in a typical mixed tumor. The center of a benign mixed tumor may

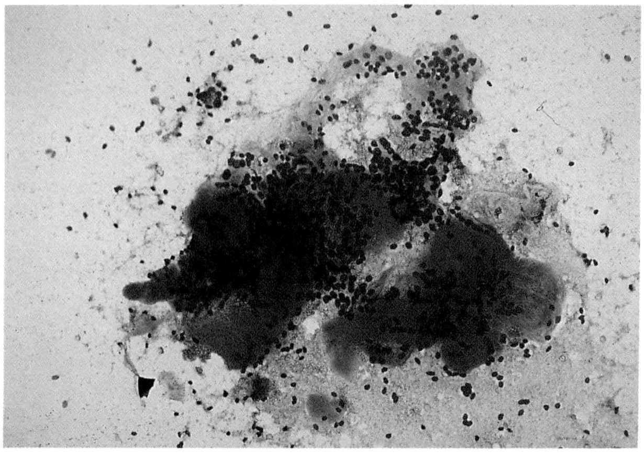

FIGURE 2.19 Parotid gland aspiration. Typical smear pattern with intimate mixture of sheets of epithelial cells embedded in a dense metachromatic stroma. Nuclei of the epithelial cells are uniform and evenly spaced. Diff-Quik® 250×.

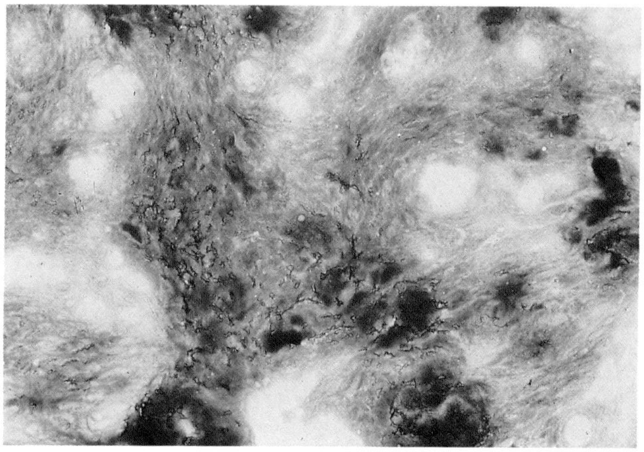

FIGURE 2.20 Parotid gland aspiration. Dominant pattern of metachromatic stroma is seen, which has no recognizable cells. The stroma is not as intensely staining as is usually the case in benign mixed tumor. It has a more mucoid appearance, which can stimulate low-grade mucoepidermoid carcinoma. Diff-Quik® 250×.

become cystic. In that event, an aspirate from the center will only yield fluid but will leave a residual mass. Occasional cases may have tyrosine crystals present in the smears, a feature supporting the diagnosis of mixed tumor.[34]

BENIGN MIXED TUMOR (PLEOMORPHIC ADENOMA)

Fibrillary chondromyxoid ground substance
- **–Metachromatic on Diff-Quik®**
- **–Blunt-ended spindle mesechymal cells**

Clusters, sheets and single epithelial cells
- **–Bland, uniform cells**
- **–Round nuclei, even chromatin**

****May be cystic; tyrosine crystals**

When interpreting aspiration biopsies from pleomorphic adenoma, differential diagnostic problems are low-grade mucoepidermoid carcinomas if the ground substance is loose and mucinlike and does not have the dense fibrillar or distinctly chondroid pattern of background matrix (Figure 2.20). Intracellular mucin may occur in benign mixed tumors but raises the possibility of mucoepidermoid carcinoma or a mucin-producing adenocarcinoma.[35] Metaplastic squamous cells may also be present, again leading to a misdiagnosis of mucoepidermoid carcinoma or well-differentiated squamous cell carcinoma. Spontaneous infarction in one case of benign mixed tumor resulted in a clinical and aspiration diagnosis of carcinoma (Figure 2.21).[36]

Mixed tumors may be predominantly epithelial with a limited amount of ground substance. This can result in a diagnosis of monomorphic adenoma. This is not a serious problem as both monomorphic and pleomorphic adenoma are handled surgically by simple excision. However, some pleomorphic adenomas have areas histologically indistinguishable from adenoid cystic carcinoma. An aspirate dominated by that pattern can result in diagnosis of adenoid cystic carcinoma (Figure 2.22). When areas of suspected adenoid cystic carcinoma are found on aspiration smears, look carefully at the rest of the smears for any inconsistencies in the pattern. This may be the only clue that the tumor is in reality only a pleomorphic adenoma.

Epithelial atypia in a pleomorphic adenoma, often histologically in the form of single very large nuclei, may also be found in aspiration biopsy smears. Thunnissen

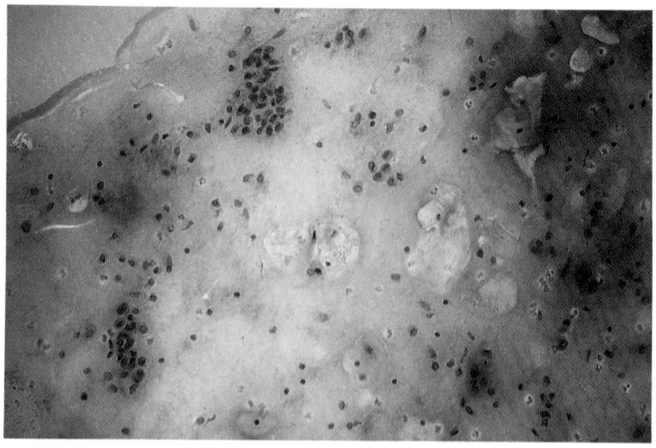

FIGURE 2.21 Parotid gland aspiration. Mucinous-like background with benign differentiated squamous cells in the center of the photomicrograph and small sheets of the epithelial cells more typical of the benign mixed tumor adjacent. Excision showed typical benign mixed tumor with areas of differentiated squamous epithelium in the center of the tumor. Papanicolaou 250×.

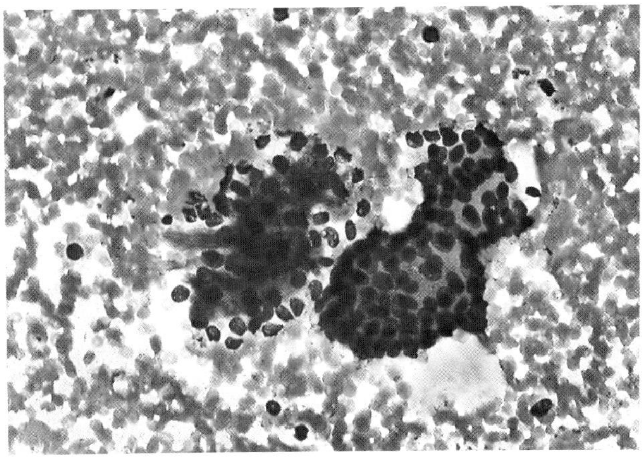

FIGURE 2.22 Submaxillary salivary gland aspirate. Smear pattern simulating adenoid cystic carcinoma in benign mixed tumor. Other areas of the smear were typical for benign mixed tumor, but it may be necessary for some examples to report as a differential diagnosis. Diff-Quik® 600×.

et al. demonstrated polyploidy by DNA cytometry in aspirates from pleomorphic adenomas with atypia. A single case of carcinoma ex-pleomorphic adenoma had a tetraploid stem line.[37] As in tissue pathology, this feature does not connote malignancy. A striking spindle cell pattern may also be found on aspiration biopsy. The clusters of spindle cells may appear in a palisade pattern and simulate a nerve sheath tumor (Figure 2.23). These pleomorphic adenomas with predominantly myoepithelial cell proliferations are only a variant on the mixed tumor pattern histologically. They have no malignant connotations. Some of these tumors may be pure myoepitheliomas. Cystic degeneration, as noted previously, may cause sampling problems and problems of differential diagnosis with other cystic salivary gland neoplasms, some of which are low-grade malignancies.[38–40]

Monomorphic Adenoma—Clinical and Cytologic Characteristics

The parotid gland is the most common site for monomorphic adenomas of the salivary gland. Patients are usually over 50 years of age. These neoplasms are often less than 3.0 centimeters in diameter and tend to lie in a superficial position in the gland where they are frequently mistaken for a lymph node. Clinically, however, this tumor is indistinguishable from pleomorphic adenoma. The most common pattern is the basal cell adenoma. A variation of the basal cell adenoma pattern, with more ground substance, has been referred to as membranous adenoma. Rarely adenomas are composed of clear or sebaceous cells. Those with sebaceous cells may also have a lymphoid component, sebaceous lymphadenoma. They are extremely rare.[41] Hurban and colleagues reported two cases diagnosed by aspiration biopsy, one an intraoral lesion in the left buccal space.[42]

The cytologic features of monomorphic adenoma include numerous clusters of cohesive cells arranged in tubules and cords. The tumor cells are uniform with round or oval nuclei and scant cytoplasm. Ground substance is minimal or absent.[43] However, when present, the ground substance is intensely metachromatic and very adherent to the clusters and trabeculae of epithelial cells. This may cause problems in differential diagnosis with adenoid cystic carcinoma, when the tumor cells cover round masses of this stroma (Figure 2.24). This pattern is generally limited in extent and inconsistent with monomorphic adenoma. The trabeculae of epithelial cells will more often have this stroma as a band or line at the periphery of the cell group (Figure 2.25). Other differential diagnostic problems are distinction from pleomorphic adenoma when there is a predominance of epithelial elements and distinction from pleomorphic adenoma when ground substance is more

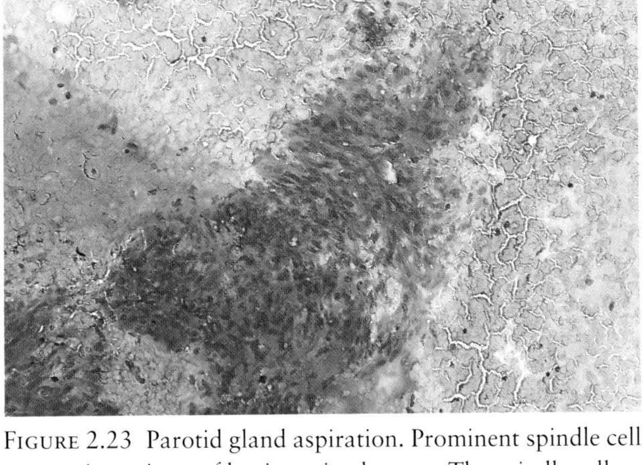

FIGURE 2.23 Parotid gland aspiration. Prominent spindle cell pattern in aspirate of benign mixed tumor. The spindle cells occur in a palisade pattern resembling neurilemomma. These cells are predominantly myoepithelial and stain by immunocytochemistry for actin and S-100 protein. Diff-Quik® 250×.

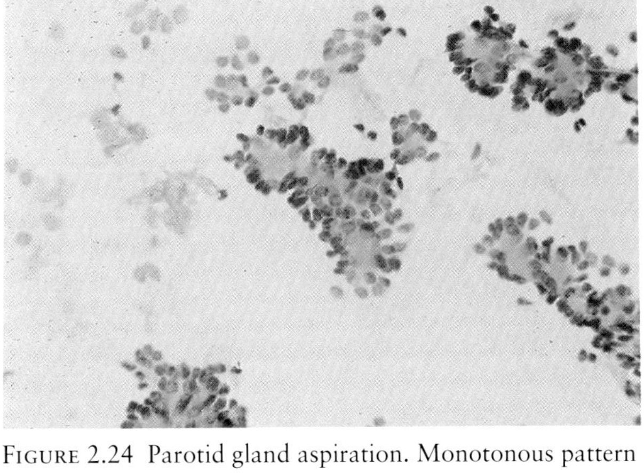

FIGURE 2.24 Parotid gland aspiration. Monotonous pattern of small cells from a monomorphic adenoma. The tumor cells have uniform oval nuclei surrounding dense homogeneous stroma simulating a pattern of adenoid cystic carcinoma. Papanicolaou 400×.

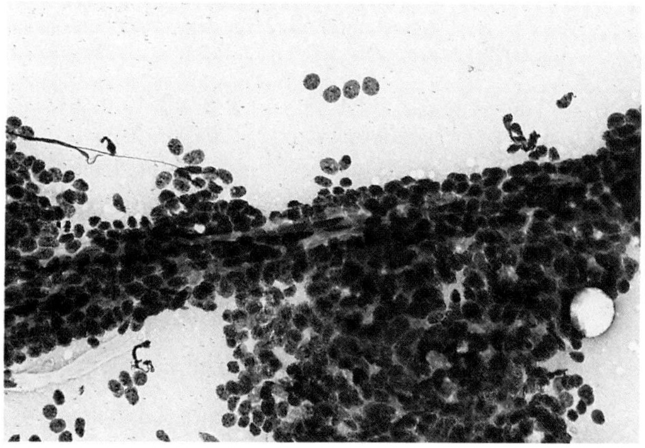

FIGURE 2.25 Parotid gland aspiration. Monomorphic adenoma with linear arrangement of cells along a band of metachromatic stroma. Diff-Quik® 400×.

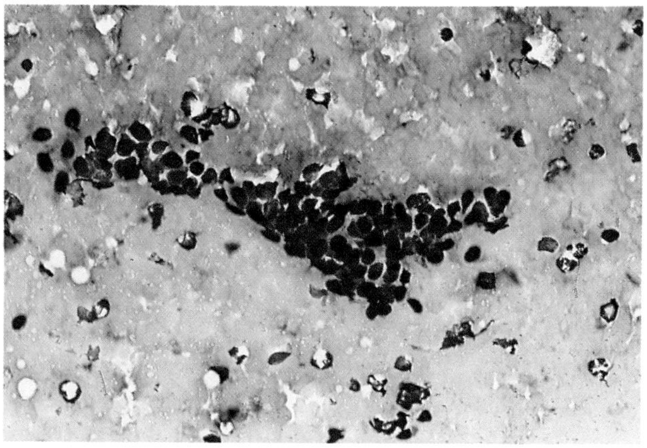

FIGURE 2.26 Submaxillary gland aspiration. Solid pattern without acinar arrangement of the cells in aspirate from adenoid cystic carcinoma. Monotonous pattern of small oval-shaped cells looks identical to that of monomorphic adenoma. Diff-Quik® 400×.

abundant, as in the membranous form. In addition to overlap with typical forms of adenoid cystic carcinoma, the solid pattern of that malignancy can be quite difficult to distinguish from monomorphic adenoma (Figure 2.26). If the mass if painful and the pain appears to follow nerve distribution in the area, then adenoid cystic carcinoma is a more likely diagnosis.[12,44–46]

MONOMORPHIC ADENOMA

Minimal ground substance

Dense metachromatic material tightly associated with cells

Cohesive cell clusters

Arranged in tubules and cords

Epithelial cells uniform
- **Round to oval nuclei**
- **Scant cytoplasm**

Adenolymphoma (Warthin's tumor)—Clinical and Cytologic Characteristics

This neoplasm is generally asymptomatic although 10 percent of patients present because of pain, pressure sensation, or rapid increase in size. Almost invariably, the mass has been present for a long time. Usually it occurs in the parotid gland where it is found most often in the lower pole. It may also arise within lymph nodes superficial or medial to the parotid. Much less commonly Warthin's tumor involves the submandibular gland. Minor salivary glands are extremely rare as a site for this tumor. Occasionally the tumor is bilateral. Clinically, adenolymphoma is well defined, soft, or fluctuant, but occasionally firm, particularly if located deep within the parotid gland. Size may range from 1.0 to 8.0 cm. This neoplasm occurs most commonly after the age of 40 and there is a 5:1 male predominance. Warthin's tumor is very rare in blacks.[47]

The cytologic picture is a background of amorphous or granular debris containing scattered sheets of oncocytic-appearing cells. These cells have a granular cytoplasm with round, slightly eccentric nuclei (Figure 2.27). The cells are quite uniform unless there have been degenerative changes. Then the cells appear much more squamous, sometimes with atypical, very dark and irregular nuclei, simulating dysplastic and degenerated squamous cells (compare with Figure 2.8). The lymphocytes usually occur dispersed on in some small aggregates. They are generally small, mature lymphoid cells, but the lymphoid tissue seen histologically does contain reactive follicles and some of the larger lymphoid cells from these follicles may be seen in the aspiration.[48] The background of the smear may also appear mucoid or mucinous and will stain quite metachromatically.

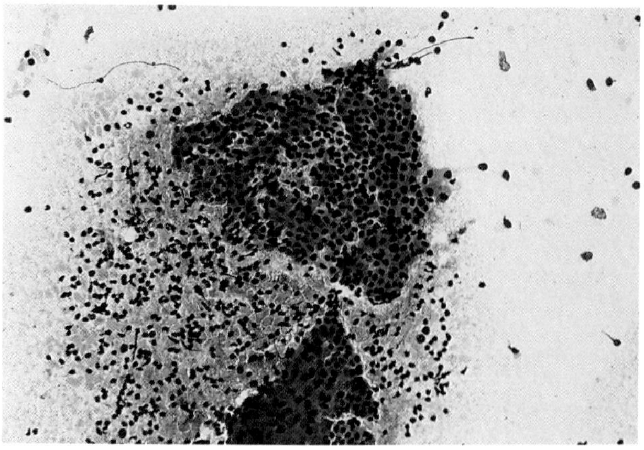

FIGURE 2.27 Parotid gland aspiration. Typical cytologic picture of Warthin's tumor composed of large, flat sheets of oncocytic cells with a background of scattered lymphocytes. Diff-Quik® 250×.

Accompanied with degenerated squamous-appearing cells this smear pattern can easily simulate a well-differentiated mucoepidermoid carcinoma (compare with Figure 2.3).[12]

WARTHIN'S TUMOR

Mucoid mucinous, or watery background +/– cholesterol crystals "machine oil"

Variable cellularity

Oncocytes arranged in cords or groups or fragments
- **–May be fragments of squamous metaplasia +/– atypia**
- **–Large cells with abundant, granular cytoplasm**
- **–Eccentric nuclei and prominent central nucleoli**

Lymphocytes
- **–Heterogeneous population especially plasma cells and small lymphocytes**
- **–Occasional germinal center fragments and DNA artifact**

Differential diagnostic problems include obtaining a suitably diagnostic aspirate from a Warthin's tumor that has become cystic; the presence of the mucoid material leading to consideration of low-grade mucoepidermoid carcinomas as described above; squamous metaplasia with atypia; a necrotic background suggesting a metastatic squamous cell carcinoma from another site; and a predominance of oncocytes that might indicate a true oncocytoma. Oncocytoma is quite rare in the salivary gland, and the aspirate of it can also be accompanied by a small number of lymphocytes. The number of abnormal cells is usually far fewer in a cystic Warthin's tumor with squamous metaplasia than in metastatic squamous cell carcinoma that has undergone necrosis with cyst formation.[49] It is not possible to find a truly large and very obvious malignant squamous cell in a cystic Warthin's tumor versus metastatic squamous cell carcinoma.

Oncocytoma—Clinical and Cytologic Characteristics

The distribution of salivary gland involvement by oncocytomas is similar to that of adenolymphomas. This lesion rarely exceeds 5.0 centimeters. Bilaterality and multicentricity are not infrequent despite the rarity of this tumor. Most patients are in their sixth decade. Growth of the tumor is slow and typically it has been present for a number of years. Oncocytic change is typical of salivary glands seen in advanced age, but one assumes that if there is a defined mass this does represent a true neoplasm. Malignant oncocytomas are extremely rare.[50]

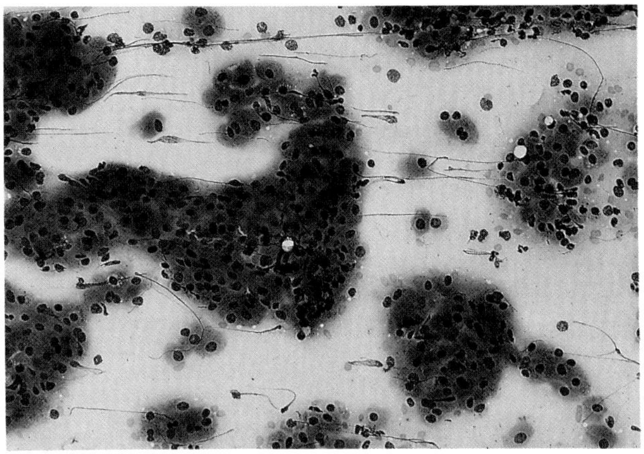

FIGURE 2.28 Parotid gland aspiration. Large sheets of oncocytic cells with a few lymphocytes in the background. One cytologic clue that may differentiate oncocytoma from Warthin's tumor are the more round and serpentine configuration of the oncocytic cells. Diff-Quik® 250×.

The smears are dominated by cohesive sheets and some three-dimensional clumps of oncocytes. There should be an absence of fluid, debris, and lymphoid cells though a few lymphoid cells may be present in the background of some aspirates from true oncocytomas (Figure 2.28). Differential diagnostic problems are that some nononcocytic tumors will have cells with abundant cytoplasm that resemble oncocytes, namely, acinous cell carcinoma, intermediate cells of mucoepidermoid carcinoma, and some adenocarcinomas that are not more specifically classifiable. Oncocytomas are also occasionally cystic and indistinguishable from an adenolymphoma.[12] While they are exceedingly rare, malignant oncocytomas can be indistinguishable cytologically from benign oncocytomas. In two reported cases, malignant oncocytomas were recognized correctly.[51,52]

ONCOCYTOMA

High cellularity

Monomorphic population of oncocytes
- **–Clusters, fragments and single cells**
- **–Large cells with abundant, granular cytoplasm**
  - **–Eccentric nuclei and prominent central nucleoli**

****Fluid, lymphocytes, and debris absent**

Hemangioma-hemangioendothelioma—Clinical and Cytologic Characteristics

Hemangioma of the salivary glands is quite rare, but it is the most common salivary gland neoplasm in childhood. The aspirates are usually just blood, but that, coupled with the clinical presence of a rather soft mass in the salivary gland of a child, is certainly supportive evidence for the diagnosis. One case reported of a hemangioendothelioma of the parotid in a teenage patient demonstrated both a very bloody aspirate and high cellularity. The FNA diagnosis was made on a recurrence of the original lesion in the preauricular area.[53] A more typical example was reported by Hilborne et al. The aspiration smears had a bloody background with only a few clusters of bland spindle-shaped cells.[54]

MALIGNANT NEOPLASMS

Malignant Mixed Tumor (Carcinoma Ex-Pleomorphic Adenoma)—Clinical and Cytologic Characteristics

Malignant mixed tumor most commonly presents in a patient with a benign mixed tumor that has been present for a considerable period of time, either due to the lack of prior treatment or following several recurrences. There is malignant transformation of the benign neoplasm (carcinoma ex-pleomorphic adenoma). Transformation is often marked clinically by sudden rapid growth of the salivary gland mass that has been present for some time. Usually the malignant element is epithelial. Much less frequently, the stromal elements are malignant, resulting in a sarcomatous or carcino-sarcomatous pattern. Rarely, a mixed tumor that is histologically and cytologically benign may metastasize, usually as a solitary mass in the lung.[55]

Cytologically, malignant mixed tumor demonstrates sheets of poorly differentiated malignant epithelial cells with either squamous or glandular features or both (Figure 2.29). Rarely the smear pattern is dominated by malignant spindle cells of a sarcoma. There is metachromatic stroma but without a particular pattern, as seen in benign mixed tumor, unless any remaining such area in the neoplasm is actually sampled by the aspiration.[56]

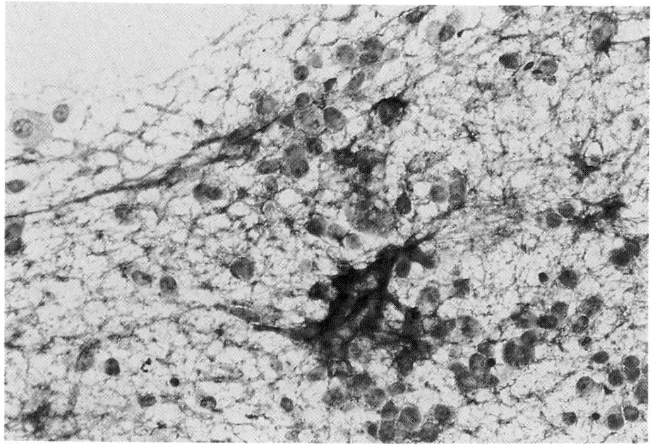

FIGURE 2.29 Parotid gland aspiration. Diffuse pattern of malignant cells forming a few small aggregates within strands of metachromatic stroma. Nuclei have somewhat coarse chromatin and variation in size. Lack of any organized pattern is the most definitive feature of carcinoma while the strands of stroma suggest the possibility of origin of this carcinoma in benign mixed tumor. Diff-Quik® 400×.

MALIGNANT MIXED TUMOR

Limited amount of metachromatic stroma

Sheets and aggregates of malignant epithelial cells

Lack of defined pattern or architecture

Rare squamous or glandular organization
- **–Scant cytoplasm and variably sized nuclei**
- **–Coarse chromatin**
- **–Visible nucleoli**

The differential diagnostic problems encountered include cases where the metachromatic stroma is not a prominent feature or is so nonspecific in pattern and composition that the tumor is identified only as a poorly differentiated or undifferentiated malignancy (Figure 2.30). Pronounced atypia in a benign mixed tumor may lead to an erroneous diagnosis of malignant transformation. This latter differential problem should not occur because the atypia is limited to a few individual cells. There is a lack of an overall abundance of clearly malignant cells as seen in most cases of malignant mixed tumor. Malignancy may not be obvious in some aspirates of carcinoma ex-pleomorphic adenoma as noted by Layfield et al. In a small series, these au-

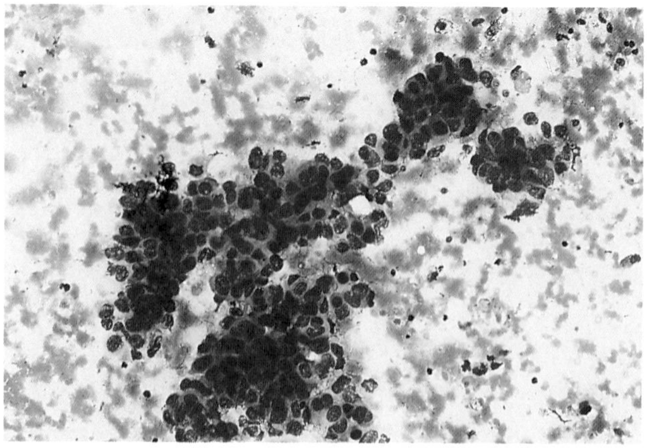

FIGURE 2.30 Parotid gland aspiration. Clusters of poorly differentiated malignant cells. Overlapping cells suggest a poorly differentiated glandular pattern. Nuclei demonstrate variation in size and shape with irregular nuclear edges. There is a slight degree of background necrosis but no definitive stroma in this field to suggest origin from a mixed tumor of the salivary gland. Diff-Quik® 250×.

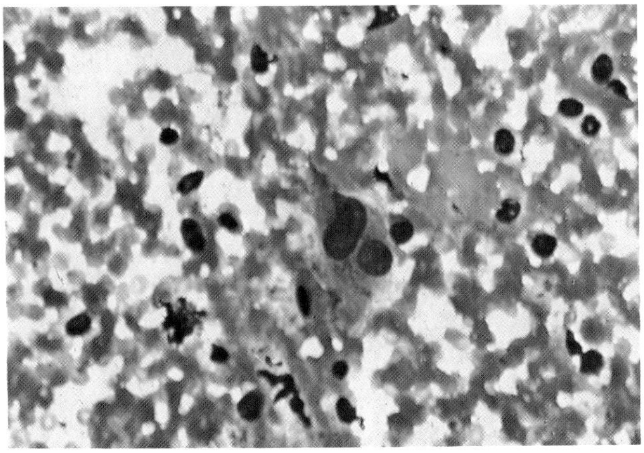

FIGURE 2.31 Parotid gland aspiration. Scattered large nuclei were seen in this aspiration smear of an otherwise typical benign mixed tumor. These cells do not indicate malignancy in a mixed tumor. Diff-Quik® 600×.

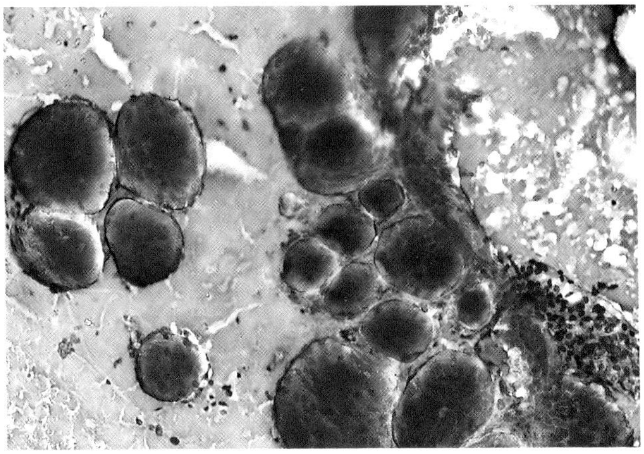

FIGURE 2.32 Submaxillary gland aspiration. Large field of round, metachromatic globular structures containing small, uniform epithelial cells at the edges of the stromal material and covering the surface in part. This feature of surrounding the basement membrane material can be appreciated by having to focus through multiple planes to see the individual epithelial cells clearly. This is the most typical feature of adenoid cystic carcinoma. Diff-Quik® 250×.

thors have reported success in the separation of benign and malignant mixed tumors with the use of digital image analysis (Figure 2.31).[57]

Adenoid Cystic Carcinoma—Clinical and Cytologic Characteristics

This neoplasm is common in the parotid gland but occurs with equal frequency in the submandibular gland. Among malignant salivary gland tumors, it is more often found in the minor salivary glands. Presentation in childhood is unusual. The mean age at the time of diagnosis is usually mid-40s. Pain is frequent because adenoid cystic carcinomas tend to invade nerves.[58] Clinically, this neoplasm is firm and often feels circumscribed. Occasionally it presents as a vague fullness in the area of a salivary gland with pain out of proportion to what is noted clinically.

The cytologic features are large, spherical globules of metachromatic material surrounded by uniform, relatively small tumor cells (Figure 2.32). Solitary, smaller, rounded stromal masses or hyaline fingerlike structures are found between neoplastic cells without spindled stromal cells embedded in this metachromatic material (Figure 2.33). The neoplastic cells are closely packed, cohesive, uniform, round or oval cells with scant cytoplasm. Nuclei are hyperchromatic but with a very uniform chromatin distribution. Nucleoli stained either by the Papanicolaou method or hematoxylin and eosin are quite inconspicuous.[59]

The differential diagnostic problems revolve around distinguishing this tumor from others with small round to oval uniform cells. This includes monomorphic adenoma, acinic cell carcinoma of the salivary gland, and dermal neoplasms of sweat glands. Distinction from monomorphic adenoma and the rare epithelial-myoepithelial carcinoma may be quite difficult if the globular bodies of basement membrane material seen in adenoid cystic carcinoma are scant or absent (Figure 2.34).[60,61] Histologically, pleomorphic adenomas may have areas within them indistinguishable from adenoid cystic carcinoma. If sampled by aspiration, this type of benign mixed tumor may appear exactly like adenoid cystic carcinoma (review Figure 2.22). One case of adenoid cystic carcinoma arising within a pleomorphic adenoma has been studied by fine needle aspiration biopsy.[62]

Some anaplastic forms of adenoid cystic carcinoma may resemble anaplastic carcinomas of other sites (Figure 2.35). Dermal sweat gland neoplasms may occur in the area of the head and neck and can resemble adenoid cystic carcinoma in aspirates including the appearance of the metachromatic globular bodies. Cylindroma, a most often benign primative cutaneous skin adenexal adenoma found most commonly on the scalp, may have the same cytologic pattern as adenoid cystic carcinoma of salivary gland origin.

ADENOID CYSTIC CARCINOMA

Large spherical globules of hyaline material
- **–Highly metachromatic on Diff-Quik®**
- **–Separate or associated with basaloid cells**
- **–Fibrillar strands with poor smear technique**

Small, spindled or basaloid cells
- **–Cohesive clusters with central globules**
- **–Cells appear to encircle central globules**
- **–Scant cytoplasm**
- **–Hyperchromatic nuclei**
- **–Even, coarse chromatin**
- **–Inconspicuous nucleoli**

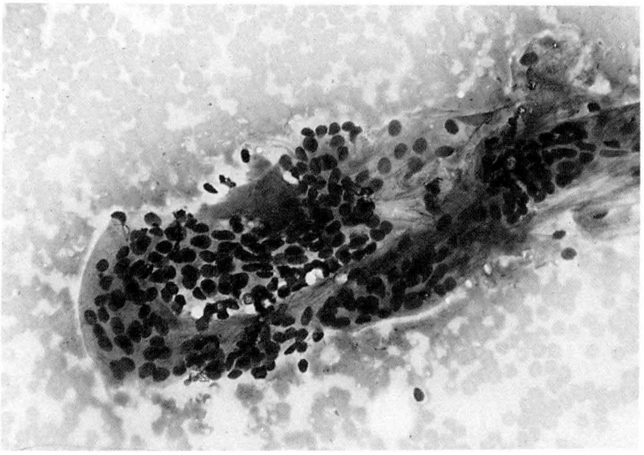

FIGURE 2.33 Submaxillary gland aspiration. Strands of dense basement membrane material have small uniform epithelial cells embedded within it. There is no typical pattern of adenoid cystic carcinoma in this field. The cell arrangement is quite similar if not identical to some aspiration smear patterns of benign mixed tumor. Diff-Quik® 400×.

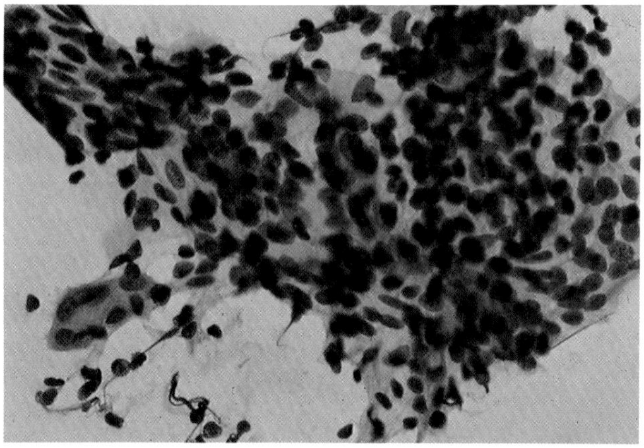

FIGURE 2.34 Submaxillary gland aspiration. Pattern of more spindle-shaped cells and only rare foci of small cells surrounding the basement membrane material (lower left of the illustration). Nuclei are uniform in size, shape, and chromasia and do not have visible nucleoli. This field is indistinguishable from aspirates of monomorphic adenoma or benign mixed tumor of the salivary gland. Papanicolaou 600×.

Acinic Cell Carcinoma—Clinical and Cytologic Characteristics

The incidence of this neoplasm outside the parotid gland is low. The second most commonly involved site is the minor salivary glands. Occasionally the tumor involves both parotid glands. While seen most frequently in patients in their fifth decade, this neoplasm also occurs in children.[63] Clinically it is firm but not hard, usually 2.0 to 4.0 cm in diameter and well circumscribed. While often solitary, the tumor may be multifocal. This tumor grows quite slowly, therefore the history of the presence of a mass may be quite long, not uncommonly several years. The author has seen one typical example that was present for 12 years before an aspiration biopsy was performed and the diagnosis revealed.

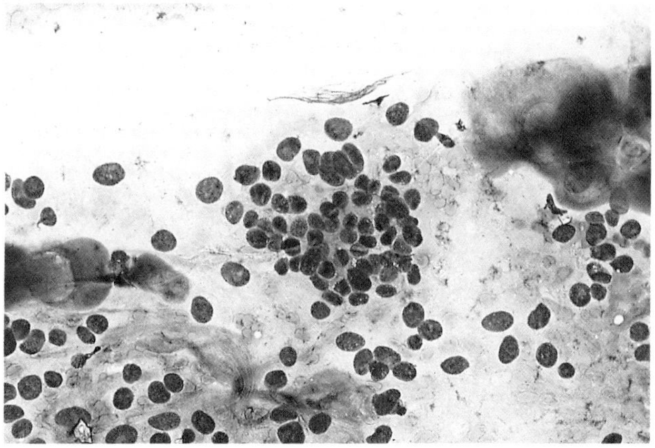

FIGURE 2.35 Submaxillary gland aspiration. Adenoid cystic carcinoma that appear solid and less differentiated. Malignancy of the individual cells is more obvious, but a consistent pattern of adenoid cystic carcinoma is lacking. Diff-Quik® 400×.

Aspirates of acinic cell carcinoma typically have a clean background with numerous tumor cells in cohesive sheets and clusters, some with visible fibrovascular cores (Figure 2.36). The cytoplasm is abundant and granular, and the cells are mildly pleomorphic and somewhat larger than the cells of adenoid cystic carcinoma or monomorphic adenoma. The nuclei of the tumor cells are small, usually round, and with distinct and also round, prominent nucleoli (Figure 2.37). The background contains bare, round lymphocyte-like tumor nuclei, and lymphocytes may be present sometimes in large numbers. This is not surprising because lymphocytes are often found in a band at the periphery of acinic cell carcinoma.[64,65]

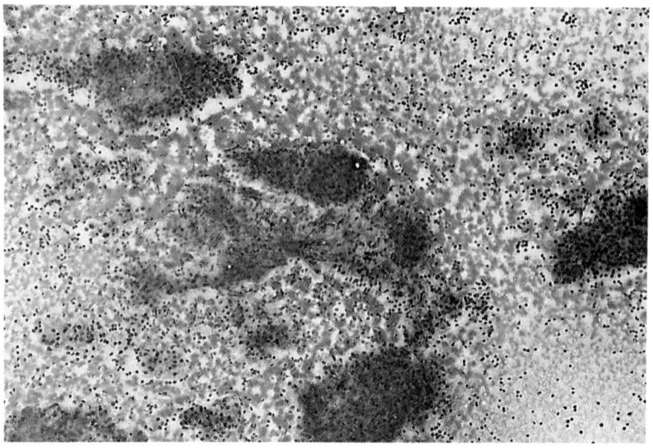

FIGURE 2.36 Parotid gland aspiration. Cellular smear with clusters and branching arrangement of cells. Some indication of fibrovascular cores of stroma can be seen in the center of the field. Diff-Quik® 100×.

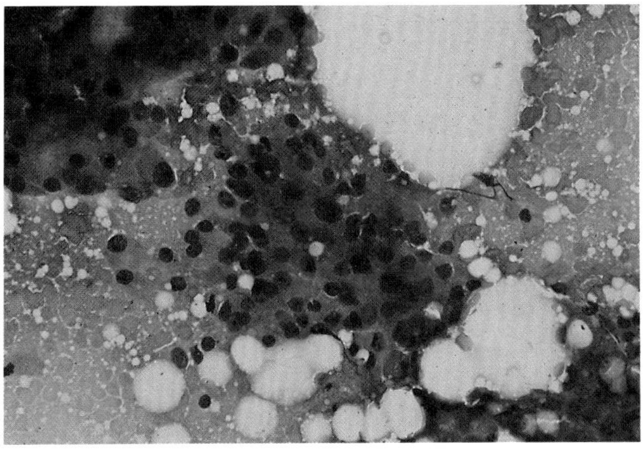

FIGURE 2.37 Parotid gland aspiration. Clusters of tumor cells from acinic cell carcinoma. Relatively abundant and granular cytoplasm is present. Nuclei are uniform, round, and larger than nuclei from cases of monomorphic adenoma and adenoid cystic carcinoma. Notice how the cell arrangement simulates an expanded version of a normal salivary gland acinous. Diff-Quik® 400×.

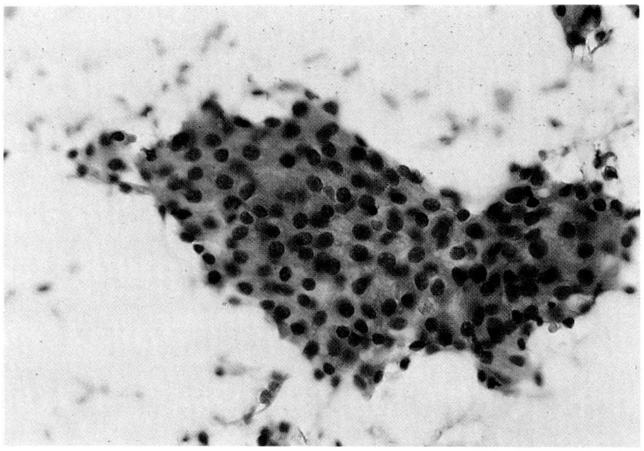

FIGURE 2.38 Parotid gland aspiration. Sheet of tumor cells from acinic cell carcinoma with both clear and granular, oncocytic appearance to the cytoplasm. The cells do not have the abundance of cytoplasm of a true oncocytoma or the consistent granularity of the cytoplasm seen in aspirates from that neoplasm. The cells lack the prominent nucleoli usually found with metastatic renal cell carcinoma. Papanicolaou 600×.

ACINIC CELL CARCINOMA

Clean background with scattered bare nuclei

High cellularity

Monomorphic cell population

Moderate size acinar cells
–Abundant granular cytoplasm
–Uniform, round nuclei

****Absent duct structures**

The differential diagnostic problems are the result of variability of the tumor cells of acinic cell carcinoma. For example, histologically this tumor may have an oncocytic appearance or be composed of clear cells. It can therefore look like an oncocytoma or Warthin's tumor on aspiration biopsy, or it can be mistaken for mucoepidermoid carcinoma or, very rarely, metastatic renal cell carcinoma because of the clear cells (Figure 2.38). Cytologically, some cases of acinic cell carcinoma look aggressive and may then be mistaken simply for nonspecific adenocarcinoma. None of these misclassifications are very significant except for Warthin's tumor or oncocytoma because at least the presence of a malignant neoplasm has been recognized in all other cases. Some very well differentiated examples may have tumor cells that look very similar to normal salivary gland acini; however, with a good aspiration sample, there are usually many more of these cells than one would expect from a hyperplastic, essentially normal or inflamed salivary gland (Figure 2.39).

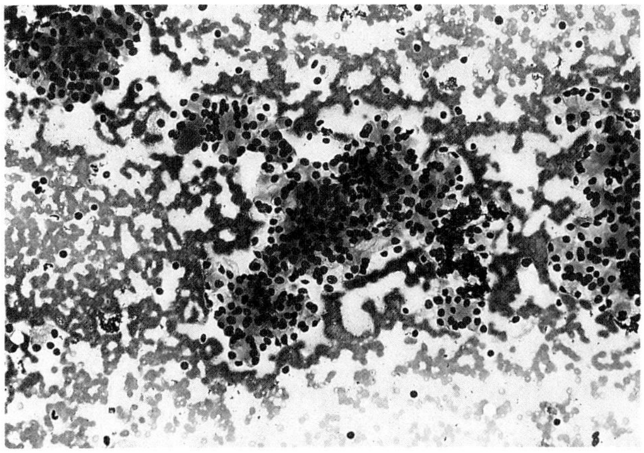

FIGURE 2.39 Parotid gland aspiration. Cells from acinic cell carcinoma that closely mimic the acinar pattern of normal salivary gland. The cells are very monotonous and there is an unusually large number for normal salivary gland. No fat is seen between the cell clusters. Diff-Quik® 250×.

Mucoepidermoid Carcinoma—Cytologic Characteristics

The majority of mucoepidermoid carcinomas arise from the epithelium of the large ducts of both major and minor salivary glands. The parotid gland is most commonly involved by this neoplasm. However, the relative incidence of this tumor is higher in the glands of the palate than in the parotid or submandibular glands. Although these tumors may occur at any age, the peak incidence is in the patient's third decade and varies little through the sixth decade. Clinically, the presentation of mucoepidermoid carcinoma varies and this variability is related to the histologic composition of the tumor. In cases of low-grade mucoepidermoid carcinoma, significant symptoms and signs of a malignant neoplasm are unusual apart from the presence of a slowly growing mass.[66] With aggressive or advanced cases, there is fixation of the mass; pain or facial paralysis may occur. The higher grade neoplasms clinically demonstrate rapid growth.

The cytologic appearance of this neoplasm is highly variable and corresponds to the histologic diversity of mucoepidermoid carcinoma.[67] The tumor can be divided into well-differentiated, moderately differentiated, and poorly differentiated groups. Cytologically, the aspiration smears of well-differentiated mucoepidermoid carcinoma have a background that may be the result of cystic degeneration with debris, foam cells, metachromatic mucinous material, and parakeratotic squamous cells (Figure 2.40). The epithelial cells are isolated or in small sheets. It is important to find sheets of juxtaposed mucinous and squamous cells to be able to either suspect or definitely indicate the diagnosis cytologically (Figure 2.41). The identification of these small, tissue-like fragments is important because there is minimal cytologic atypia of either the mucinous or squamous cells.[68]

MUCOEPIDERMOID CARCINOMA

Well-differentiated
- **–Cystic background with debris, mucinous material**
- **–Small sheets of epithelial cells**
- **–Parakeratotic and degenerating squamous cells**
- **–Clear, vacuolated cells with basal, compressed nucleus**

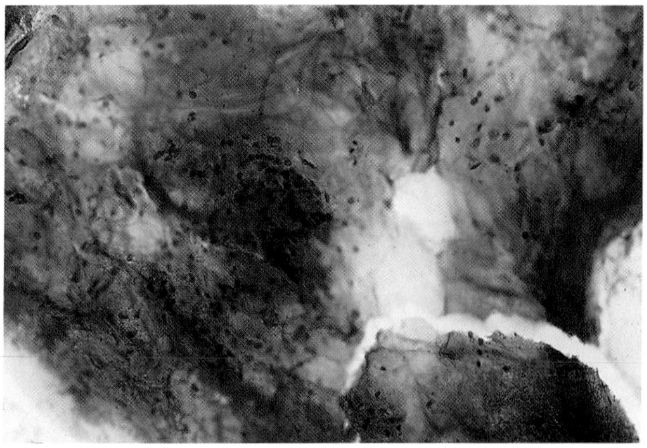

FIGURE 2.41 Parotid gland aspiration. Smear with juxaposed mucinous and squamous cells, the former dominating. There is an extensive mucinous background. The mucinous cells, which make up the majority of the tumor cells in this illustration, have the same color cytoplasm as the background to the smear. Papanicolaou 250×.

Cytologically and sometimes histologically, low-grade mucoepidermoid carcinoma can be confused with any lesion of the salivary glands that undergoes squamous metaplasia, namely, pleomorphic adenoma, adenolymphoma, and chronic sialadenitis. Likewise, both neoplasms that have mucinous changes, namely, pleomorphic adenoma, adenolymphoma, and mucinous adenocarcinoma, may be mistaken for low-grade mucoepidermoid carcinoma (Figure 2.42). Chronic sialadenitis may also exhibit a great amount of mucinous degeneration, presenting a cytologic pitfall with respect to mucoepidermoid carcinoma. Both cystic degeneration of other neoplasms or the presence of an actual cystic lesion, namely, retention cysts or branchial cleft

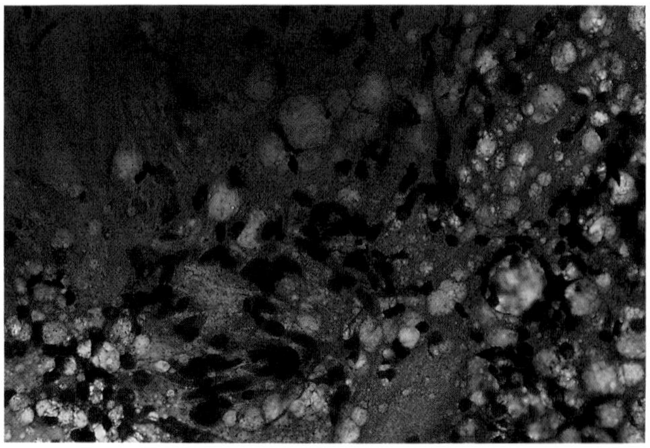

FIGURE 2.40 Parotid gland aspiration. Smears from low-grade mucoepidermoid carcinoma demonstrating metachromatic background of mucin with a sheet of cells having some squamous characteristics, chiefly a dense blue cytoplasm adjacent to some clear vacuolated cells. The vacuoles, which compress the tumor cell nucleus, also stain lightly metachromatic. Diff-Quik® 400×.

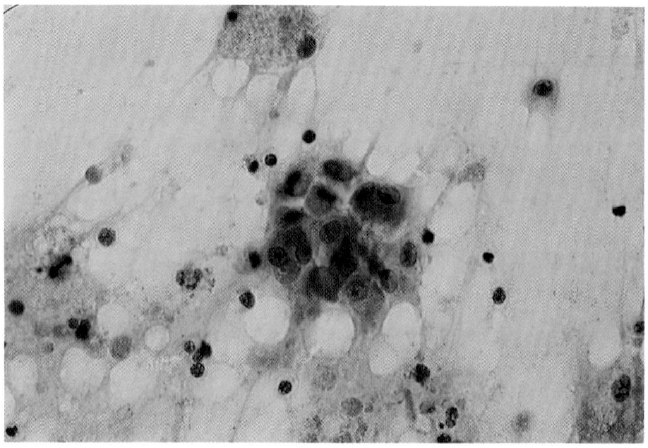

FIGURE 2.42 Parotid gland aspiration. Small sheets of cells with squamous features and atypia within a mucinous-like background. This smear is from a Warthin's tumor with cystic degeneration and squamous metaplasia that simulates, to some degree, low-grade mucoepidermoid carcinoma. Papanicolaou 600×.

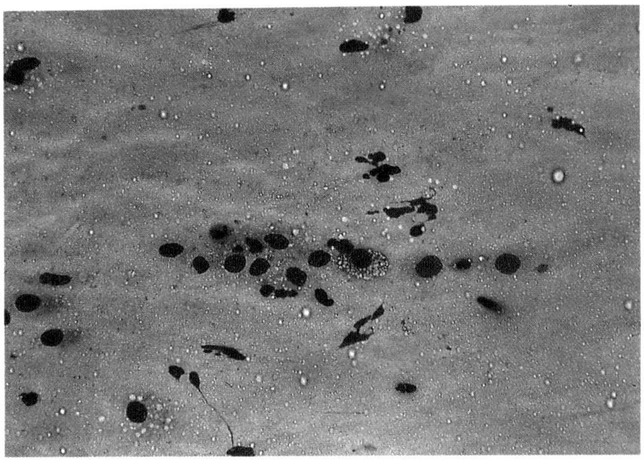

FIGURE 2.43 Aspirate of a mass in the buccal mucosa. Mucocele demonstrating mucinous background of the smear with a few bland cells showing small degenerative vacuoles in the cytoplasm. The smear lacks the usual cellularity of a salivary gland neoplasm and does not show a clear separation of cell types—mucinous and squamous cell—that one expects with well-differentiated mucoepidermoid carcinoma. Diff-Quik® 400×.

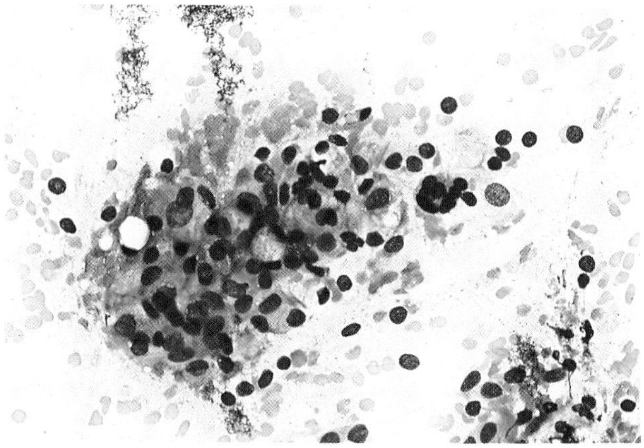

FIGURE 2.44 Parotid gland aspiration. Intermediate-grade mucoepidermoid carcinoma. Two cell types, squamous and mucinous, are present, but the malignant features of both are much more evident here in comparison to low-grade mucoepidermoid carcinoma. Diff-Quik® 400×.

cysts that contain mucin and squamous cells, fall into the differential diagnosis of aspirates from low-grade mucoepidermoid carcinoma (Figure 2.43).[12]

The cytologic features of moderately differentiated mucoepidermoid carcinoma still demonstrate two type of cells—mucinous and/or cells with a clear cytoplasm and squamous cells—that in Diff-Quik®-stained smears, have a deep blue, dense cytoplasm. Both types of cells are more obviously malignant, as evidenced by increase in nuclear size, more pleomorphism of the nuclei, and more prominent nucleoli. The contrast between the two cell types is not as definitive, reflecting the same lack of striking contrast histologically with this neoplasm (Figure 2.44).

MUCOEPIDERMOID CARCINOMA

Moderately differentiated
- **–Often two cell types—less contrast between them**
- **–Mucinous with clear cytoplasm**
- **–Squamous with hard, dense cytoplasm**
  - **–Nuclear: cytoplasmic ratio increased in both cell types**
  - **–Increased pleomorphism**
  - **–Prominent nucleoli**

Differential diagnostic problems occur when one cell type predominates. When mucin-containing cells are few in number, the aspirate will look like squamous cell carcinoma, a distinctly rare neoplasm of the salivary glands. The opposite cytologic pattern may occur with a dominance of mucinous cells that will be mistaken for an adenocarcinoma or even carcinoma ex-pleomorphic adenoma, a much more common, primary malignant tumor of the salivary glands. If the clear cells predominate and there is not too much pleomorphism, then the cytologic pattern mimics an acinic cell carcinoma with clear cells or conceivably raises the possibility of a clear cell carcinoma metastasized from the kidney. Intermediate-grade mucoepidermoid carcinoma may also undergo cystic degeneration yielding only fluid on the initial aspiration. The caveat of reexamination for any residual mass is important, necessitating repeat aspiration of such a mass for a more definitive diagnosis. The author has seen one example in which the cystic mass completely disappeared following aspiration, but the fluid contained clearly malignant cells. Exploration found a small, residual salivary gland tumor in the parotid that proved histologically to be a moderately differentiated mucoepidermoid carcinoma.

The aspiration smear pattern of poorly differentiated mucoepidermoid carcinoma is highly cellular with sheets, some clusters, and isolated tumor cells showing typical malignant features of a poorly differentiated carcinoma (Figure 2.45). There is frequently a lack of sufficient differentiation of these malignant cells to actually classify this tumor as mucoepidermoid carcinoma, specifically. Use of mucicarmine stain may demonstrate mucin secretion and aid in the diagnosis, but the high-grade nature of the cytologic features is sufficient to indicate the presence of an aggressive carcinoma. Therefore, the exact classification is unimportant. Essentially, the only differential diagnostic problem is the lack of sufficient differentiation of the malignant glandular and squamous cells to allow distinction from other types of poorly differentiated or undifferentiated tumors.

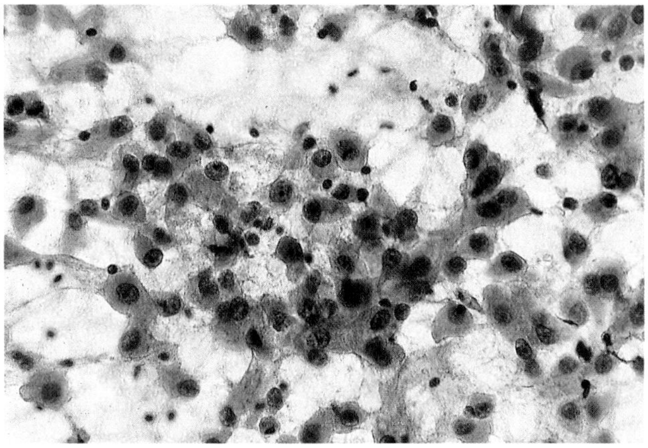

FIGURE 2.45 Parotid gland aspiration. Cellular aspirate with a loose, irregular arrangement of tumor cells. There is little evidence of contrast between squamous and mucous-producing cells. Nuclei are variable in size and shape and have very coarse chromatin and prominent nucleoli. Papanicolaou 400×.

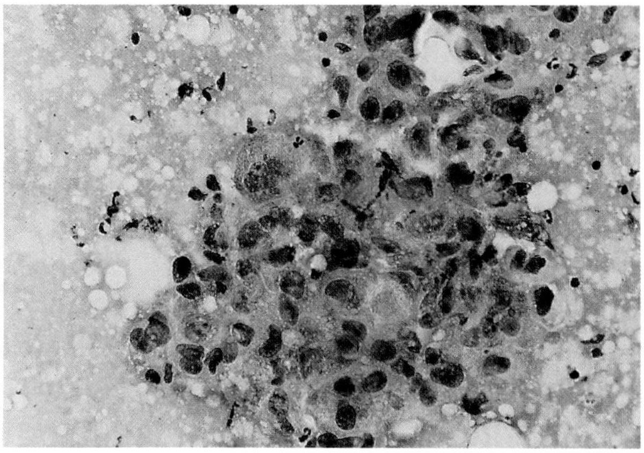

FIGURE 2.46 Parotid gland aspiration. Large sheet of malignant squamous cells that are poorly differentiated. Cytoplasm is eosinophilic and relatively dense. Hematoxylin and eosin 400×.

MUCOEPIDERMOID CARCINOMA

Poorly differentiated

High cellularity

Epithelial cells in sheets and clusters and isolated singly
- **–Obvious malignant features**
- **–Little distinction between squamous and glandular cells**
- **–Pleomorphic nuclei, coarse chromatin**
- **–Prominent nucleoli**

Squamous Cell Carcinoma—Cytologic Characteristics

Primary squamous cell carcinoma of the salivary gland is rare. Many of these neoplasms represent mucoepidermoid carcinomas in which the squamous element predominates. Other examples are metastases to the salivary glands from other sites, the lung and oral cavity. Determining that squamous cell carcinoma actually arises in the salivary gland rather than being metastatic to the gland can be quite difficult.[69]

The cytologic characteristics of this tumor depend on the degree of differentiation. The smears are cellular and composed of sheets and isolated, often pleomorphic-shaped tumor cells. Clusters of neoplastic cells are infrequent. The more differentiated examples have orangeophilic, keratinized tumor cells demonstrated with the Papanicolaou stain. These same tumor cells will have very dense and deep-blue cytoplasm with well-defined cell boundaries as seen on air-dried smears and with Romanowsky staining methods. The keratinizing squamous cell carcinomas have a background of necrosis and acute inflammation. The poorly differentiated examples retain the dense cytoplasm, which is basophilic with the Papanicolaou stain but is still a deep blue with the Diff-Quik® stain. The nuclei of poorly differentiated neoplastic cells have very coarse chromatin and very visible nucleoli (Figure 2.46). The sheets of tumor cells will still demonstrate sharp cell boundaries and some cytoplasmic attachments—general cytologic features of squamous cell carcinoma.

SQUAMOUS CELL CARCINOMA

Cytology dependent on differentiation

High cellularity

Background of necrosis and cell debris

Acute inflammation

Sheets and irregular fragments of pleomorphic cells
- **–Well-defined boundaries (orangeophilic on Papanicolaou; deep blue on Diff-Quik®)**
- **–Cytoplasmic keratinization**
- **–Pleomorphic nuclei, coarse chromatin**
- **–Distinct nucleoli**

Differential diagnostic problems include cases of well-differentiated squamous cell carcinoma, which can be mistaken for inflamed branchial cleft cysts or an abscess if only necrosis or inflammation with a few very degenerated tumor cells is present.[12] It will be necessary to screen such smears quite carefully for a very few recognizable neoplastic cells. Sometimes a cell block is useful in this circumstance to identify the pleomorphic, anucleated and intensely orangeophilic ghosts of squamous cells that are, at the very least, suspicious for the presence of squamous cell carcinoma. As previously described, examples of poorly differentiated mucoepidermoid carcinomas may be considered pure squamous cell carcinoma, an error of no clinical significance.

Adenocarcinoma, Not Otherwise Specified—Cytologic Characteristics

Adenocarcinomas that are not otherwise specifically categorized are quite uncommon. They show a wide age distribution. Clinically, they usually present as a palpable mass.[70,71] They vary in size, are firm to hard and are often somewhat attached to adjacent tissue. The tumors may be papillary or nonpapillary and mucin or nonmucin producing. The nonpapillary forms resemble mammary duct carcinomas cytologically and histologically.[72] The papillary examples have been segregated more specifically in the past few years and are usually of low-grade malignancy and correspondingly less clinically aggressive.[73]

The aspirates are usually cellular with neoplastic cells in papillary, adenomatous, or acinar arrangement. There are variable numbers of isolated cells in these smears. The tumor cells are columnar with rather obvious cytologic features of malignancy (Figure 2.47). Intra- and/or extracellular mucin may be present. The nuclear chromatin is distinct and fine with the nuclei having small but distinct nucleoli in the papillary and better-differentiated forms (Figure 2.48). Those that are less differentiated have the expected prominent nucleoli and coarse chromatin. The papillary clusters are truly three-dimensional and depth of focus is required to see the individual tumor cells clearly.[74]

The common differential diagnostic problems are metastatic adenocarcinomas from other sites, such as lung and the gastrointestinal tract, and examples of mucoepidermoid carcinoma with few squamous cells.

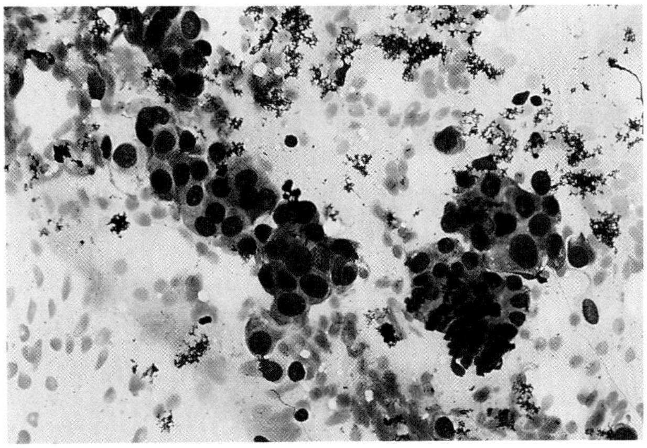

FIGURE 2.47 Parotid gland aspiration. Clusters of poorly differentiated tumor cells. Note variation in nuclear size and shape and granularity of nuclear chromatin. There is no specific pattern. The cells have some finely vacuolated cytoplasm, but there are also some cells with relatively dense cytoplasm and well-defined cell boundaries, features of mucoepidermoid carcinoma. Diff-Quik® 400×.

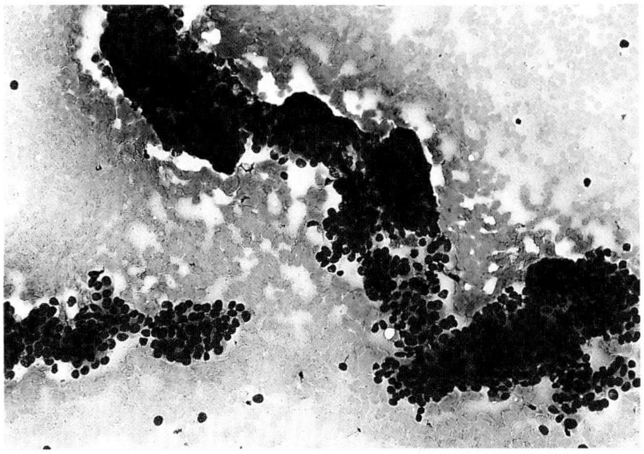

FIGURE 2.48 Submaxillary gland aspiration. Serpentine clusters of uniform cells in the aspirate from polymorphous low-grade adenocarcinoma that was metastatic to the submaxillary lymph node. The original primary occurred in the minor salivary glands of the floor of the mouth. Diff-Quik® 250×.

ADENOCARCINOMA, NOT OTHERWISE SPECIFIED

High cellularity

Isolated cells plus acinar, papillary, or glandular arrangements
- **Columnar cells with moderate, finely vacuolated cytoplasm**
- **Variability in nuclear size, chromatin granularity**
- **Small distinct nucleoli**

Intra- or extracellular mucin may be present

Undifferentiated Carcinoma—Cytologic Characteristics

Undifferentiated carcinoma usually presents clinically with signs of malignancy and may be primary or metastatic to the salivary gland. Because primary undifferentiated carcinomas of the salivary gland are quite rare, metastatic carcinoma, particularly from undifferentiated primary carcinomas of the lung, is often the first consideration.[75] It has not been possible to differentiate primary, small-cell carcinoma of the parotid from metastasis from a lung primary by the use of immunohistochemistry or electron microscopy.[76] Lymphoepithelial carcinoma, the carcinoma arising in benign lymphoepithelial lesions, is included in the undifferentiated group of salivary gland neoplasms. It is the most common malignant salivary gland tumor in Eskimos and also among Orientals in Asia.[77]

Cytologically, there is no distinctive pattern of these undifferentiated carcinomas. The aspirates are cellular with sheets, groups, and many isolated tumor cells.

The cells have obvious malignant features but lack any suggestion of differentiation (Figure 2.49). When the tumor cells are small, there is individual tumor cell necrosis and a necrotic background with degenerated nuclear DNA, a pattern identical to small-cell carcinoma of the lung. This is the major differential diagnostic problem. Necrosis and small cell size with fragmentation of the cytoplasm may also mimic malignant lymphoma, simulated by a background of lymphoglandular bodies (Figure 2.50). Immunohistochemical stains, employing the leukocyte common antigen, CD45, will help to arrive at the correct diagnosis.

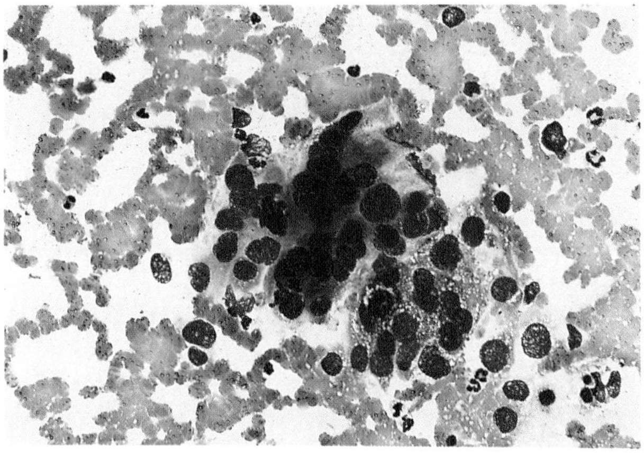

FIGURE 2.49 Parotid gland aspiration. Sheet of very undifferentiated large tumor cells. The cytoplasm forms a syncytia without cell boundaries, and the nuclear overlap is a feature that can be seen with poorly differentiated adenocarcinomas. Diff-Quik® 400×.

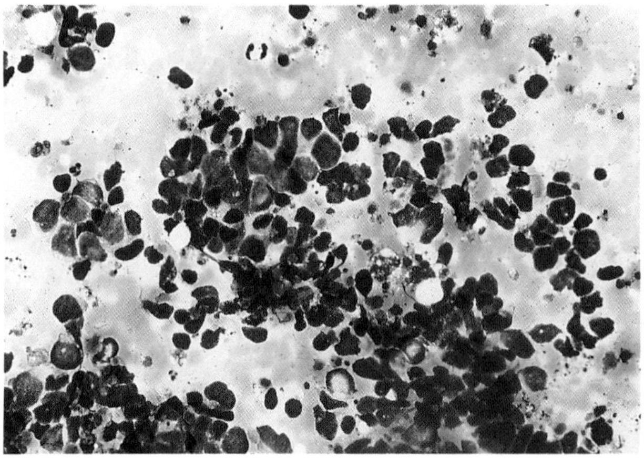

FIGURE 2.50 Parotid gland aspiration. Sheets of undifferentiated, small tumor cells with extensive nuclear molding. Note the two cell populations and necrotic smaller cells and better-preserved large cells, a classic cytologic picture of small-cell carcinomas, regardless of site. There are some cytoplasmic fragments in the background that suggest these cells might be lymphoid, but the extreme degree of molding and the two cell populations are definitely against that diagnosis. Diff-Quik® 400×.

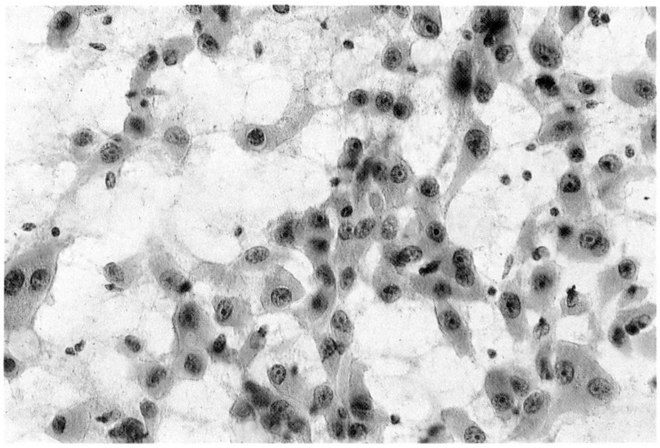

FIGURE 2.51 Parotid gland aspiration. Sheets of spindle-shaped undifferentiated tumor cells from metastatic cutaneous melanoma. Nuclei have coarse chromatin and prominent nucleoli. One cell with double mirror-image nuclei is seen to the right. No pigment is present. Papanicolaou 400×.

Carcinoma Metastatic to the Salivary Gland—Cytologic Characteristics

The majority of tumors metastatic to the salivary gland are of regional origin from primary sites of involvement, such as the scalp, face, external ear and nose, eyelids and lacrimal glands, and the sinonasal, nasopharyngeal, or oropharyngeal areas.[78] Metastases from more distant sites are most commonly from lung, breast, and cutaneous melanoma (Figure 2.51). Occasionally, metastases occur from primary tumors in the kidney and gastrointestinal tract. Cytologic characteristics depend on the site of the primary and may be recognized from a specific pattern or from ancillary studies, immunohistochemistry, and/or electron microscopy. Comparison of the smear pattern with histologic sections from any known primary can be very informative. Two cases of metastatic Merkle cell carcinoma of the skin that metastasized to the parotid gland and were diagnosed on aspiration biopsy have been reported. The resemblance to metastatic small-cell carcinoma from other sites, primarily the lung, is quite close. [79,80]

Lymphomas—Cytologic Characteristics

Lymphomas may occur in the salivary glands, particularly in the parotid gland, either as a primary manifestation or later in the course of disseminated disease. *For more specific examples and cytologic criteria refer to Chapter 4.* Any subtype of non-Hodgkin's lymphoma may be found, although the most frequent forms are small-cell and small cleaved-cell lymphoma followed by rare, large-cell lymphomas. Those arising within mucosa-associated lymphoid tissue (MALT) are predominantly small lymphocytic lymphoma with plasmacytoid differentiation and monocytoid B-cell lymphoma. The latter may progress to large-cell lymphoma, but the clinical course of the MALT lymphomas is prolonged.[81]

Hodgkin's disease may invade salivary glands from contiguous structures, but it is very rare for it to arise *de novo* in salivary gland tissue. The incidence is reported at between 3% and 7% of primary lymphomas of the salivary glands.[81]

Lymphoma may arise from a benign lymphoepithelial lesion, although this is quite rare.[81] Lymphomas usually present as a painless mass. Large-cell lymphomas may increase rapidly in size. The age distribution of lymphoma correlates with the subtype. Small-cell and small cleaved-cell lymphomas are rare in patients under the age of 40 while large-cell lymphoma has a wider age range. Lymphoblastic lymphoma or leukemia may involve the salivary glands and is seen primarily in children and young adults.

Cytologically, the aspirates are quite cellular. They have a relatively monomorphic population composed of mature or immature lymphocytes depending upon the basic morphology of the lymphoma (Figure 2.52). The presence of lymphoglandular bodies on Romanowsky stains aids in the identification of the cells as lymphoid. Immunohistochemical staining of the aspirate, usually a Cytospin preparation, can confirm that the cells are lymphoid (positive CD45) and may be used to type the lymphoma as B or T cell or determine the presence of monoclonality. Molecular biologic techniques may be used to identify gene rearrangements indicating clonality. These studies can also be performed on aspiration biopsy samples.

The differential diagnostic problems are chronic sialadenitis with a heavy lymphoid infiltrate; reactive intra- or paraglandular lymph nodes; a benign lymphoepithelial lesion; and undifferentiated carcinoma (indistinguishable from large-cell lymphoma). Lymphomas may also present initially as a totally infarcted lymph node, particularly in the head and neck area and the submaxillary triangle. The aspirate will demonstrate many necrotic cells, usually small, and with fragments of cytoplasm that can simulate lymphoglandular bodies in the background. The preservation is usually so poor that immunostains are not reliable and may in fact give a positive result for both epithelial and lymphoid antigens. Metastatic tumor to the lymph nodes seldom presents with a totally necrotic enlarged lymph node. Table 2.1 lists the important microscopic differential diagnoses of lesions based on a dominant feature of FNA of the major salivary glands.

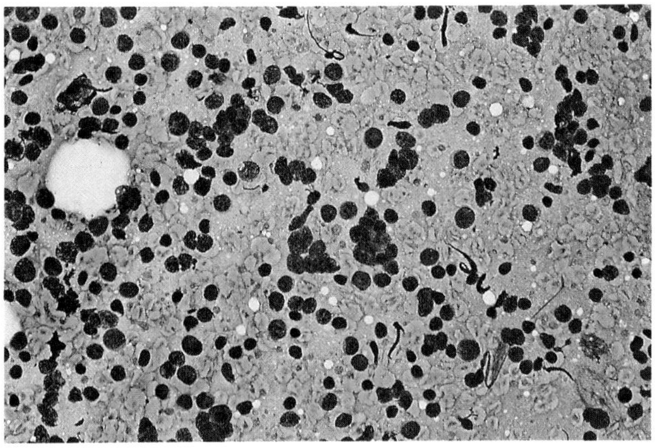

FIGURE 2.52 Parotid gland aspiration. Cellular aspirate with monotonous pattern of immature lymphocytes with a tendency to form small aggregates. The chromatin pattern is open and metachromatic. More mature lymphocytes are present in the background. Numerous lymphoglandular bodies identify the aspirate as being from lymphoid tissue. Diff-Quik® 400×.

COMPLICATIONS

Complications of aspiration biopsy of the salivary gland are quite rare. The author has had a single case of a small hematoma that developed shortly after aspiration biopsy. It was clinically of no concern. Two cases have been reported in which hematomas resulted in transient clinical symptoms that quickly resolved. In both cases, the FNAB was of a vascular lesion. Kameswaran[82] reported an unusual case in which aspiration of a parotid hemangioma resulted in a large hematoma causing transient facial palsy. A related report[83] documented the development of Kasabach-Merrit syndrome (rapidly expanding hemangiomas complicated by thrombocytopenia) following FNAB (20 gauge) of a hemangioma overlying the parotid gland.

Needle tract seeding as a potential complication in aspiration biopsy of salivary gland masses is seldom realized but seems to be much feared. Yamaguchi et al. reported a case of needle tract seeding of a poorly differentiated mucoepidermoid carcinoma of the parotid, but it is important to note that a Vim-Silverman needle, not a fine needle, was used.[84] Several studies have addressed the issue of tumor implantation from FNAB of salivary gland neoplasms. Qizilbash et al. tattooed and excised their needle tracts in an effort to document needle tract seeding. They were unable to do so and concluded that there is no risk of needle tract implantation by fine (less than 22-gauge) needles.[85] Damage to the facial nerve from FNA of the salivary gland has, to the author's knowledge, been reported only in the case noted above. The size of the aspirating needle was not reported in that case.[82]

Histologic alterations from FNAB are of current interest as reflected in the surgical pathology literature. There is concern that FNAB may cause tissue damage that hinders or precludes subsequent histologic interpretation. Based on the literature, this has occurred in relatively few cases.[86,87] The majority of histologic alterations that occur following superficial aspiration biopsy of any site are not dramatic. There are two changes that seem to predominate: (1) a reactive tissue proliferation that eventually leads to a fibrous tract or region and (2) infarction/hemorrhage that may result in more widespread

TABLE 2.1 FNA of the Salivary Gland—Quick Microscopic Reference

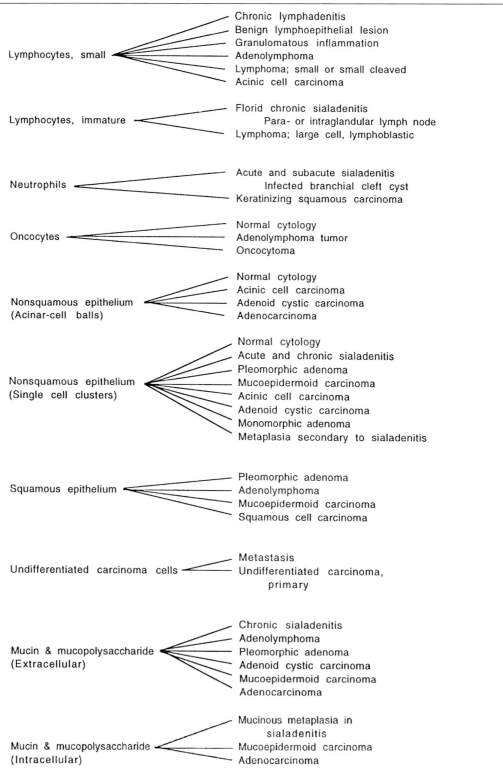

Lymphocytes, small	Chronic lymphadenitis
	Benign lymphoepithelial lesion
	Granulomatous inflammation
	Adenolymphoma
	Lymphoma; small or small cleaved
	Acinic cell carcinoma
Lymphocytes, immature	Florid chronic sialadenitis
	Para- or intraglandular lymph node
	Lymphoma; large cell, lymphoblastic
Neutrophils	Acute and subacute sialadenitis
	Infected branchial cleft cyst
	Keratinizing squamous carcinoma
Oncocytes	Normal cytology
	Adenolymphoma tumor
	Oncocytoma
Nonsquamous epithelium (Acinar-cell balls)	Normal cytology
	Acinic cell carcinoma
	Adenoid cystic carcinoma
	Adenocarcinoma
Nonsquamous epithelium (Single cell clusters)	Normal cytology
	Acute and chronic sialadenitis
	Pleomorphic adenoma
	Mucoepidermoid carcinoma
	Acinic cell carcinoma
	Adenoid cystic carcinoma
	Monomorphic adenoma
	Metaplasia secondary to sialadenitis
Squamous epithelium	Pleomorphic adenoma
	Adenolymphoma
	Mucoepidermoid carcinoma
	Squamous cell carcinoma
Undifferentiated carcinoma cells	Metastasis
	Undifferentiated carcinoma, primary
Mucin & mucopolysaccharide (Extracellular)	Chronic sialadenitis
	Adenolymphoma
	Pleomorphic adenoma
	Adenoid cystic carcinoma
	Mucoepidermoid carcinoma
	Adenocarcinoma
Mucin & mucopolysaccharide (Intracellular)	Mucinous metaplasia in sialadenitis
	Mucoepidermoid carcinoma
	Adenocarcinoma

tissue damage and a total or near total loss of microscopic features needed to identify a true neoplasm.[88]

Spontaneous infarction of lymph nodes and some thyroid and salivary gland lesions have been documented. It is usually not a localized phenomenon. Although attributed temporarily to FNAB, it has usually occurred prior to the procedure as judged by the necrotic nature of the aspirate. Such changes may make the interpretation of the FNAB quite difficult and much less diagnostically specific.

TABLE 2.2 Algorithm to Evaluate FNA of the Salivary Gland Mass

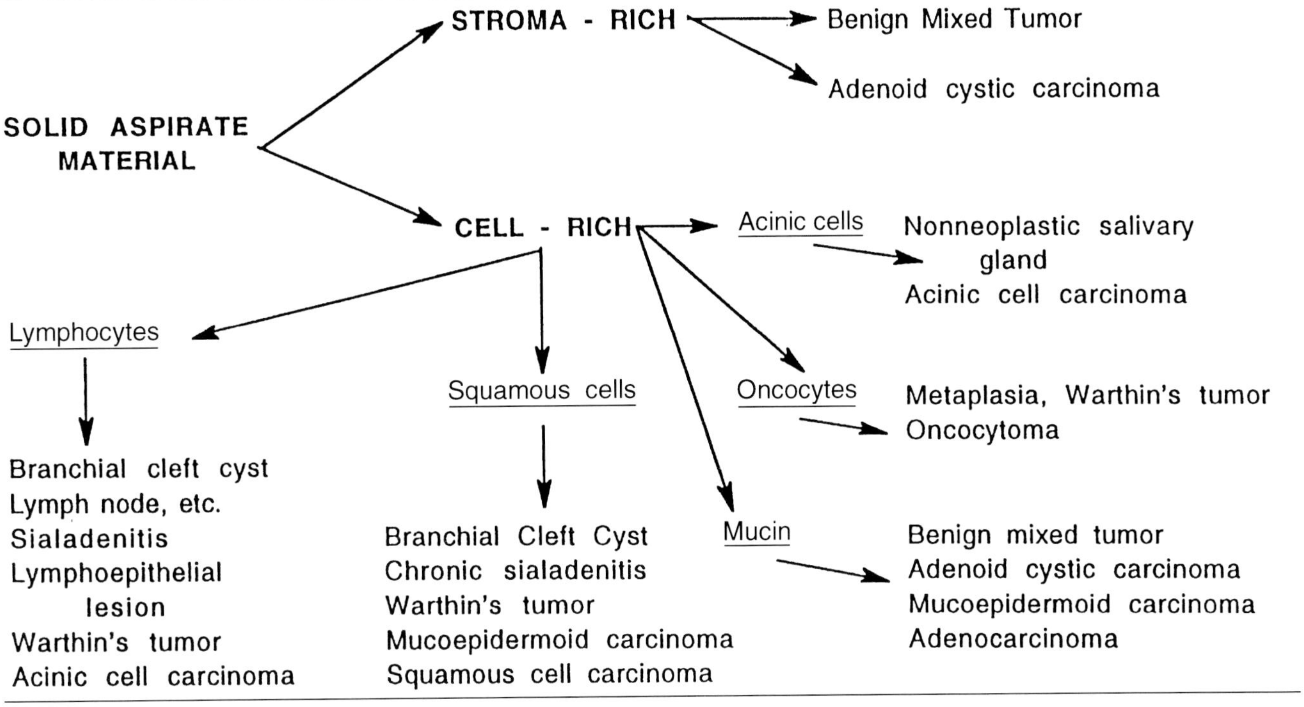

Adapted from Cohen MB, Reznicek MJ, Miller TR. Fine-needle aspiration biopsy of the salivary glands. *Pathol Ann* 1992;2:240. Used with permission.

UTILITY OF SALIVARY GLAND FINE NEEDLE ASPIRATION BIOPSY

There is still some controversy over the utility of FNAB in the workup of patients with salivary gland masses.[38,86,89] There are also numerous reports in the literature that support the efficacy of this technique if utilized in the proper clinical setting.[4,85,90–92] Cohen et al. have provided a valuable algorithm for the analysis of aspirate of salivary gland masses as presented in Table 2.2.[93]

These large series have also shown that clinical complications are virtually nonexistent, with the occasional development of a small hematoma.[12,94] Aspiration biopsy can effectively and efficiently answer some questions about a salivary gland neoplasm: Is it a neoplasm? Is it benign or malignant, primary metastatic or recurrent? This information is quite valuable in directing the next step in evaluation and appropriate treatment of a salivary gland mass.

REFERENCES

1. Martin HE, Ellis EB. Biopsy by needle puncture and aspiration. *Ann Surg* 1930;92:169–181.
2. Eneroth CM, Franzen S, Zajicek J. Cytologic diagnosis on aspirates from 1000 salivary gland tumours. *Acta Otolaryngol* (Suppl.) 1967;224:168–171.
3. Eneroth CM, Zajicek J. Aspiration biopsy of salivary tumors. III. Morphological studies on smears and histologic sections from 368 mixed tumors. *Acta Cytol* 1966;10:440–454.
4. Frable MA, Frable WJ. Fine needle aspiration biopsy of salivary glands. *Larnygoscope* 1991;101: 245–249.
5. Layfield LJ, Tan P, Glasgow BJ. Fine-needle aspiration of salivary gland lesions. *Arch Pathol Lab Med* 1987;11:346–353.
6. Abad MM, G-Macias C, Alonso MJ, Munoz E, Paz JI, Galindo P, Herrero A, Bullon A. Statistical evaluation of the predictive power of fine needle aspiration (FNA) of salivary glands. Results and cytohistological correlation. *Pathol Res Pract* 1992;188:340–343.
7. Pitts DB, Hilsinger RL Jr., Karandy E, Ross JC, Caro JE. Fine needle aspiration in the diagnosis of salivary gland disorders in the community hospital setting. *Arch Otolaryngol Head Neck Surg* 1992;118:479–482.
8. Nettle WJ, Orell SR. Fine needle aspiration in the diagnosis of salivary gland lesions. *Aust NZJ Surg* 1989;59:47–51.
9. Orell SR, Nettle WJS. Fine-needle aspiration biopsy of salivary gland tumours. Problems and pitfalls. *Pathology* 1988;20:332–337.
10. Chan MKM, McGuire LJ. Cytodiagnosis of lesions presenting as salivary gland swellings: A report of seven cases. *Diagn Cytopathol* 1992;8:439–443.
11. Layfield LJ, Glasgow BJ. Diagnosis of salivary gland tumors by fine-needle aspiration cytology: A review of clinical utility and pitfalls. *Diagn Cytopathol* 1991;7:267–272.

12. MacLeod CB, Frable WJ. Fine needle aspiration biopsy of the salivary gland: Problem cases. *Diagn Cytopathol* 1993;9:216–225.

13. Frable WJ. Thin-needle aspiration biopsy. In Bennington JL (ed.), *Major problems in pathology,* Vol. 14. Philadelphia: W.B. Saunders Co., 1983, pp. 119–151.

14. Abad MM, G-Macias C, Alonso MJ, Munoz, Paz JI, Galindo P, Herrero A, Bullon A. Statistical evaluation of the predictive power of fine needle aspiration (FNA) of salivary glands: Results and cytohistological correlation. *Path Res Pract* 1992;188:340–343.

15. Zajdela A, Zillhardt P, Voillemot N. Cytologic diagnosis by fine needle sampling without aspiration. *Cancer* 1987;59:1201–1205.

16. Thackray AC, Lucas RB. Tumors of the major salivary glands. *Atlas of tumor pathology,* 2nd Series, Fascicle 10. Washington, DC: Armed Forces Institute of Pathology, 1974, pp. 1–5.

17. Batsakis JG. Sialadenosis. *Ann Otol Rhinol Laryngol* 1988;97:94–95.

18. Ascoli V, Albedi FM, DeBlasiis R, et al. Sialadenosis of the parotid gland: Report of four cases diagnosed by fine-needle aspiration cytology. *Diagn Cytopathol* 1993;9:151–155.

19. Frierson HF Jr., Fechner RE. Chronic sialadenitis with psammoma bodies mimicking neoplasia in a fine-needle aspiration specimen from the submandibular gland. *Am J Clin Path* 1991;95:884–888.

20. Koss LG, Woyke S, Wlodzimierz Olszewski W. *Aspiration biopsy. Cytologic interpretation and histologic bases,* 2nd ed. New York: Igaka-Shoin, 1992, p. 323.

21. Advisory Council for the elimination of tuberculosis. Centers for Disease Control and Prevention. Initial therapy for tuberculosis in the era of multidrug resistance. *MMWR* 1993;42(RR-7)1:8.

22. Maygarden SJ, Flanders E. Mycobacteria can be seen as "negative images" in cytology smears from patients with acquired immunodeficiency syndrome. *Mod Pathol* 1989;2:239–243.

23. Mair S. Curschmann's spirals and actinomycosis in a fine needle aspirate of the parotid. *Acta Cytol* 1989;33:903–906.

24. Verbin RS, Barnes L. Cysts and cyst-like lesions of the oral cavity, jaws and neck. In Barnes L (ed.), *Surgical pathology of the head and neck.* New York: Marcel Dekker, 1985, pp. 1285–1287.

25. Finfer MD, Gallo L, Perchick A, Schinella RA, Burstein DE. Fine needle aspiration biopsy of cystic benign lymphoepithelial lesion of the parotid gland in patients at risk for the acquired immune deficiency syndrome. *Acta Cytol* 1990;34:821–826.

26. Tao L-C, Gullane PJ. HIV infection-associated lymphoepithelial lesions of the parotid gland: Aspiration biopsy cytology, histology, and pathogenesis. *Diag Cytol* 1991;7:158–162.

27. Labouyre E, Merlio JPH, Beylot-Barry M, DeLord B, Vergier B, Broussard G, LaCoste D, Beylot J, Leng B, Fleury H, Bloch B, deMascarel A. Human Immunodeficiency virus type 1 replication within cystic lymphoepithelial lesion of the salivary gland. *Am J Clin Pathol* 1993;100:41–46.

28. Gunhan O, Celasun B, Dogan N, et al. Fine needle aspiration cytologic findings in a benign lymphoepithelial lesion with microcalcifications. A case report. *Acta Cytol* 1992;36:744–747.

29. Sciubba JJ, Batsakis JG. The major salivary glands. In Silverberg SG (ed.), *Principles and practice of surgical pathology,* 2nd ed. New York: Churchill Livingstone, 1990, pp. 923–925.

30. Cleary KR, Osborne BM, Butler JJ. Lymph node infarction foreshadowing malignant lymphoma. *Am J Surg Pathol* 1982;6:435–442.

31. Auclair PL, Ellis GL, Gnepp DR. *Surgical pathology of the salivary glands: Vol. 25. Major problems in pathology.* Philadelphia: W.B. Saunders Co., 1991, pp. 135–146.

32. Eneroth CM. Salivary gland tumors in the parotid gland, submandibular gland, and palate region. *Cancer* 1971;27:1415–1418.

33. Waldron CA. Mixed tumor (Pleomorphic adenoma and myoepithelioma). In Ellis GL, Auclair PL, Gnepp DR (eds.), *Surgical pathology of the salivary glands: Vol. 25. Major problems in pathology.* Philadelphia: W.B. Saunders Co., 1991, pp. 165–167.

34. Bottles K, Ferrell LD, Miller TR. Tyrosine crystals in fine needle aspirates of a pleomorphic adenoma of the parotid gland. *Acta Cytol* 1984;28:490–492.

35. Stanley MW, Lowhagen T. Mucin production by pleomorphic adenomas of the parotid gland; A cytologic spectrum. *Diagn Cytopathol* 1990;6:49–52.

36. Layfield LF, Reznicek M, Lowe M, Bottles K. Spontaneous infarction of a parotid gland pleomorphic adenoma. Report of a case with cytologic and radiographic overlap with a primary salivary gland malignancy. *Acta Cytol* 1992;36:381–386.

37. Thunnissen FB, Peterse JL, Buchholtz R, et al. Polyploidy in pleomorphic adenomas with cytological atypia. *Cytopathology* 1992;3:101–109.

38. Cramer H, Layfield L, Lampe H. Fine needle aspiration of salivary gland lesions. In Schmidt WA (ed.), *Cytopathology annual.* Baltimore: William and Wilkins, 1993, pp. 181–188.

39. Orell SR, Sterrett GF, Walter Max N-I, et al. *Manual and atlas of fine needle aspiration cytology,* 2nd ed. New York: Churchill Livingstone, 1992, pp. 46–50.

40. Bhatia A. Fine needle aspiration cytology in the diagnosis of mass lesions of the salivary gland. *Indian J Cancer* 1993;30:26–30.

41. Kratochvil FJ. Canalicular adenoma and basal cell adenoma. In Ellis GL, Auclair PL, Gnepp DR (eds.),

Surgical pathology of the salivary glands, Vol. 25. Major problems in pathology. Philadelphia: W.B. Saunders Co., 1991, pp. 202–224.

42. Hruban RH, Erozan YS, Zinreich SJ, et al. Fine-needle aspiration cytology of monomorphic adenomas. *Am J Clin Pathol* 1988;90:46–51.

43. Layfield L. Fine needle aspiration cytology of a trabecular adenoma of the parotid gland. *Acta Cytol* 1985;29:999–1002.

44. Hood IC, Qizilbash AH, Salama SS, et al. Basal-cell adenoma of parotid. Difficulty of differentiation from adenoid cystic carcinoma on aspiration biopsy. *Acta Cytol* 1983;27:515–520.

45. Lopez JI, Ballestin C. Fine-needle aspiration cytology of a membranous basal cell adenoma arising in an intraparotid lymph node. *Diagn Cytopathol* 1993; 9:668–672.

46. Sparrow SA, Frost FA. Salivary monomorphic adenomas of dermal analog type: Report of two cases. *Diagn Cytopathol* 1993;9:300–303.

47. Warnock GR. Papillary cystadenoma lymphomatosum (Warthin's tumor) In Ellis GL, Auclair PL, Gnepp DR (eds.), *Surgical pathology of the salivary glands, Vol. 25. Major problems in pathology.* Philadelphia: W.B. Saunders Co., 1991, pp. 187–201.

48. Eneroth CM, Zajicek J. Aspiration biopsy of salivary gland tumors: II, Morphologic studies on smears and histologic sections from oncocytic tumors. *Acta Cytol* 1965;9:355–361.

49. Olsen KD, Goellner JR. False-positive cytologic findings in Warthin's tumor: A report of two cases. *Ear Nose Throat J* 1992;1:417–421.

50. Goode RK. Oncocytoma. In Ellis GL, Auclair PL, Gnepp DR (eds.), *Surgical pathology of the salivary glands, Vol. 25. Major problems in pathology.* Philadelphia: W.B. Saunders Co., 1991, pp. 225–237.

51. Austin MB, Frierson HF Jr., Feldman PS. Oncocytoid adenocarcinoma of the parotid gland: Cytologic, histologic and ultrastructural findings. *Acta Cytol* 1987;31:351–356.

52. Abdul-Karim FW, Weaver MG. Needle aspiration cytology of an oncocytic carcinoma of the parotid gland. *Diagn Cytopathol* 1991;7:420–422.

53. Jayaram G. Cytology of hemangioendothelioma. *Acta Cytol* 1984: 28:153–156.

54. Hilborne LH, Glasgow BJ, Layfield LJ. Fine-needle aspiration cytology of juvenile hemangioma of the parotid gland: A case report. *Diagn Cytopathol* 1987;3:152–155.

55. Gnepp DR, Wenig BM. Malignant mixed tumors. In Ellis GL, Auclair PL, Gnepp DR (eds.), *Surgical pathology of the salivary glands, Vol. 25. Major problems in pathology.* Philadelphia: W.B. Saunders Co., 1991, pp. 350–368.

56. Qizilbash AH, Young JEM. *Guides to clinical aspiration biopsy. Head and neck.* New York: Igaku-Shoin, 1988, pp. 79–86, 92–94.

57. Layfield LJ, Hall TL, Fu YS. Discrimination of benign versus malignant mixed tumors of the salivary gland using digital image analysis. *Cytometry* 1989; 10:217–221.

58. Tomich CE. Adenoid cystic carcinoma. In Ellis GL, Auclair PL, Gnepp DR (eds.), *Surgical pathology of the salivary glands, Vol. 25. Major problems in pathology.* Philadelphia: W.B. Saunders Co., 1991, pp. 333–349.

59. Eneroth CM, Zajicek J. Aspiration biopsy of salivary gland tumors: IV, Morphologic studies on smears and histologic sections from 45 cases of adenoid cystic carcinoma. *Acta Cytol* 1969;13:59–63.

60. Carrillo R, Poblet E, Rocamora A, et al. Epithelial-myoepithelial carcinoma of the salivary gland. Fine needle aspiration cytologic findings. *Acta Cytol* 1990;34:243–247.

61. Kocjan G, Milroy C, Fisher EW, Everson JW. Cytological features of epithelial-myoepithelial carcinoma of salivary gland: Potential pitfalls in diagnosis. *Cytopathology* 1993;4:173–180.

62. Geisinger KR, Reynolds GD, Vance RP, et al. Adenoid cystic carcinoma arising in a pleomorphic adenoma of the parotid gland. An aspiration cytology and ultrastructural study. *Acta Cytol* 1985;29:522–526.

63. Ellis GL, Auclair PL. Acinic cell adenocarcinoma. In Ellis GL, Auclair PL, Gnepp DR (eds.), *Surgical pathology of the salivary glands, Vol. 25. Major problems in pathology.* Philadelphia: W.B. Saunders Co., 1991, pp. 299–317.

64. Eneroth CM, Jakobsson P, Zajicek J. Aspiration biopsy of salivary gland tumors: V, Morphologic investigations on smears and histologic sections of acinic cell carcinoma. *Acta Radiol* (Suppl.) 1971;310:85–93.

65. Palma O, Torri AM, deCristofaro JA, Fiaccavento S. Fine needle aspiration cytology in two cases of well-differentiated acinic-cell carcinoma of the parotid gland: Discussion of diagnostic criteria. *Acta Cytol* 1985;29:516–521.

66. Auclair PL, Ellis GL. Mucoepidermoid carcinoma. In Ellis GL, Auclair PL, Gnepp DR (eds.), *Surgical pathology of the salivary glands, Vol. 25. Major problems in pathology.* Philadelphia: W.B. Saunders Co., 1991, pp. 269–298.

67. Zajicek J, Eneroth CM, Jakobsson P. Aspiration biopsy of salivary gland tumors: VI, Morphologic investigation on smears and histologic sections of 24 cases with mucoepidermoid carcinoma. *Acta Cytol* 1976;20:35–41.

68. Kumar N, Kapila K, Verma K. Fine needle aspiration cytology of mucoepidermoid carcinoma. A diagnostic problem. *Acta Cytol* 1991;35:357–359.

69. Auclair PL, Ellis GL. Primary squamous cell carcinoma. In Ellis GL, Auclair PL, Gnepp DR (eds.), *Surgical pathology of the salivary glands, Vol. 25. Major problems in pathology.* Philadelphia: W.B. Saunders Co., 1991, pp. 369–378.

70. Everson JW, Cawson RA. Salivary gland tumours: A review of 2410 cases with particular reference to histological types, site, age and sex distribution. *J Pathol* 1985;146:51–58.

71. Auclair PL, Ellis GL. Adenocarcinoma, not otherwise specified. In Ellis GL, Auclair PL, Gnepp DR (eds.), *Surgical pathology of the salivary glands, Vol. 25. Major problems in pathology.* Philadelphia: W.B. Saunders Co., 1991, pp. 318–332.

72. Gal R, Strauss M, Zohar Y, et al. Salivary duct carcinoma of the parotid gland. Cytologic and histopathologic study. *Acta Cytol* 1985;29:454–456.

73. Wenig BM, Gnepp DR. Polymorphous low-grade adenocarcinoma of minor salivary glands. In Ellis GL, Auclair PL, Gnepp DR (eds.), *Surgical pathology of the salivary glands, Vol. 25. Major problems in pathology.* Philadelphia: W.B. Saunders Co., 1991, pp. 390–411.

74. Frierson HF, Covell JL, Mills SE. Fine-needle aspiration cytology of terminal duct carcinoma of minor salivary gland. *Diagn Cytopathol* 1987;3:159–162.

75. Mair S, Phillips JI, Cohen R. Small cell undifferentiated carcinoma of the parotid gland: Cytologic, histologic, immunohistochemical and ultrastructural features of a neuroendocrine variant. *Acta Cytol* 1989;33:164–168.

76. Cameron WR, Johansson L, Tennvall J. Small cell carcinoma of the parotid: Fine needle aspiration and immunochemical findings in a case. *Acta Cytol* 1990;34:837–841.

77. Eversole LR, Gnepp DR, Eversole GM. Undifferentiated carcinoma. In Ellis GL, Auclair PL, Gnepp DR (eds.), *Surgical pathology of the salivary glands, Vol. 25. Major problems in pathology.* Philadelphia: W.B. Saunders Co., 1991, pp. 422–440.

78. Gnepp DR. Metastatic disease to the major salivary glands. In Ellis GL, Auclair PL, Gnepp DR (eds.), *Surgical pathology of the salivary glands, Vol. 25. Major problems in pathology.* Philadelphia: W.B. Saunders Co., 1991, pp. 560–569.

79. Gattuso P, Castelli MJ, Shah PA, et al. Fine needle aspiration cytologic diagnosis of metastatic Merkel cell carcinoma in the parotid gland. *Acta Cytol* 1988;32:576–578.

80. Gherardi G, Marveggio C, Stiglich F. Parotid metastasis of Merkel cell carcinoma in a young patient with ectodermal dysplasia. Diagnosis by fine needle aspiration cytology and immunocytochemistry. *Acta Cytol* 1990;34:831–836.

81. Sciubba JJ, Auclair PL, Ellis GL. Malignant lymphomas. In Ellis GL, Auclair PL, Gnepp DR (eds.), *Surgical pathology of the salivary glands, Vol. 25. Major problems in pathology.* Philadelphia: WB. Saunders Co., 1991, pp. 528–543.

82. Kameswaran M, Abu-Eshy S, Hamdi J. Facial palsy following fine needle aspiration biopsy of parotid hemangioma: A case report and review of literature. *Ear Nose Throat J* 1991;70:801–803.

83. Karabocuglo M, Basarer N, Aydogan U, Demirkol M, Kurdoglu G, Neyzi O. Development of Kasabach-Merrit syndrome following needle aspiration of a hemangioma. *Pediatr Emerg Care* 1992;8:218–220.

84. Yamaguchi KT, Strong MS, Shapshay SM, et al. Seeding of parotid carcinoma along Vim-Silverman needle tract. *J Otolaryngol* 1979;8:49–52.

85. Qizilbash AH, Sianos J, Young JEM, et al. Fine needle aspiration biopsy cytology of major salivary glands. *Acta Cytol* 1985;29:503–512.

86. Batsakis JG, Sneige N, El-Naggar AK. Fine-needle aspiration of salivary glands: Its utility and tissue effects. *Ann Otol Rhinol Laryngol* 1992;101:185–188.

87. Kern SB. Necrosis of a Warthin's tumor following fine needle aspiration. *Acta Cytol* 1988;32:207–208.

88. Powers CN. Fine needle aspiration biopsy: Perspectives on complications: The reality behind the myths. In *Cytopathology annual.* Chicago: ASCP Press, 1995, In Press.

89. Olsen KD. The parotid lump—don't biopsy it! An approach to avoiding misadventure. *Postgrad Med* 1987;81:225–234.

90. Webb AM. Cytologic diagnosis of salivary gland lesions in adult and pediatric surgical patients. *Acta Cytol* 1985;29:503–512.

91. Lindberg LG, Akerman M. Aspiration cytology of salivary gland tumors: Diagnostic experience from 6 years of routine laboratory work. *Laryngoscope* 1976;86:584–594.

92. Kline T, Merriam JM, Shapshay SM. Aspiration biopsy cytology of the salivary gland. *Am J Clin Pathol* 1981;76:263–269.

93. Cohen MB, Reznicek MJ, Miller TR. Fine-needle aspiration biopsy of the salivary glands. *Pathol Ann* 1992;2:213–245.

94. Mavec P, Eneroth CM, Franzen S, Moberger G, Zajicek J. Aspiration biopsy of salivary gland tumors: I, Correlation of cytologic reports from 652 aspiration biopsies with clinical and histologic findings. *Acta Otolaryngol* 1964;58:471–484.

CHAPTER

3 Thyroid and Parathyroid

THYROID

One of the most accessible organs that is frequently selected for FNAB is the thyroid gland; indeed, FNAB has become integral in the workup of patients with thyroid nodules.[1–8] In addition to surgeons and cytopathologists, endocrinologists also perform thyroid aspirations, which in some institutions exceed aspiration biopsies of the breast as the most commonly performed superficial aspiration biopsy.

Although thyroid nodules are frequent, developing at a rate of 0.06% to 0.08% per year in the United States, only a small percentage are actually cancerous (25 cancers per million people per year).[9] Because the vast majority of thyroid nodules are benign, representing nonneoplastic conditions such as goiter or thyroiditis, patients can be managed conservatively with follow-up and/or suppression therapy. Prior to FNAB, surgery was the only specific diagnostic procedure available to these patients. Currently, FNAB is an excellent, minimally invasive, low-risk procedure that easily and rapidly and with high accuracy differentiates individuals with benign disease from those with suspicious or malignant nodules. The other predominant use for FNAB is documentation of thyroid malignancy in those patients on whom surgery is not advised or considered the treatment of choice (Table 3.1). No longer the exclusive province of the academic medical center, FNAB, when used appropriately, has been proven very effective in the community hospital setting.[10]

The Examination

Prior to FNAB, evaluation of clinical information as well as laboratory and radiologic studies is necessary. It is important to be aware of any past or ongoing treatment for thyroid disease. Although still of low incidence, prior neck irradiation sufficiently increases the risk of cancer over the baseline (0.5 percent per year increasing to 5 percent at 20 years)[11] to warrant close follow-up and evaluation of any nodules. Other important information to obtain is the duration and rapidity of growth of the nodule as well as any complaints of hoarseness, dysphagia, or fullness. From a practical standpoint, it is also useful to know if the patient is on any medication or has any health problems that may interfer with the aspiration biopsy, namely, anticoagulants. Historical information should be evaluated in conjunction with any radiologic studies, ultrasonography, and radioiodine uptake studies available. Ultrasonography is extremely useful in determining whether the lesion has a cystic component, a common occurrence in benign nonneoplastic conditions and in less frequently encountered papillary carcinomas. Radioiodine studies can also distinguish hyperfunctioning "hot" nodules of thyrotoxicosis from "cold" or hypofunctioning nodules that have a higher probability of malignancy.

Most patients referred for FNAB have a readily identifiable nodule or nodules or obvious diffuse enlargement. Physical examination should begin with the patient in a sitting position. A visual examination of the anterior neck for any obvious lesions is followed by palpation of the thyroid from the front and then from behind. It is often useful to have the patient take sips of water, swallowing on demand to clearly demarcate the nodule(s). Movement of the palpable nodule during swallowing confirms its presence within the thyroid gland. FNAB can be performed in this position if the patient is comfortable and the mass stabilized. More often the patient is placed in the supine position with a pillow

TABLE 3.1 Clinical Indications for Fine Needle Aspiration Biopsy

Nodule
Solitary nodule in normal thyroid
Dominant nodule in multinodular goiter
Rapid enlargement in solitary or dominant nodule
Nodule in patient with family history of medullary carcinoma
Diffuse Enlargement
Confirm
Chronic lymphocytic thyroiditis
Hyperplasia (Graves' disease)
Acute or subacute thyroiditis
Rapid diagnosis and treatment
Malignant lymphoma
Anaplastic carcinoma

or towel placed under the shoulderblades to hyperextend the neck. This often causes the nodule to become more prominent and easier to isolate for the aspiration biopsy. It is important to ask patients, especially older individuals, if they suffer from vertigo, arthritis, or problems with the cervical spine that make it quite uncomfortable, if not impossible, for them to lie supine with the neck in hyperflexion (Figure 3.1).

The Technique

Although the FNAB technique is the same for the thyroid as for other masses in the head and neck, it is important to remember that as an endocrine organ the thyroid is highly vascular. For this reason, the smaller the needle gauge the better, preferably 23- or 25-gauge needles that can be used with or without negative pressure. A more comprehensive discussion of FNAB technique can be found in Chapter 1. Typically one or two passes should ensure collection of an adequate sample, but this is obviously dependent upon the size of the nodule and the quantity and type of material obtained during the initial FNAB. Hamburger[12–14] suggests that at least six groups of follicular epithelium on two slides is the minimum required to be considered adequate. This guideline is less useful in the case of cystic lesions. Often, physical examination can suggest the possibility of a cyst; a nodule that is smooth, round, and tense. Typically, cystic fluid contains abundant histiocytes with scant follicular epithelium. It is recommended that the area be reaspirated even if no residual mass is palpable.[7,15] If a cystic lesion is suspected, FNAB with an aspiration gun and 10- to 20-mL syringe should be used to collect fluid. This fluid can be transported to the laboratory directly in the capped syringe or can be transferred or rinsed into a tube of balanced salt solution. For solid or semisolid masses, material should be smeared onto slides and/or rinsed into balanced salt solution for cytospins.

Following each FNAB, an assistant or the patient should keep firm pressure on the site of needle puncture for a few minutes to prevent bruising and bleeding. Only a few patients will require an adhesive bandage following the procedure. Significant bleeding within the thyroid may result in a hematoma. Fortunately, if FNAB is properly performed, this is a rare occurrence. In this situation, application of ice to the affected area will rapidly reduce the swelling.

The Diagnosis

Algorithms are step-by-step procedures that can be referred to for appropriate clinical management following categorization of thyroid disease as diffuse or localized (Table 3.2).[16–18] These decision trees can also be useful in the cytologic characterization of thyroid aspiration smears (Table 3.3). However, assessment of any thyroid aspiration begins with the question, has adequate material been obtained? If diagnostic material is available for analysis, then the algorithm can be initiated. Overall cellularity and pattern of the cytopreparations, assessed at low magnification, is the first step. This is followed by evaluation of the individual components of the smears: colloid, follicular cells, lymphocytes, macrophages, and so forth. It has been well documented that the presence of colloid substantially decreases the likelihood that the nodule sampled represents a neoplasm (Figure 3.2). The exception to this generalization is the presence of ropy or bubblegum colloid associated with papillary carcinoma. Neoplasms, whether benign or malignant, are typically highly cellular and monomorphic as opposed to inflammatory, hyperplastic, and nonneoplastic nodules with variable cellularity and smear patterns. Overall architectural pattern as seen with low-power objectives (4× and 10×) should be used in the initial categorization of these lesions.

Normal Cytology

FNAB of normal thyroid often yields scant material and is composed predominantly of scattered follicular cell nuclei and small fragments of thyroid parenchyma that retain their follicular structure, often with remnants of central colloid visible as dark, dense acellular material (Figure 3.3). The three-dimensional nature of the thyroid follicle is best appreciated on the Papanicolaou stain where different focal planes are available (Figure 3.4). On Romanowsky-stained preparations, the nuclei are deep purple, round, and sharply defined; nucleoli are typically not visible with any stain (Figure 3.5A). As with other endocrine organs, variability in nuclear size is normal. Cytoplasm, when intact, has a gray-blue tinge with Romanowsky stains, and pastel, almost translucent green on Papanicolaou stain (Figure 3.5B). At times, lysosomal (paravacuolar) granules may be prominent, staining intensely cobalt blue

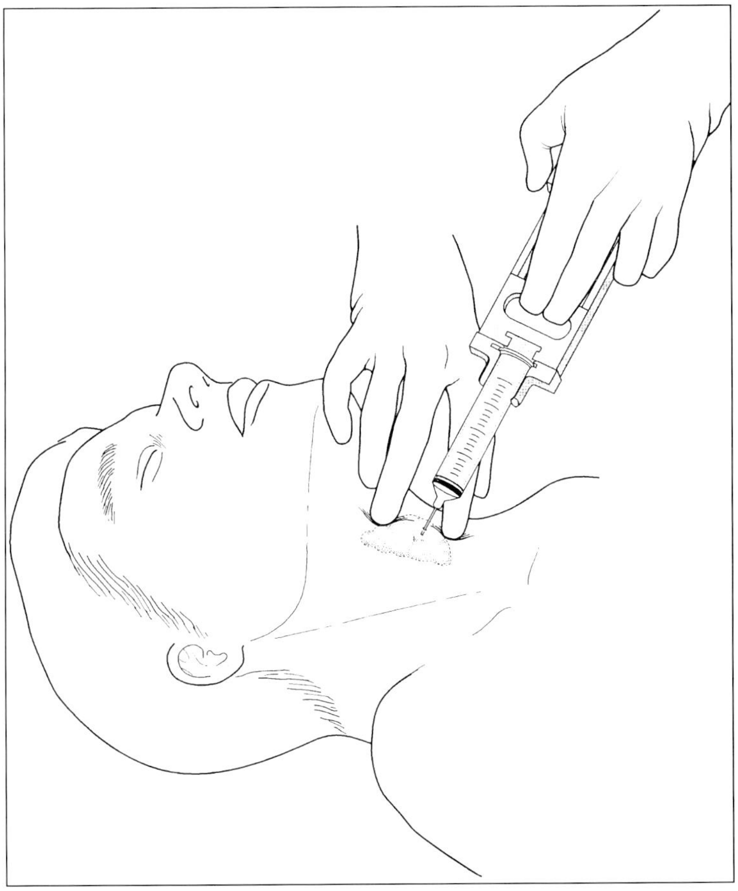

A

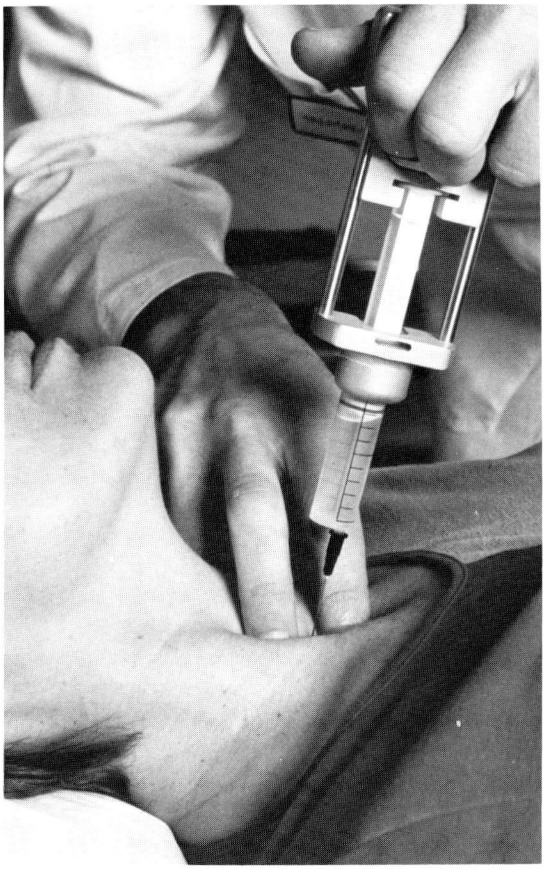

B

FIGURE 3.1 (A and B) FNAB of thyroid nodule. The use of an aspiration gun or syringe holder allows the aspirator to use fingers of nondominant hand to stabilize the mass. Reprinted with the permission of M. Stanley and T. Löwhagen, *Fine Needle Aspiration of Palpable Masses*. Butterworth–Heinemann: Boston (1993), p. 74.

TABLE 3.2 Algorithm of the Clinical Management of Thyroid Disease

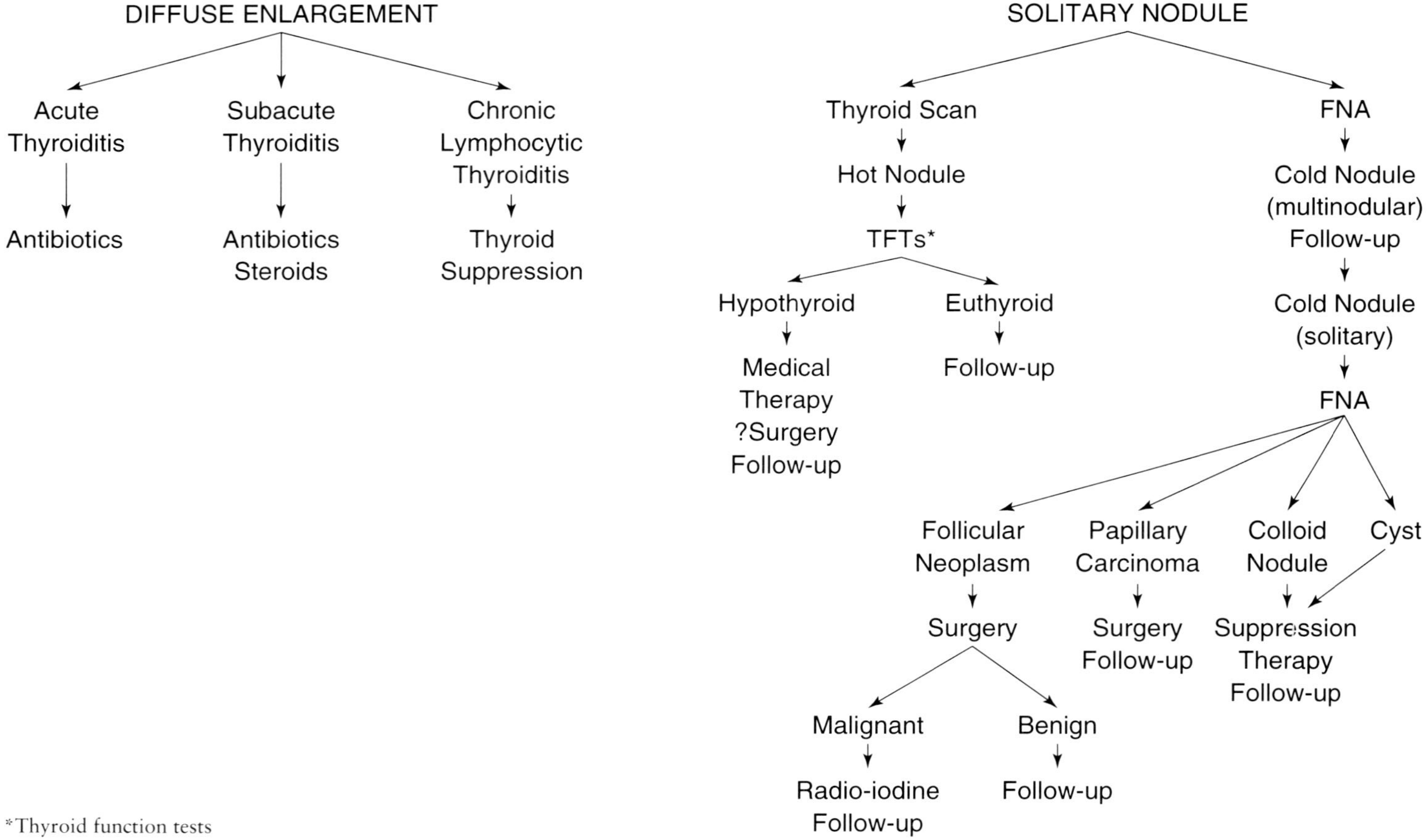

*Thyroid function tests

Table 3.3 Algorithm of Diagnosis of Thyroid Disease Based on Cytologic Features

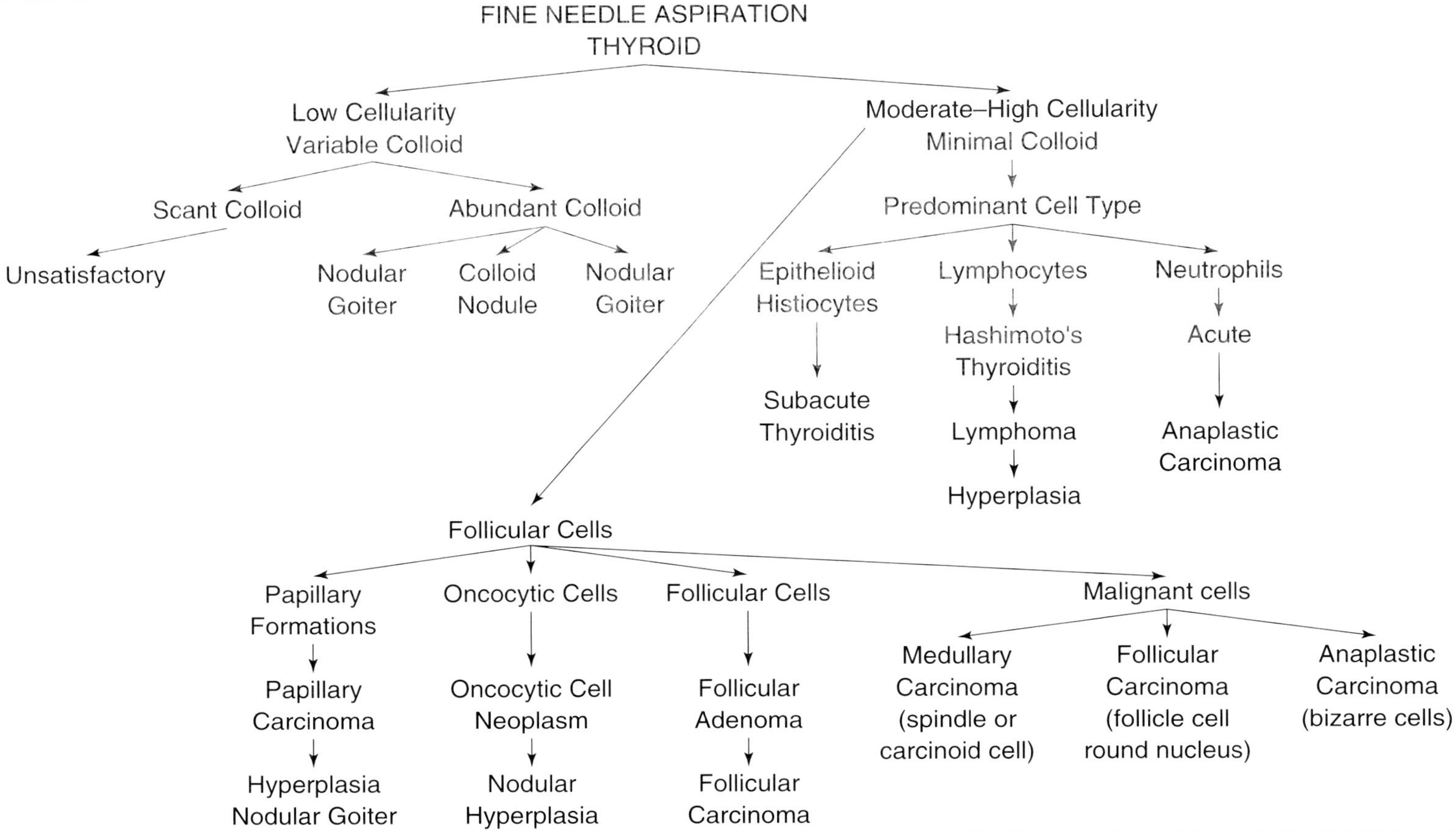

FINE NEEDLE ASPIRATION THYROID
Low Cellularity Variable Colloid
Moderate–High Cellularity Minimal Colloid
Scant Colloid
Abundant Colloid
Unsatisfactory
Nodular Goiter
Colloid Nodule
Nodular Goiter
Predominant Cell Type
Epithelioid Histiocytes
Lymphocytes
Neutrophils
Subacute Thyroiditis
Hashimoto's Thyroiditis
Lymphoma
Hyperplasia
Acute
Anaplastic Carcinoma
Follicular Cells
Papillary Formations
Papillary Carcinoma
Hyperplasia Nodular Goiter
Oncocytic Cells
Oncocytic Cell Neoplasm
Nodular Hyperplasia
Follicular Cells
Follicular Adenoma
Follicular Carcinoma
Malignant cells
Medullary Carcinoma (spindle or carcinoid cell)
Follicular Carcinoma (follicle cell round nucleus)
Anaplastic Carcinoma (bizarre cells)

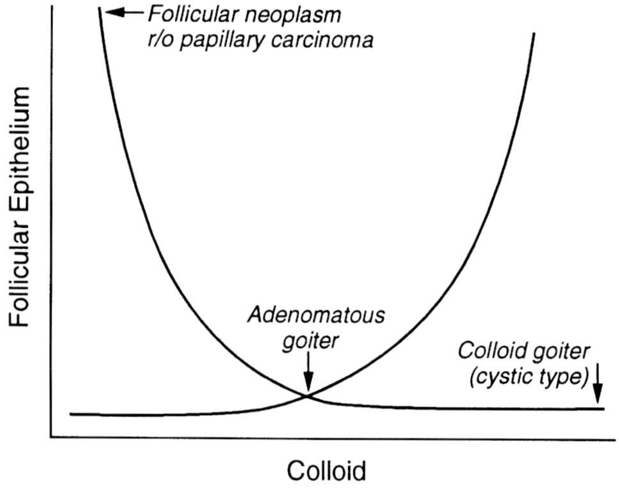

FIGURE 3.2 Relationship of colloid and follicular epithelium to diagnosis of thyroid FNAB. As the amount of colloid increases, the likelihood of a neoplasm decreases.

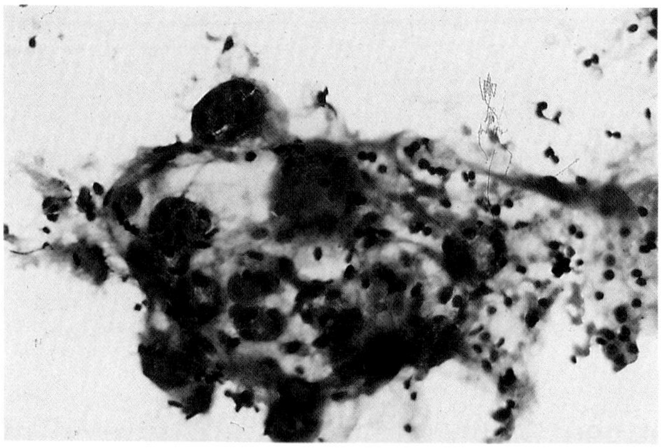

FIGURE 3.3 Variably sized follicles in normal thyroid. Diff-Quik® 250×.

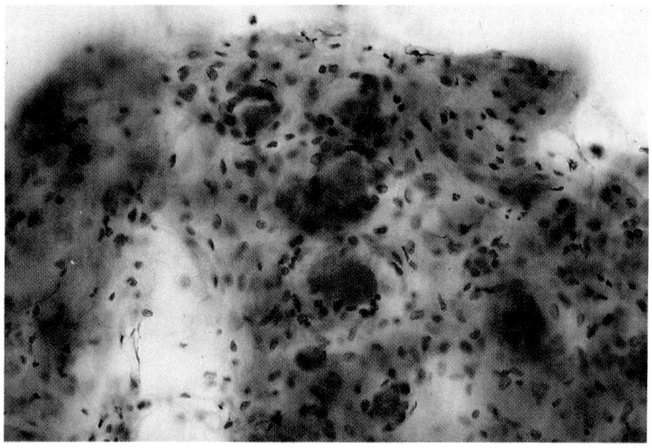

FIGURE 3.4 Normal thyroid showing several follicles with dense central colloid. Papanicolaou 250×.

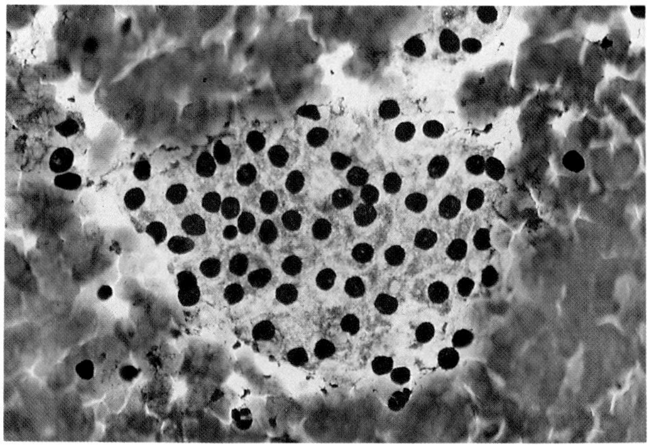

A

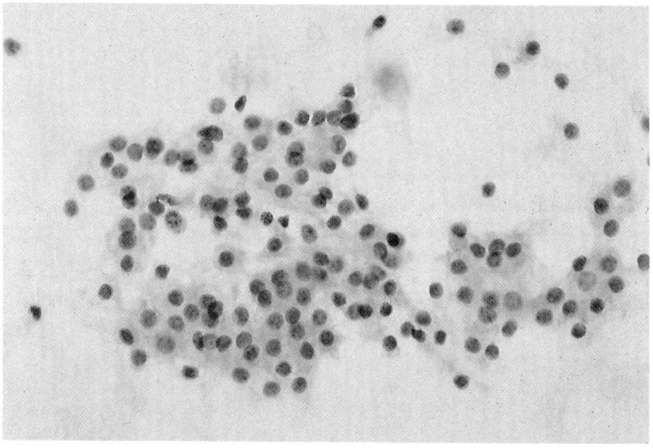

B

FIGURE 3.5 Sheet of normal thyroid epithelium showing relatively uniform nuclei and pale cytoplasm. (A) Diff-Quik® 600×; (B) Papanicolaou stain 600×.

with Romanowsky stain. Colloid occurs as a viscous fluid that smears as a sheet that sometimes "cracks"—the result of aspiration of a large collection of colloid—or as very dense collections of inspissated colloid (Figure 3.6). Fragments of normal thyroid parenchyma are often encountered in aspirations of nonneoplastic lesions, such as goiter.

Nonneoplastic Lesions

Multinodular Goiter

Diverse terminology is used by clinicians when discussing the most common thyroid condition: multinodular goiter (MNG). A dominant nodule within MNG also represents the most frequent thyroid nodule sampled by FNAB. Patients with MNG, as the name implies, may develop several nodules of varying size and consistency during the course of their disease. This nonspecific term is also used by pathologists to indicate the benign cytology/histology of these nodules. A diagnosis of MNG usually guides the clinician toward more con-

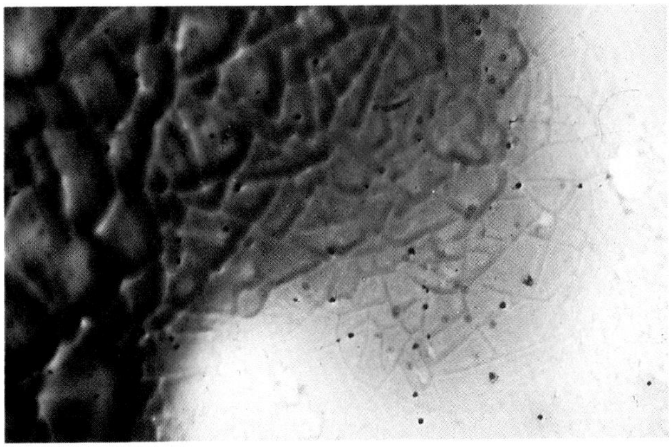

FIGURE 3.6 Colloid goiter. "Cracked" colloid seen on air-dried, Romanowsky-stained preparations. Diff-Quik® 100×.

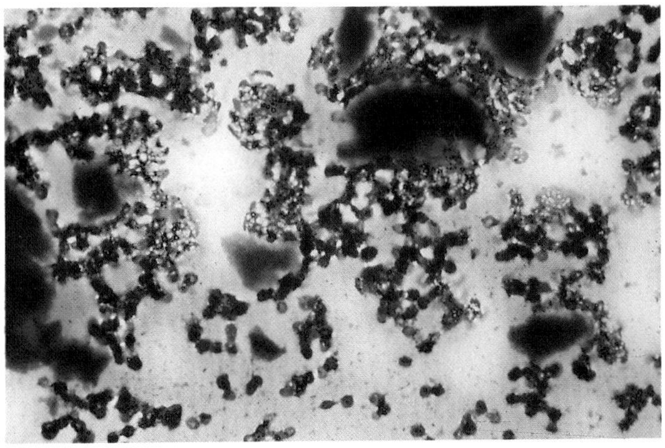

FIGURE 3.8 Colloid goiter. Free, dense colloid scattered in a background of blood. Diff-Quik® 250×.

servative management. Nonneoplastic goiter is another frequent, generic phrase. The most common reason for this broad categorization is the diversity of cytologic patterns present in MNG. Nodules of MNG may be solid, cystic, or complex and vary in size from less than 1 centimeter to greater than 10 centimeters. Occasionally, hemorrhage may cause these nodules to enlarge rapidly, prompting patients to seek treatment. The complete cytomorphologic spectrum may be seen in MNG. There is remarkable variation in cellularity, colloid, and blood. Benign follicular cells may be arranged in irregular, flat sheets, papillary clusters, and/or follicles (Figure 3.7). Abundant colloid may be present as a diffuse background or as scattered dense fragments, sometimes referred to as *inspissated colloid* (Figure 3.8). Evidence of cystic change—debris, cholesterol crystals, and histiocytes/macrophages—can often be identified. Further classification of these benign nodules is often attempted if one particular pattern predominates.

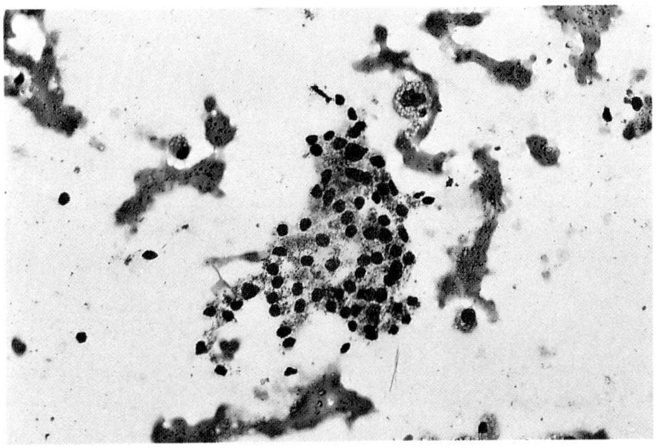

FIGURE 3.7 Multinodular goiter with loosely cohesive sheet of follicular epithelium, rare macrophages in a background of blood. Diff-Quik® 400×.

Colloid nodules, as the name implies, show abundant colloid with minimal numbers of follicular cells. Colloid may be thin and watery and may smear smoothly onto slides, or it may be inspissated and dense. Colloid nodules that have been present for a long duration may be very difficult to sample, and little material may be obtained despite vigorous aspiration. Conversely, adenomatous nodules are composed predominantly of bland follicular epithelium arranged in sheets, loose follicles, and/or single cells. These single cells are often stripped of their cytoplasm and look like lymphocytes. Hurthle cells—enlarged follicular cells with abundant granular cytoplasm, large nuclei, and prominent, centrally placed nucleoli—may be present. In adenomatous nodules, colloid is present but may vary significantly in amount. Smears with numerous follicular cells that show overlapping and scanty colloid are often worrisome, resulting in a recommendation for surgery to exclude a follicular neoplasm.

Cystic degeneration is a common finding in these nonneoplastic nodules resulting in the recovery of thin, watery brown fluid during aspiration. Cytocentrifugation is the best method for analysis of this fluid. The hallmark of cystic degeneration/hemorrhage is the presence of numerous hemosiderin-laden macrophages (Figure 3.9). Hemosiderin appears as dark blue granules of varying sizes on Diff-Quik® and golden brown, slightly refractile granules on Papanicolaou stains. Cholesterol crystals may be seen in older lesions that are aspirated. Although usually dissolved during staining by the Papanicolaou method, they are easily visible against the gray-blue background of the Diff-Quik® stain. Degenerating nodules will show benign follicular cells with frayed cytoplasm and indistinct nuclear features in a background of watery colloid. Repair in the form of squamous metaplasia and spindle cell proliferation may also occur within these nodules and result in cytologic atypia (Figure 3.10).

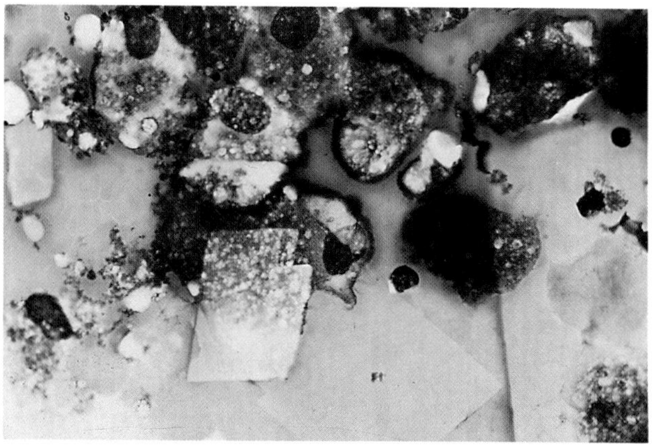

FIGURE 3.9 Cystic degeneration of nodular goiter. Macrophages with cobalt-blue hemosiderin pigment and cholesterol crystals predominate in the smear. Stripped nuclei of degenerated follicular epithelium may be seen. Diff-Quik® 200×.

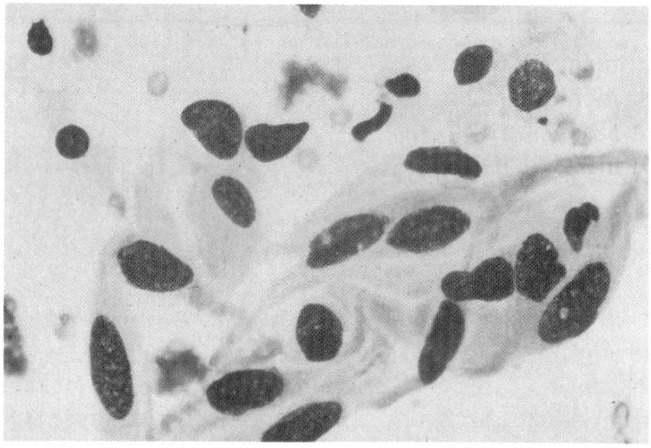

FIGURE 3.10 Regressive changes in nodular (cystic) goiter. Spindle cells with mild nuclear atypia are often associated with a resolving cyst. These atypical cells are few in number. Diff-Quik® 600×.

NONNEOPLASTIC GOITER—CYTOLOGIC FEATURES

Colloid
- **Inspissated or smooth/cracked: light green—Papinicolaou (Pap); purple—Diff-Quik® (DQ)**

Follicular cells
- **May be arranged as follicles, sheets, or single cells**
- **Bland nuclear features**
- **Indistinct nucleoli/chromocenters**
- **Frayed cytoplasm (degeneration)**

Hemosiderin-laden macrophages

Inflammatory Disease

There are three distinct conditions considered in the category of inflammatory disease of the thyroid: subacute (granulomatous), acute (suppurative), and chronic lymphocytic (Hashimoto's) thyroiditis. Patients with these conditions will most likely present with diffuse enlargement, but both granulomatous and Hashimoto's thyroiditis may present clinically as a solitary nodule.

Acute Thyroiditis

Although acute thyroiditis is a rare condition of the thyroid, an accurate diagnosis can be made by FNAB. Patients will present with fever and diffuse, painful swelling of one or, more commonly, both lobes of the thyroid. The thyroid will be very tender to palpation and the patient will experience pain on aspiration. The aspiration may yield frank pus; alternatively, aspirates may show scattered neutrophils associated with degenerating tissue fragments with few identifiable follicular cells (Figure 3.11). It is important to adequately sample the gland because the major differential diagnosis is high-grade or anaplastic carcinoma with necrosis and inflammation. Sterile material should be sent for culture and smears made for bacterial (Gram) stains.

ACUTE THYROIDITIS—CLINICAL AND CYTOLOGIC FEATURES

Pain during aspiration

Purulent exudate
- **Neutrophils, fibrin, and blood**
- **Bacteria rarely identified (Gram-stained smears)**

Rare to absent follicular cells

Histiocytes and fibroblasts (resolution phase)

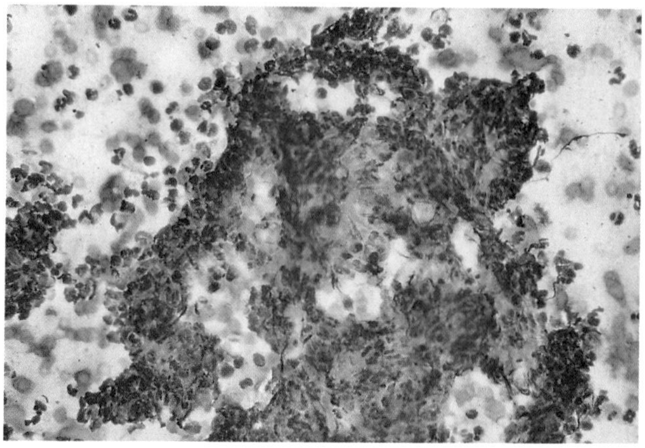

FIGURE 3.11 Acute thyroiditis. Scattered neutrophils admixed with fragments of very degenerated follicular epithelium. Diff-Quik® 400×.

In addition to bacterial thyroiditis, it is anticipated that mycotic thyroiditis will be reported more frequently due to the increasing prevalence of immunocompromised patients. *Cryptococcus, Aspergillus,* and *Candida* have been implicated in mycotic thyroiditis cases.[19–21] Stains for fungal organisms, Gomori methenamine silver (GMS), Mucicarmine, and Periodic Acid-Schiff (PAS) are indicated for confirmation.

Subacute Thyroiditis. Subacute (granulomatous; de Quervain's) thyroiditis is another rare condition of the thyroid that typically manifests as an asymmetric swelling of the gland. Most patients are women, 30 to 50 years old. As in acute thyroiditis, the patient presents with fever, an elevated sedimentation rate, and a tender gland. FNAB tends to be painful, with pain often manifested as radiating neck pain. This disease is usually self limited, resolving over several weeks. Aspiration smears reflect this time course. They are paucicellular with scattered inflammatory cells initially (Figure 3.12) followed by a typical granulomatous reaction that leads to fibrosis (Figure 3.13).

SUBACUTE THYROIDITIS—CLINICAL AND CYTOLOGIC FEATURES

Pain during aspiration

Limited numbers of follicular cells
- **Degenerative changes:vacuolization**

Acute and chronic inflammation

Epithelioid histiocytes
- **Loose aggregate "granulomas"**
- **Langhans' multinucleate giant cells**

Debris

Colloid

Fibrosis

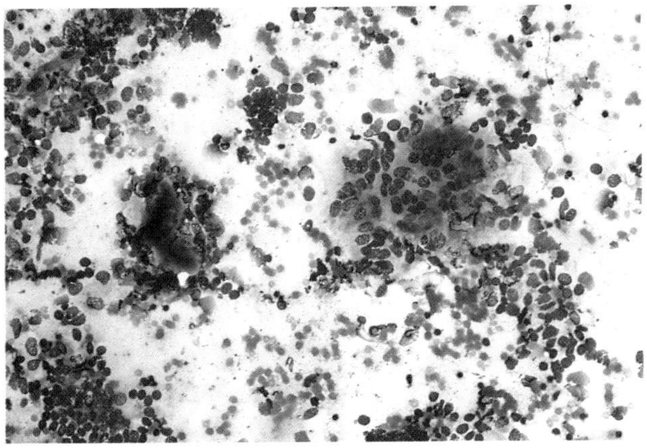

FIGURE 3.12 Early stage of granulomatous thyroiditis with inflammatory cells associated with disrupted, reactive follicular epithelium. Diff-Quik® 100×.

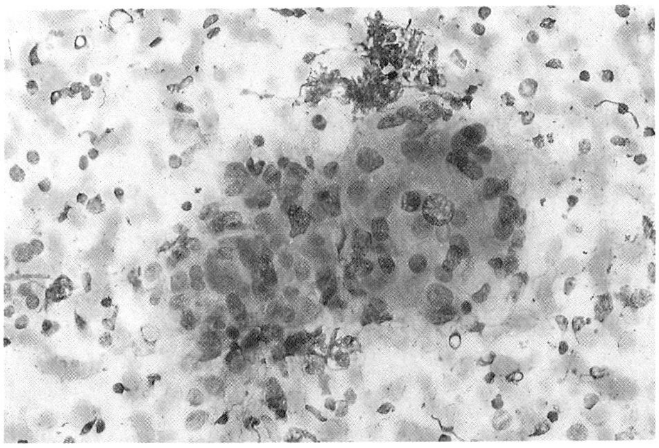

FIGURE 3.13 Later stage of granulomatous thyroiditis with multinucleated giant cells and epithelioid histiocytes forming a granuloma, scattered follicular cells and bare nuclei, and scattered small mature lymphocytes. Diff-Quik® 400×.

Chronic Lymphocytic Thyroiditis. Chronic lymphocytic thyroiditis, or Hashimoto's thyroiditis, is an autoimmune process that is the most commonly encountered inflammatory condition of the thyroid examined by FNAB. Clinically, patients present with hypothyroidism and a diffuse enlargement of the thyroid gland. Presumptive inflammatory conditions of the thyroid, particularly Hashimoto's thyroiditis, represent one of the few exceptions to the rule that superficial FNAB should be used only for diagnosis of discrete, palpable masses. Patients present with diffuse, painless asymmetric thyroid enlargement that, on physical examination, has a firm, slightly nodular consistency. For most patients, FNAB is performed concurrently with the confirmation of the serologic findings (increased antithyroid antibodies). Lymphocytic thyroiditis has a fairly characteristic pattern on FNAB smears. These smears are dominated by a heterogeneous population of lymphocytes, often including germinal centers, scattered among follicular cell arrays. The thin rim of basophilic cytoplasm (Diff-Quik®) distinguishes the inflammatory cells from the stripped nuclei of follicular cells (Figure 3.14). Colloid is minimal or absent. Follicular cells may show reactive changes including small nucleoli and loss of follicular arrangement (Figure 3.15). Follicular cells often show Hurthle cell change (Figure 3.16). The lymphocytic component may dominate the smears suggesting the possibility of lymphoma; or Hurthle cells may be present in abundance, suggesting a Hurthle cell tumor. This dominant Hurthle cell pattern will lead to some false-positive diagnosis of Hurthle cell neoplasm. Patients with Hashimoto's thyroiditis have an increased incidence of lymphoma.[22,23] If cytomorphology alone is not sufficient to distinguish between these entities, immunocytochemistry and/or flow cytometry can be used to characterize the lymphoid populations.

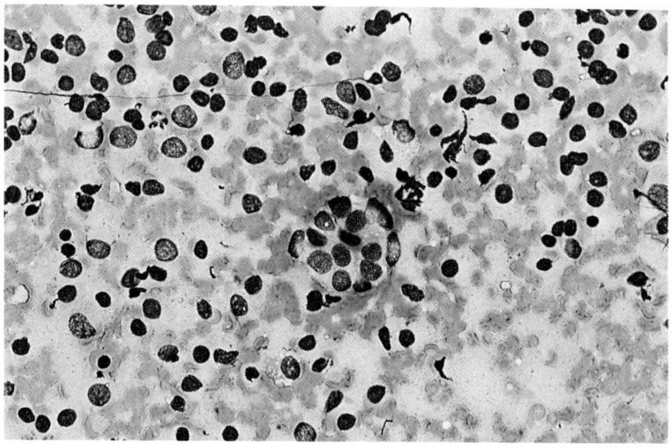

FIGURE 3.14 Hashimoto's thyroiditis. Follicle surrounded by heterogeneous population of mature lymphocytes. Diff-Quik® 400×.

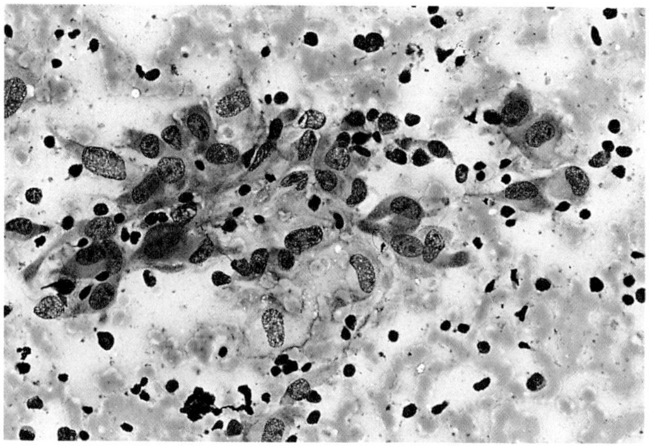

FIGURE 3.15 Hashimoto's thyroiditis. Loose aggregate of reactive follicular cells with small, distinct nucleoli surrounded by lymphocytes. Diff-Quik® 400×.

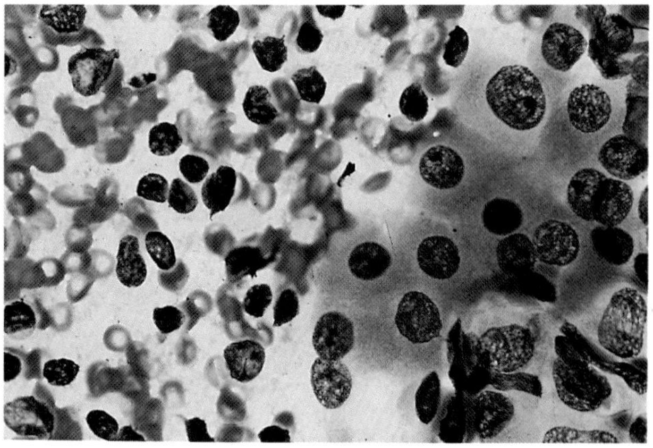

FIGURE 3.16 Hashimoto's thyroiditis. Hurthle cell metaplasia is frequently associated with thyroiditis. Prominent nuclei and granular cytoplasm of Hurthle cells will distinguish these fragments from germinal centers. Diff-Quik® 400×.

HASHIMOTO'S THYROIDITIS—CYTOLOGIC FEATURES

Scant colloid

Few follicle cells
- **–Hurthle cell change**

Heterogeneous population of lymphocytes
- **–Reactive lymphocytes, especially plasma cells**
- **–Germinal center fragments**

Fibrosis

Hyperthyroidism

Clinical and radiologic studies, rather than FNAB, are the usual procedures used to diagnose hyperthyroidism (Graves' disease). Patients are "hyperactive" with increased appetite but without concomitant weight gain. Other signs include tachycardia and exophthalmos. Radiologic evidence of increased uptake of radioactive iodine completes the diagnosis. If the patient has had radiologic studies with the identification of a "hot" nodule prior to FNAB, then the FNAB becomes a safe, rapid confirmatory test. More often, this condition is found *de novo* as a localized form of hyperplasia, the "toxic nodule." These nodules may be encountered unexpectedly when FNAB is used as the first step in the diagnostic workup of a solitary thyroid nodule. Hyperplasia is easily recognized when characteristic follicular cells are demonstrated on Romanowsky-stained smears.[24,25] These hyperplastic follicular cells show distinctive cytoplasmic changes variously referred to as marginal vacuoles and frayed or blebbing cytoplasmic edges ("colloid suds") that have a magenta tinge ("fire flares") (Figures 3.17 and 3.18). This cytomorphologic clue is not present on Papanicolaou-stained preparations.

HYPERTHYROIDISM—CYTOLOGIC FEATURES

Abundant blood

Minimal free colloid

Moderate to high cellularity
- **–Follicular cells**
  - **–Occasional Hurthle cell change**
  - **–Loose groupings; papillary excrescences**
  - **–Fire flares/colloid suds/marginal vacuoles**

Neoplastic Lesions

Follicular Neoplasms

The category of follicular neoplasms represents not only follicular adenomas, including the Hurthle cell vari-

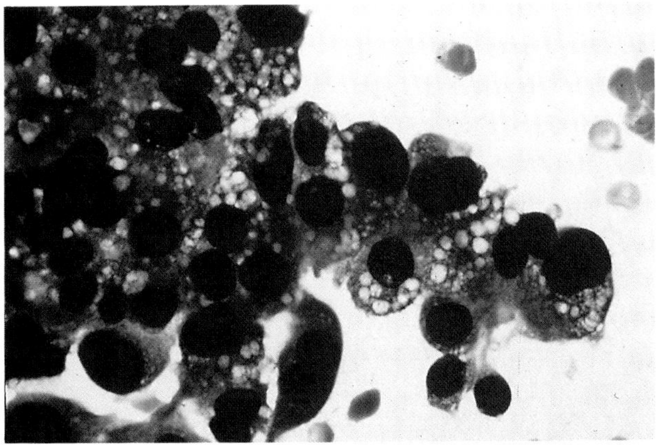

FIGURE 3.17 Hyperplasia. Marginal vacuoles and "fire flares" identified as violet or magenta cytoplasmic edges. Diff-Quik® 400×.

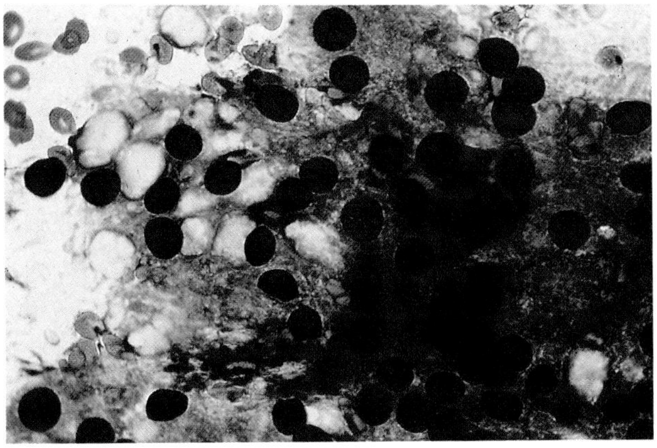

FIGURE 3.18 Hyperplasia. "Colloid suds" seen as cytoplasmic vacuoles with thick, magenta borders. Diff-Quik® 600×.

ant, but follicular carcinomas as well. One of the arguments used by detractors of FNAB is the inability of this technique to distinguish between follicular lesions: adenomatous nodules of goiter, follicular adenomas, and follicular carcinomas. It is certainly true that it is difficult to consistently distinguish between adenomas and low-grade follicular carcinomas by FNAB alone.[26] Histologic evaluation for capsular and vascular invasion is still the gold standard. However, the utility of FNAB rests in its ability to select patients who need surgical excision. In this respect, aspiration biopsy represents a screening rather than a diagnostic procedure.[27,28] Follicular carcinomas represent between 15% and 20% of thyroid malignancies; the majority of patients are women over 40 years of age. These neoplasms, typically long-standing, often come to clinical attention when patients notice a sudden increase in the size of the mass, usually due to hemorrhage. While metastases are common, less than 10 percent of patients will present with obvious regional metastases. Radiologic studies will usually confirm the presence of a well-demarcated cold lesion.

As Figure 3.2 illustrates, the distinction between a follicular lesion and nonneoplastic goiter is based predominantly on the ratio between follicular cells and colloid. Hypercellular aspirates composed of follicular cells arranged in follicular arrays, often with scalloped edges without colloid, are suspicious for follicular neoplasia (Figures 3.19 and 3.20). Certainly, nuclear characteristics commonly associated with malignant behavior (increased nuclear to cytoplasmic ratio, coarse chromatin, and distinct nucleoli) may suggest carcinoma. However, this cannot be relied upon because low-grade follicular carcinomas are cytologically very bland. FNAB final diagnosis of these neoplasms are best phrased to suggest the possibility of carcinoma with surgery recommended for definitive diagnosis. Our experience as well as Layfield's indicate that over 80 percent of thyroid nodules diagnosed as follicular neoplasms by FNAB are correctly diagnosed.[29] Histologic evaluation of these nodules indicates that the majority are adenomas with a small but significant percentage representing well-differentiated follicular carcinomas. Nodular (adenomatous) goiter represents the remaining nodules. Misclassification of these nodules into a neoplastic category is a pitfall that even experienced cytopathologists will sometimes encounter.

The rare colloid adenoma will have a cytologic picture identical in most aspirates to nonneoplastic goiter. These are true adenomas but they are composed of large colloid-filled follicles. They do not show clustering of cells with nuclear overlap in aspiration biopsy smears and do not demonstrate scalloping of the outer border of the follicular cell groups. One of the authors (WJF) has been able to diagnose correctly only 1 of 19 cases of this type of adenoma in a series of several thousand thyroid aspiration biopsies. The true neoplastic nature of colloid adenomas comes to clinical attention when they do not respond to suppression therapy and are eventually excised.

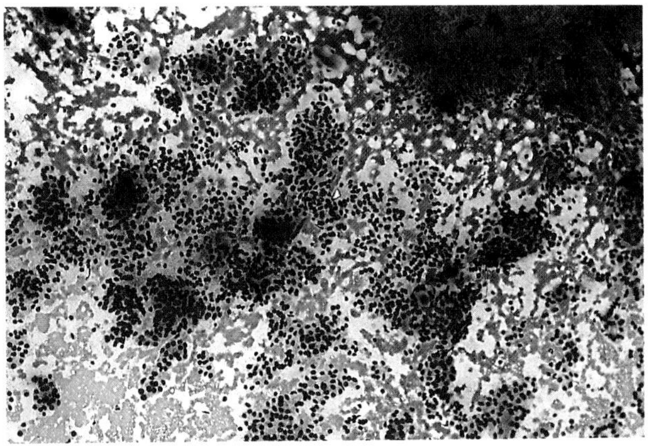

FIGURE 3.19 Follicular neoplasm. Hypercellular aspirate showing follicular cells in dense arrays in a background of blood admixed with scant amounts of colloid. Diff-Quik® 50×.

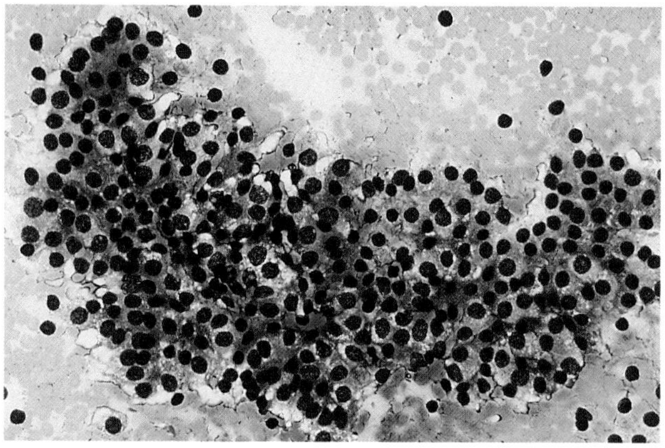

A

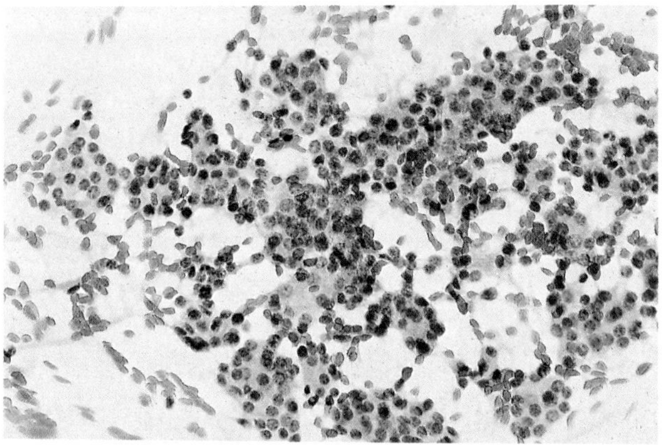

B

FIGURE 3.20 Follicular neoplasm. Monomorphic follicular cells arranged in groups with (A) scalloped edges (Diff-Quik® 400×) and (B) as microfollicles (Papanicolaou 400×). Colloid is absent.

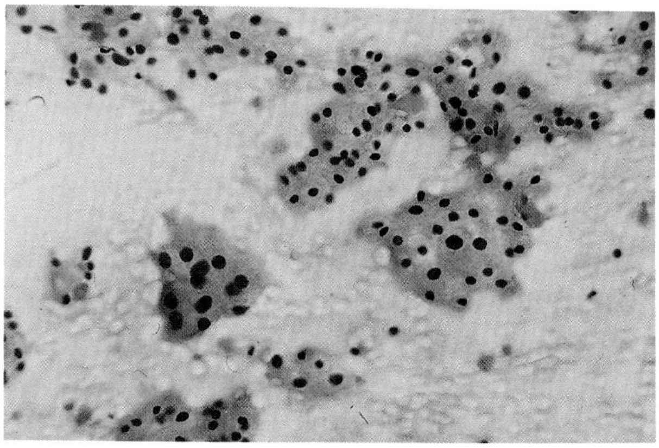

A

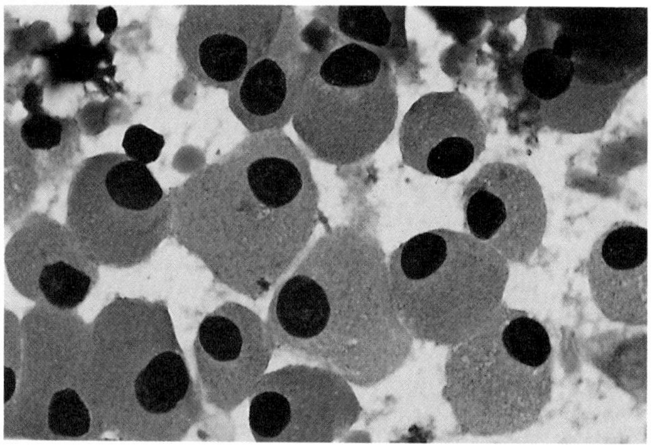

B

FIGURE 3.21 Hurthle cell tumor. (A) Monomorphic population of Hurthle cells in clusters or sheets. Variation of nuclear size is not an indication of biologic behavior. Papanicolaou 200×. (B) Large cells with abundant granular cytoplasm, eccentric nuclei, and prominent nucleoli (nucleoli may appear indistinct on some Diff-Quik® preparations). Diff-Quik® 1000×.

FOLLICULAR NEOPLASM—CYTOLOGIC FEATURES

Scant to absent colloid

Hypercellularity
- **–Monotonous follicular cells**
  - **–Micro- or macrofollicles, trabeculae, syncytial fragments, scalloping**
  - **–Enlarged, bland nuclei, overlapping (except in higher grade carcinomas)**
  - **–Fine to coarse, dispersed chromatin**
  - **–Distinct nucleoli**

Hurthle Cell Tumor

A common variant of the follicular neoplasms is the Hurthle cell tumor (HCT). As discussed above, Hurthle cell change, or metaplasia, is a common finding in many thyroid lesions: adenomatous nodules in MNG, hyperplasia, chronic lymphocytic thyroiditis, Graves' disease, and papillary carcinoma. Differentiating these entities from HCT may be difficult if an area of Hurthle cell metaplasia is sampled. Cytomorphologic clues include the percentage of Hurthle cells in conjunction with their arrangement (Figure 3.21A). Hurthle cells that are present as small, cohesive clusters and/or isolated cells typically represent metaplasia, particularly common in Hashimoto's thyroiditis and MNG. Aspiration smears from HCT will reflect a highly cellular, monomorphic population of discohesive cells or syncytia coupled with the absence of lymphoplasmacytic inflammatory cells and macrophages.[30,31] Colloid is usually very scant or inspissated. Interestingly, the recognition of Hurthle cells is not color-dependent. These cells may stain blue, green, or orange by the Papanicolaou method and appear blue, gray, or purple on Romanowsky preparations (Figure 3.21B). Abundant granular cytoplasm with large, eccentric nuclei and prominent nucleoli are the clues to correct identification of this cell.

An uncommon papillary variant of HCT has been reported by Kaur et al.[32] In their study, five cases of a papillary variant of HCT were encountered on FNAB and subsequently determined histologically to represent carcinomas. This variant was composed entirely of Hurthle cells in papillary arrays. True papillae with fibrovascular cores were present but there were no nuclear features of classic papillary carcinoma. Differentiating these cases from papillary carcinomas will be quite difficult because the characteristic nuclear features are sparse or absent in such cases.

As in "generic" follicular neoplasms, the malignant potential of HCTs is best assessed histologically. Unlike follicular carcinomas that can be deceptively bland, making the distinction from adenomas challenging, the opposite problem, cytologic atypia, makes the precise diagnosis of HCT difficult. Cytologic pleomorphism and atypia are frequently encountered in HCTs that are subsequently classified histologically as adenomas.

HURTHLE CELL TUMORS—CYTOLOGIC FEATURES

Hypercellularity

Monomorphic population of Hurthle cells
- **–Large polygonal cells**
- **–Granular cytoplasm**
- **–Enlarged nuclei, binucleation**
- **–Prominent nuclei**

Scant to absent colloid

Absent inflammation

Papillary Carcinoma

The most frequently occurring carcinoma that is the easiest to identify cytologically is papillary carcinoma. Patients present with a solitary, often cold nodule that may feel hard or more firm than the palpable nodules of nonneoplastic goiter. This tumor may undergo cystic degeneration with significant distortion of the usual cytologic picture of papillary carcinoma. A distinctive "scritching" sound may accompany FNAB of firm nodules. Histologic correlations of these papillary carcinomas suggest the needle is in contact with either psammoma bodies and/or firm fibrous tissue (sclerotic papillary carcinomas). This noise is very similar to that encountered occasionally in breast carcinomas. Interestingly, psammoma bodies, often alluded to in the histopathologic diagnosis of papillary carcinoma, are not nearly as frequently encountered in FNAB specimens.

Numerous cytologic clues have been elucidated that allow excellent diagnostic accuracy and rapid triage of patients with papillary carcinoma.[33–35] A clue at low magnification is, of course, the presence of papillary fragments. However, the foremost cytomorphologic criteria are nuclear—the presence of nuclear grooves and/or intranuclear cytoplasmic inclusions.[36–38] Nuclear grooves should transect the nucleus, usually along the longitudinal axis, and they are best seen on Papanicolaou preparations. Incomplete grooves, if abundant, should not be discounted but should be accompanied by other criteria for a diagnosis of papillary carcinoma (Figure 3.22). Intranuclear inclusions are invaginations of cytoplasm into the nucleus and therefore should stain quite similarly to the cytoplasm (Figure 3.23). Although both Diff-Quik® and Papanicolaou stains highlight this feature, the authors prefer the Diff-Quik® for rapid, low-magnification identification due to the contrast of color within the nucleus (Figure 3.24). The optically clear nuclei, a strong criterion in hematoxylin and eosin (H&E) stained tissue is less obvious in cytologic preparations. The nuclei may appear quite uniformly bland in Papanicolaou-stained smears. The presence of true papillae, overlapping clusters of cells with fibrovascular cores, when combined with the presence of at least one nuclear feature allows a rapid diagnosis of papillary carcinoma (Figure 3.25). Because the smear technique tends to shear the papillae away from the core, follicular cells appear unfurled as

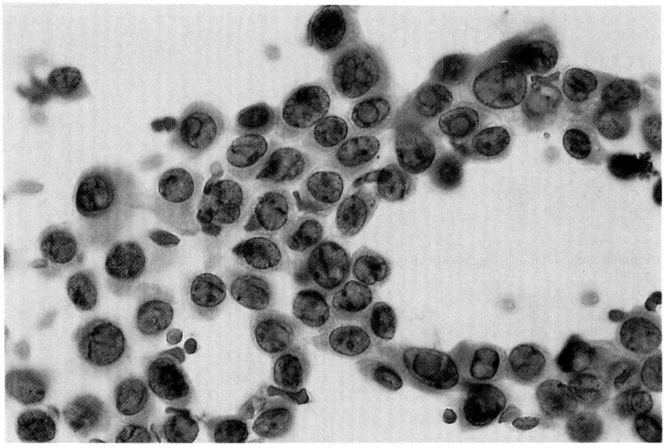

FIGURE 3.22 Papillary carcinoma. Loosely cohesive follicular cells with enlarged nuclei and variably prominent longitudinal nuclear grooves and small intranuclear cytoplasmic inclusions. Papanicolaou 400×.

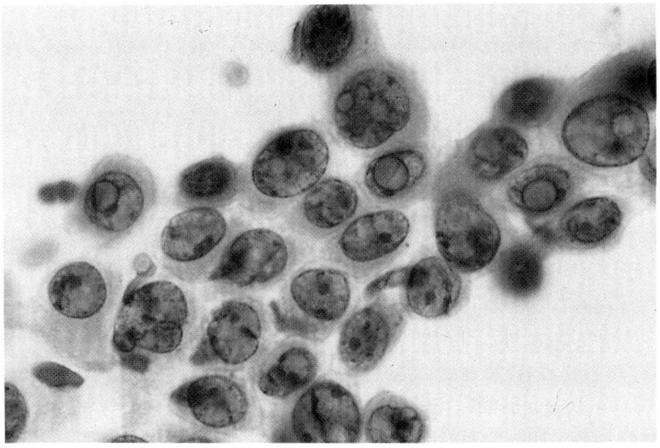

FIGURE 3.23 Papillary carcinoma. Follicular cells with prominent small nucleoli and nuclear inclusions. Papanicolaou 1000×.

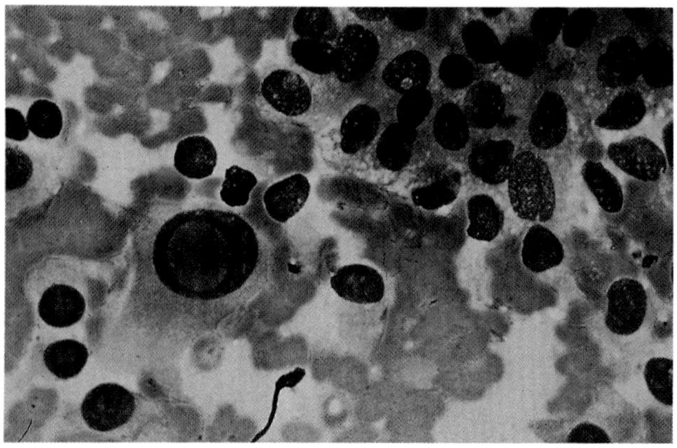

FIGURE 3.24 Papillary carcinoma. Large intranuclear, cytoplasmic inclusion in Hurthle cell as well as smaller inclusions with follicular fragment. Diff-Quik® 400×.

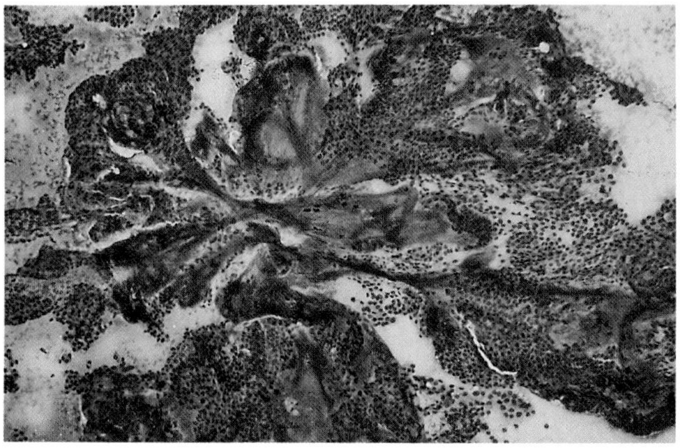

FIGURE 3.25 Papillary carcinoma. Fibrovascular cores appearing as splayed, pink fingerlike projections surrounded by sheets of neoplastic follicular cells. Diff Quik® 100×.

sheets adjacent to the fingerlike fibrovascular cores. Close evaluation of this homogeneous material should reveal vessels or at least elongate, oval nuclei of the endothelial cells (Figure 3.26).

Ropy or bubblegum colloid is often present as clumps of metachromatic material (Diff-Quik®). While not a strong indicator of papillary carcinoma, its presence should result in a careful search for the diagnostic nuclear features (Figure 3.27). Psammoma bodies, frequently identified in histologic preparations of papillary carcinomas, are much less often encountered on aspirate smears (Figure 3.28). This may be due in part to the inability of the needle to either accommodate the entire psammoma body or to fracture it into smaller fragments.

PAPILLARY CARCINOMA—CYTOLOGIC FEATURES

Smear Composition
- **–Cellular**
- **–Monolayered cell sheets**
- **–Three-dimensional tissue fragments**
- **–Multinucleated giant cells (follicular variant)**
- **–Ropy (bubblegum) colloid**
- **–Psammoma bodies (infrequent)**

Cytoplasm
- **–Metaplastic cytoplasm (oncocytic)**
- **–Distinct cell borders**

Nuclei
- **–Pale nuclei (Papanicolaou stain)**
- **–Definitive nucleoli**
- **–Intranuclear inclusions**
- **–Nuclear grooves**
- **–Variation in nuclear size**
- **–Enlarged nuclei**

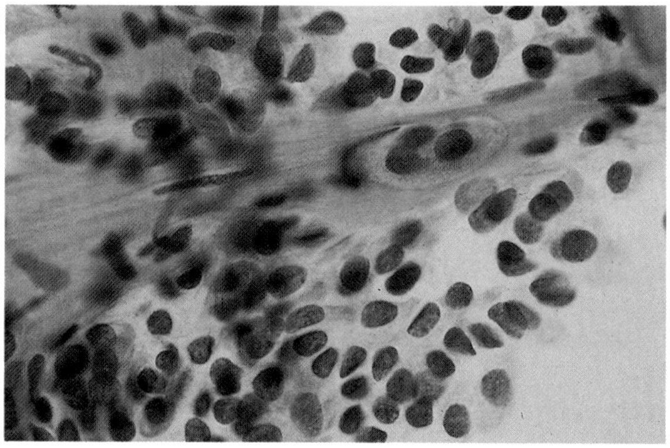

FIGURE 3.26 Papillary carcinoma. Oval, elongate nuclei of endothelial cells within the "stroma" help confirm this as a true fibrovascular core. Papanicolaou 400×.

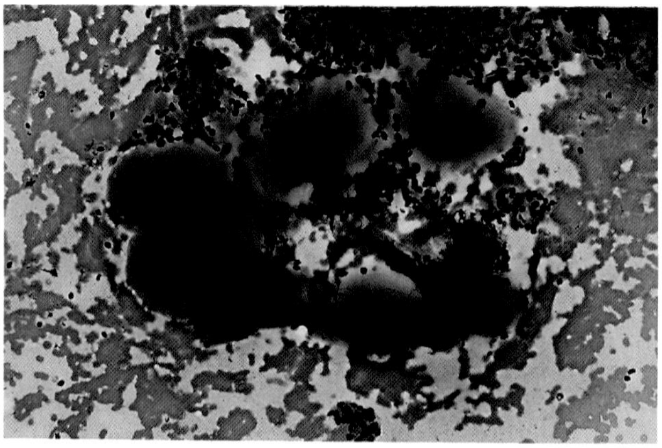

FIGURE 3.27 Papillary carcinoma. Thick, metachromatic ropy or bubblegum colloid is a distinct subset of colloid that is associated with papillary carcinoma. Diff-Quik® 200×.

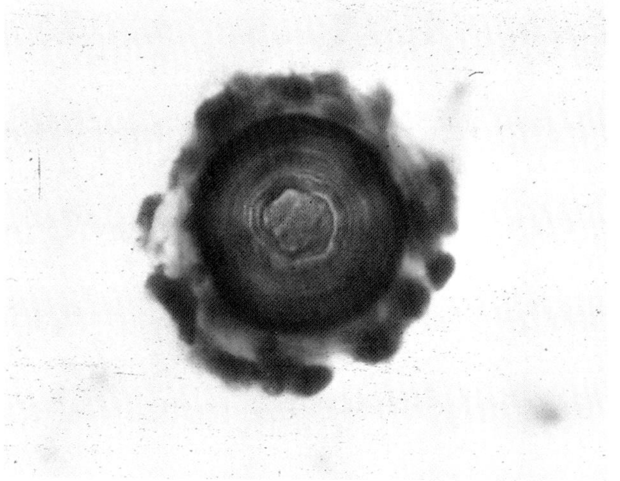

FIGURE 3.28 Psammoma body. These refractile spherules are infrequent in FNAB of papillary carcinoma and can be distinguished from dystrophic calcification by their distinct concentric lamellar rings. Papanicolaou 1000×.

Papillary carcinoma has a number of histologic variants. All represent departures from the standard cytologic criteria listed above. Difficulties arise in separating these variants from other thyroid lesions that have some of the cytologic criteria of papillary carcinoma. The most frequent subtype of papillary carcinoma encountered during thyroid FNAB is the follicular variant. The recognition that this nodule is a neoplasm is not as difficult as classifying it as a follicular neoplasm or papillary carcinoma. Substantial reliance must be placed on the identification of nuclear inclusions and grooves. Most of these patients will be triaged to surgery for definitive classification of the nodule by histology.

Cystic papillary carcinoma is a low-cellularity lesion difficult to distinguish from cystic degeneration within benign nodules. Once again, nuclear changes are key to the diagnosis but clinical clues may be even more important. A thyroid cyst that refills immediately after FNAB or a cyst with gross blood are suspicious for cystic papillary carcinoma. Just as a papillary variant of HCT occurs, so does the Hurthle cell variant of papillary carcinoma. Cells in the aspirate from this neoplasm occur as sheets and have granular cytoplasm and some of the nuclear pleomorphism found in true Hurthle cell neoplasms (Figure 3.29). This variant of papillary carcinoma may have few or no intranuclear inclusions or nuclear grooves to help identify it correctly on FNAB.

The dedifferentiated forms of follicular and papillary carcinoma are rare malignancies that have cytologic features similar to anaplastic carcinoma. They are quite easy to recognize as malignant on FNAB though their exact classification may be more of a problem. However, that is of little clinical consequence because these carcinomas are all treated aggressively.

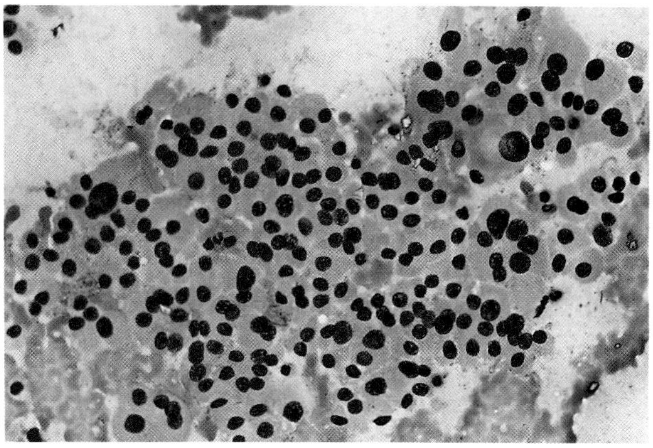

FIGURE 3.29 Hurthle cell variant of papillary carcinoma showing flat sheet of Hurthle cells indistinguishable from other lesions in which Hurthle cells predominate. Diff-Quik® 200×.

Medullary Carcinoma

FNAB is often employed to evaluate new thyroid nodules in individuals with a family history of medullary carcinoma. Medullary carcinoma may also arise sporadically. Several criteria have been developed for diagnosis of medullary carcinoma. The majority of medullary carcinomas are composed of distinctive neoplastic C cells—large, polygonal cells with ample cytoplasm and one or more nuclei and prominent nucleoli. The cells can resemble plasma cells, Hurthle cells, cells of malignant melanoma, carcinoid tumors, and anaplastic carcinomas. Romanowsky stains are extremely useful to highlight the cytoplasmic neurosecretory red granules characteristic of this endocrine neoplasm (Figure 3.30). Amyloid is also highlighted by these stains; it appears dense, acellular, and somewhat fibrillary. On

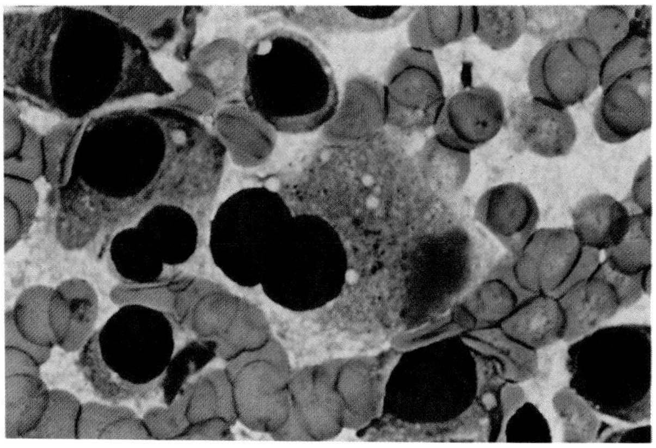

FIGURE 3.30 Medullary carcinoma. Large neoplastic follicular cells, occasionally bi- or multinucleated with characteristic red granules within cytoplasm. These may be distinct and perinuclear or form a vague blush at the cytoplasmic periphery. Diff-Quik® 400×.

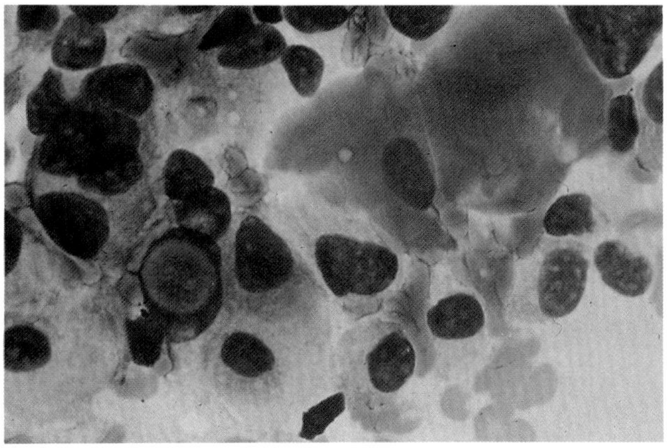

FIGURE 3.31 Medullary carcinoma. Amyloid is identified as an amorphous, acellular pink material often intimately associated with the neoplastic cells. Note the intranuclear inclusion and multinucleation. Diff-Quik® 400×.

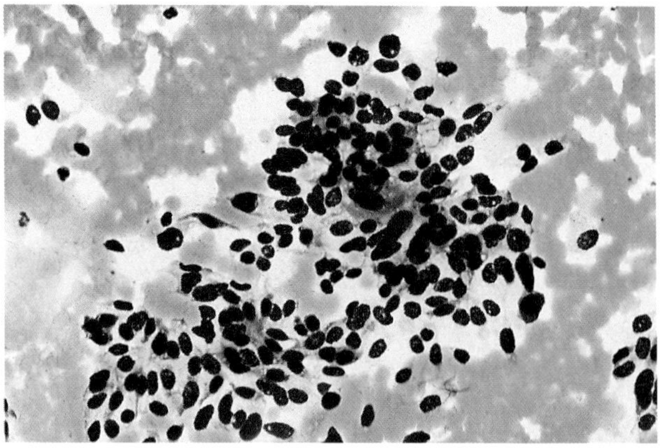

FIGURE 3.33 Medullary carcinoma. Loosely cohesive fragment of neoplastic cells with elongate (spindle) nuclei in a background of blood. Diff-Quik® 200×.

Diff-Quik®, amyloid is seen as ill-defined pink to violet masses easily noticed at low magnification (Figure 3.31). On Papanicolaou-stained preparations, it is light green, almost cyanophilic, and as such easily blends into the background (Figure 3.32). Special stains such as Congo red and/or crystal violet are useful to confirm the presence of amyloid. At times medullary carcinoma can resemble papillary and follicular carcinoma, particularly the insular carcinoma, HCT, and even myeloma/lymphoma. Recognition of the spindle cell variant of medullary carcinoma as a thyroid primary is also quite difficult (Figure 3.33). Although the differential diagnosis encompasses extrathyroidal tumors, immunocytochemistry panels that include calcitonin will readily confirm the diagnosis of medullary carcinoma.

MEDULLARY CARCINOMA—CYTOLOGIC FEATURES

Scant to absent colloid

Moderate to high cellularity

Monomorphic population of C cells
- **–Discohesive or loosely cohesive (plasmacytoid)**
- **–Polygonal cell shape; ample, finely granular cytoplasm**
- **–Neurosecretory granules (DQ)**
- **–Bi- and multinucleation**
- **–Eccentric nuclei**
- **–Coarse chromatin**
- **–Intranuclear inclusions**
- **–Nucleoli**

Amyloid

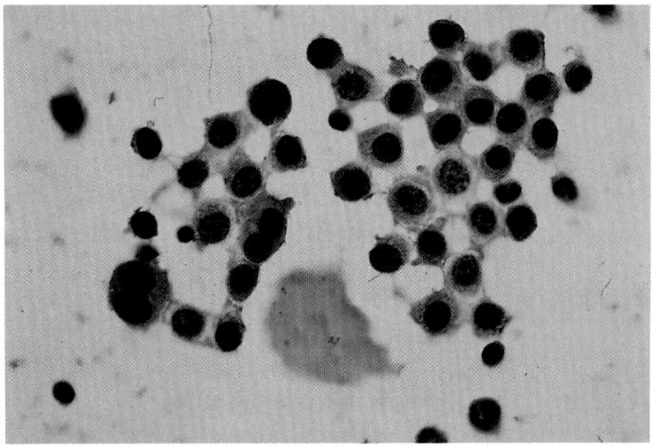

FIGURE 3.32 Medullary carcinoma. Discohesive large cells with occasional binucleation, coarse chromatin, and small, round nucleoli are adjacent to a dense acellular fragment of amyloid. Papanicolaou 400×.

Anaplastic Carcinoma

Anaplastic carcinoma occurs in older patients who may present emergently with the history of a growing mass in the neck. This is a very aggressive, rapidly enlarging carcinoma that may, over a short period of time, compromise the patient's ability to breathe by compressing and invading the trachea. FNAB allows a rapid diagnosis, in the Emergency Room if necessary. In the past, clinicians often have instituted treatment prior to a definitive histologic diagnosis because the differential diagnosis is usually limited to malignant lymphoma or anaplastic carcinoma. Fortunately, both malignancies are responsive to radiation therapy. Smears of this carcinoma, variably termed anaplastic or giant cell, are dominated by large, often bizarre cells with background necrosis and inflammation. Neutrophils are often seen

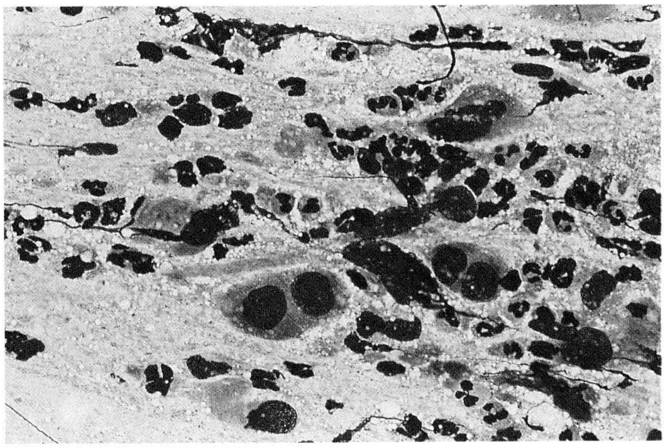

FIGURE 3.34 Anaplastic carcinoma. Large pleomorphic and bizarre cells in a background of acute inflammation and cell debris. Neutrophils may be seen within the cytoplasm of the tumor cells. Diff-Quik® 200×.

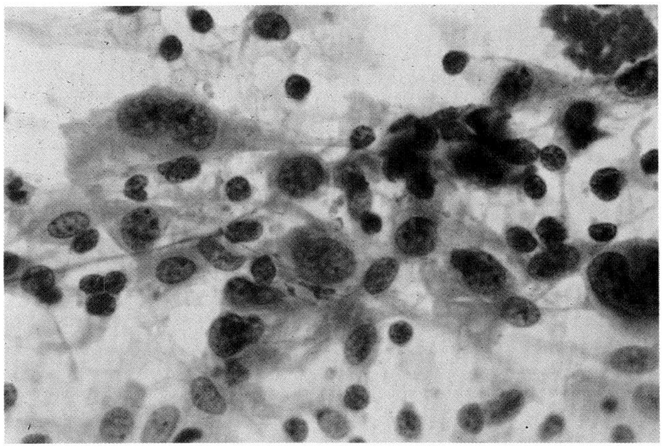

FIGURE 3.35 Anaplastic carcinoma. Large, pleomorphic cells with nuclei characteristic of malignant cells. Diff-Quik® 400×.

within the cytoplasm of the tumor cells (Figure 3.34). The presence of enlarged, pleomorphic nuclei with coarse chromatin and prominent nucleoli clearly identify these cells as a high-grade malignancy (Figure 3.35).

ANAPLASTIC CARCINOMA—CYTOLOGIC FEATURES

Absent colloid

High cellularity

Acute inflammation

Necrosis

Bizarre, pleomorphic/giant cells
- **–Isolated cells, syncytial fragments**
- **–Sarcomatoid appearance**
- **–Neutrophils within the cytoplasm**
- **–Coarse chromatin**
- **–Macronucleoli—often multiple**
- **–Mitoses, many atypical**

Insular Carcinoma

Insular thyroid carcinoma (ITC), described in 1984 by Carcangiu and Rosai[39] has been shown to represent a relatively aggressive tumor whose morphology and biologic behavior may be characterized as intermediate between well-differentiated tumors and aggressive anaplastic carcinomas.[39] It has been sporadically encountered in FNAB and its cytomorphologic characteristics have been studied.[40–42] While a specific diagnosis of ITC remains difficult, important cytologic features include high cellularity and cells occurring singly and in clusters, nests, and trabeculae (Figure 3.36). A low grade of cytologic atypia; grooved nuclei; intranuclear inclu-

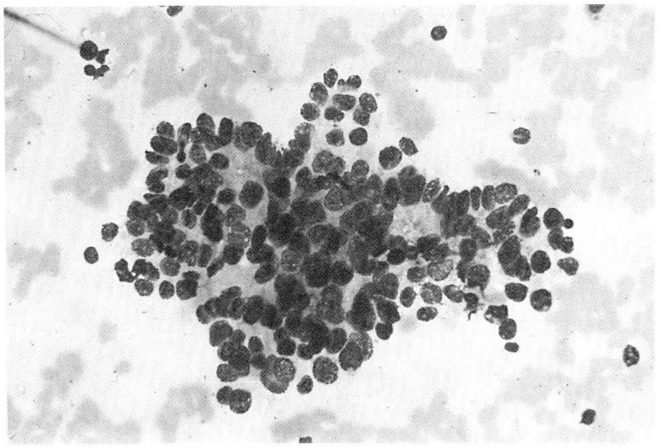

FIGURE 3.36 Insular carcinoma. Loosely arranged nests of follicular cells with minimal nuclear atypia. Variation in nuclear shape, nuclear compression, and irregular nuclear edges indicate this is not an ordinary follicular neoplasm. Diff-Quik® 200×.

sions; and thyroglobulin-positive cytoplasmic vacuoles are usually found, but this tumor may have many cytologic features that overlap with variants of medullary carcinoma of the thyroid.

Malignant Lymphoma

Malignant lymphomas that occur *de novo* within the thyroid gland are rare. As in anaplastic carcinoma, lymphoma often presents as a rapidly growing mass causing tracheal compression and may also represent a clinical emergency. The majority of these lymphomas appear as a monomorphic population of cells on aspirate smears and are usually high-grade, large cell, B cell type (Figure 3.37). A small but significant percentage of malignant lymphomas arise within chronic lymphocytic

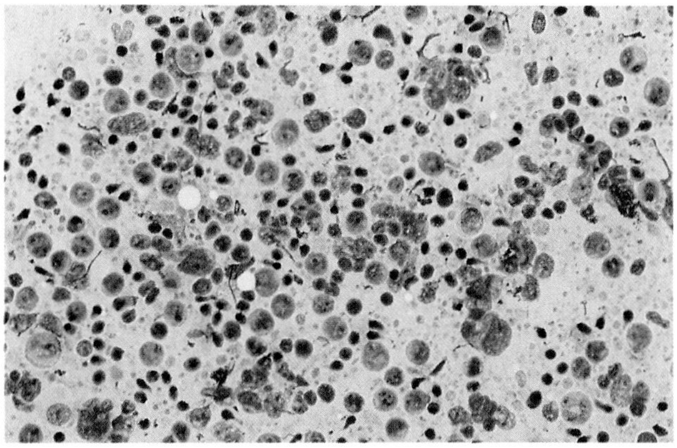

FIGURE 3.37 Malignant lymphoma, large cell type. Highly cellular aspirate containing large neoplastic lymphocytes and bare malignant appearing nuclei in a background of lymphoglandular bodies, scattered small benign lymphocytes and blood. Diff-Quik® 400×.

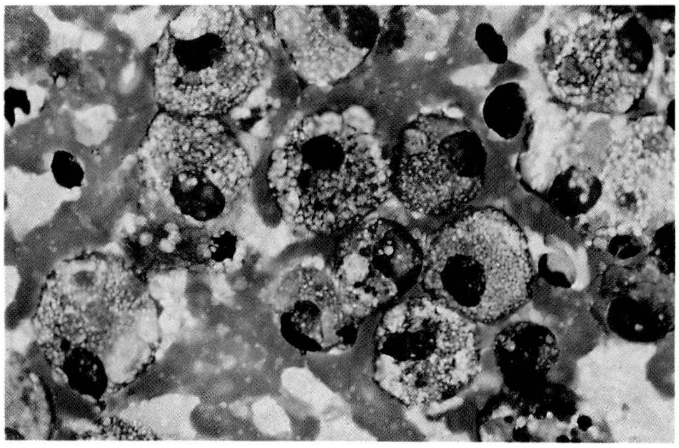

FIGURE 3.38 Metastatic renal cell carcinoma. Monomorphic population of rather bland cells with abundant, vacuolated cytoplasm and round nuclei with minimal atypia. (A) Diff-Quik® 400×; (B) Diff-Quik® 1000×.

thyroiditis. This is heralded by a relatively rapid enlargement of one part of the thyroid that is already enlarged and multinodular as the result of long-standing Hashimoto's thyroiditis. Aspirates in these situations may show a mixture of atypical or neoplastic lymphocytes within in a reactive lymphoid population that may contain germinal center fragments. In these situations, ancillary studies such as flow cytometry and immunocytochemistry will be useful. Rarely malignant lymphomas of the thyroid may be well differentiated and have a follicular pattern. This can be quite difficult to diagnose with FNAB.

Uncommon Malignancies and Metastases

Rarely, malignancies not normally associated with the thyroid will be encountered on FNAB. Scattered reports of mucoepidermoid carcinoma[43] and liposarcoma[44] have been documented. Although these tumors are primary to the thyroid, their cytologic and histologic characteristics are no different from those used in the diagnosis of these neoplasms elsewhere. Renal cell carcinoma (RCC) and squamous cell carcinoma represent the most frequent metastases encountered in the thyroid. Usually the primary carcinoma will have been located and diagnosed previously. Comparison of the primary tumor's cytology/histology with smears obtained from the thyroid mass will confirm metastatic disease. RCC will often appear as discohesive cells with only slightly increased nuclear to cytoplasmic ratio and minimal nuclear atypia. Recognition of the possibility of an RCC is often due to the presence of slightly atypical cells with abundant clear, vacuolated, or granular cytoplasm (Figure 3.38). Vigorous smearing may result in cytoplasmic disruption, releasing cytoplasmic vacuoles into the smear background. Histochemical stains for glycogen may be useful.

Accuracy

Various studies have addressed the sensitivity, specificity, and diagnostic accuracy of thyroid FNAB. It is important to realize that there are several degrees of accuracy to be considered. Does FNAB reliably distinguish between benign and malignant conditions? Can it accurately classify lesions within these two broad categories? A combined study detailing the breakdown of FNAB of the thyroid indicates that a benign diagnosis is rendered in 67% to 80% of cases, a malignant diagnosis in 5% to 20% and an inconclusive diagnosis in 17 percent.

Akerman et al. addressed the sensitivity and specificity of FNAB related to definitive diagnoses.[45] In their study, the sensitivity for papillary and follicular carcinoma was only 58% and 42%, respectively. Reasons given for these low sensitivities included occult tumors, microscopic misinterpretation, and indeterminate diagnoses. However, their study did demonstrate high specificities indicating FNAB was very useful in selecting patients for surgical evaluation and intervention. In 1988, Bedrossian et al. summarized the sensitivity and specificity reported in 13 series from 1975 to 1986. The mean sensitivity was 94 percent, specificity 96 percent, and positive predictive value 93 percent.[46] In his 1994 review, Gharib[18] also reported a high accuracy rate (95 percent). Clearly, statistical data is influenced by the definition of false positive and false negative. If one includes those lesions called "suspicious" as positive, then sensitivity will be increased, specificity decreased, and the percentage of false positives will also increase. The converse is true if suspicious findings are not included as a positive diagnosis.

Limitations to FNAB include sampling problems (inadequate aspiration technique and the biologic nature of the lesion) and inexperience (misdiagnosis). Because FNAB is not infallible, some suggest that it should be used as a screening technique. Therefore, overcalling nonneoplastic lesions as neoplasms would ensure a high sensitivity and positive predictive value.[47]

Pitfalls and Complications

Pitfalls

Interpretation of FNAB cytology of most thyroid lesions is straightforward if

1. there is adequate material and good cytopreparations,
2. the cytologic criteria for diagnoses of various lesions are understood, and
3. appropriate and accurate clinical and radiologic information are available.

Despite the best preparations, an impressive fund of knowledge, and an overabundance of clinical information, pitfalls are still present. The literature is replete with discussions of difficult cases that both experts and the unwary alike may encounter.[48–55] Awareness of these diagnostic problems in FNAB interpretation of the thyroid is the first step toward their avoidance.

Overlapping Criteria

Perhaps the most difficult error to avoid is the placement of too much emphasis on any one cytologic criterion for a specific diagnosis. Cytodiagnosis of thyroid lesions, perhaps more than for any other organ, is hampered by overlapping cytologic criteria. Almost any cytologic feature associated with a specific diagnosis can be found to a lesser extent in other thyroid lesions. There is no single criterion that allows for the distinction between benign and malignant. Table 3.4 provides a list of useful criteria and diagnoses that can be associated with them. Perhaps the most formidable challenge is the problem of papillary formations.

In addition to papillary carcinoma, papillary formations can be seen in other thyroid conditions. Unfortunately, fibrovascular cores, the hallmark of true papillae, are found in both neoplastic and nonneoplastic lesions. Papillary variants of HCT have been described. Papillary formations can also be identified in follicular and medullary carcinomas. FNAB of nonneoplastic goiter can sample areas of hyperplasia that may show exuberant papillary formations. Cellularity, the presence of other cell types, and careful examination of the nuclear features of the cells comprising the papillae are keys to distinguishing among these thyroid diseases.

It is well known that pregnancy can exacerbate some neoplasms, result in worrisome alterations in organs such as breast and cervix, and is an essential piece of clinical information whenever FNAB diagnoses are rendered. Enlargement of the thyroid resulting from an elevation of the basal metabolic rate during pregnancy is not uncommon. Hyperplasia of the thyroid may manifest as hypercellular smears with exuberant papillary formations that mimic the architectural pattern seen in papillary carcinomas. Fortunately, the nuclear features of enlargement, inclusions, and grooves are not found in abundance (Figure 3.39).[56] Although thyroid carcinomas can occur during pregnancy, their incidence does not appear to be higher than in the nonpregnant woman of similar age.[57] Caution should be employed in the diagnosis of papillary carcinoma in pregnant women.

TABLE 3.4 Pitfalls in Diagnoses: Overlapping Cytologic Criteria

Cystic Change
Degeneration in nodular goiter
Papillary carcinoma
Follicular carcinoma
Thyroglossal duct cysts
Metastatic carcinomas
Papillary Formations
Papillary carcinoma
Papillary hyperplasia in nodular goiter
Pregnancy-induced hyperplasia
Hurthle cell tumor—papillary variant
Follicular carcinoma
Hurthle Cells
Hurthle cell tumor
Hashimoto's thyroiditis
Nodular goiter
Papillary carcinoma
Hyperplasia
Intranuclear Inclusions
Papillary carcinoma
Medullary carcinoma
Hurthle cell tumor
Follicular neoplasm
Metastatic malignant melanoma

Histologic Alterations

One area of current interest reflected in the surgical pathology literature is the potential for FNAB to cause tissue damage that hinders or precludes subsequent histologic interpretation. The majority of these cases focus on histologic alterations in thyroid, lymph node, and salivary glands—organs easily sampled using FNAB techniques. Two types of histologic alterations may occur following superficial aspiration biopsy: (1) a reactive proliferation that eventually leads to a fibrous

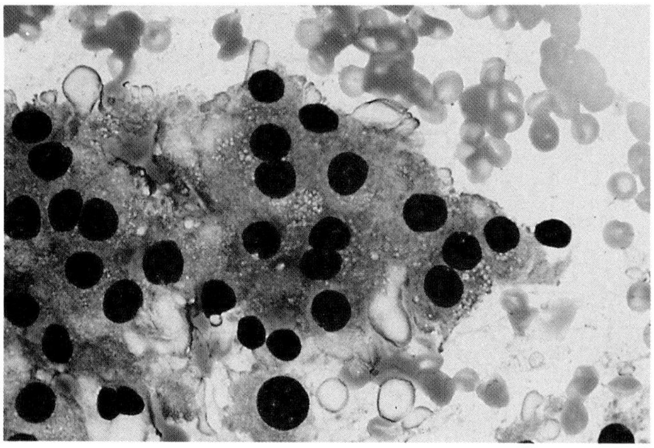

FIGURE 3.39 Fragment of enlarged follicular cells with slight variation in nuclear size and cytologic vacuolization (colloid suds), evidence of hyperplasia in pregnancy. Diff-Quik® 1000×.

tract or region and (2) infarction/hemorrhage that may result in necrosis.

LiVolsi[58] has characterized the spectrum of changes that can occur following FNAB of the thyroid. The temporal sequence of morphologic changes observed in postaspiration thyroid histology is similar to that of a healing wound. Reactive proliferation and hemorrhage may be seen in the acute phase (1 to 3 weeks post-FNAB); while fibrosis, metaplasia, and hemosiderin-laden macrophages characterize the chronic phase (3 to 12 weeks post-FNAB). Obviously, a potential concern to the pathologist interpreting follicular lesions is the presence of follicular cells within an altered capsule, usually the result of multiple passes during FNAB. In this rare event, these areas are usually associated with an obvious needle tract.[58] The author is familiar with two cases in which follicular cells were detected within and just outside of the capsule of the follicular adenoma. However, the break in the capsule was obviously associated with the needle tract and presented no problem in histologic interpretation (Ardao, G., personal communication to WJF).

Additional tissue alterations encountered in the thyroid include partial or complete infarction or necrosis as well as regression of thyroid neoplasms.[59–64] While a compromised vascular supply may be the proximate cause of FNAB-related infarction or necrosis, it may be preceded or induced by other factors. The size and type of needle, the vigor of the aspiration, and especially the number of passes are important variables as are the size, type, and location of the neoplasm. Hurthle cell tumors seem prone to infarction.[60,62,65] The reason for this is still obscure, but oncocytic tumors are prone to undergoing spontaneous necrosis not related to any procedure. An additional, though rarely encountered, morphologic change in the thyroid that may mimic angiosarcoma is extravascular papillary endothelial hyperplasia.[66,67] These alterations, while exuberant, are considered an unusual response in an organizing hematoma and can be distinguished from vascular neoplasms. In LiVolsi's series of histologic alterations, nearly all cases are from the FNABs of one clinician. This suggests faulty technique (LiVolsi, VA, personal communication to WJF). The author (WJF) has seen only one infarcted adenoma of Hurthle cell type and has identified the needle tract histologically in an excised thyroid on only one occasion following FNAB in a series of several thousand cases, using 22- and 23-gauge needles.

FNAB represents the best technique for initial workup of thyroid masses, despite the pitfalls associated with their diagnosis. The importance of clinico-radiologic-pathologic correlation cannot be overemphasized. As in other body sites, if the cytomorphology of the lesion does not "fit" with the clinical information, further workup, including surgery, should be pursued.

Complications

The number of minor complications—local bleeding, vasovagal episodes, and tracheal puncture—are insignificant when compared to the sheer numbers of FNABs performed. Most bleeding can be controlled by the application of slight pressure to the puncture site. Rarely, delayed bleeding within the thyroid may cause some enlargement and patient anxiety, but this resolves within a relatively short period of time. The potential for tracheal puncture is greatest when aspirating midline lesions. It is detectable by loss of negative pressure within the syringe barrel and is confirmed by the presence of bronchial cells on the aspiration smears. Typically, patients feel nothing at all or minimal discomfort of a tickling sensation that may induce a cough response.

There have been only three reports of acute enlargement of the thyroid gland[68,69] (Frable, WJ, personal communication) and delayed swelling of the prethyroidal soft tissues.[70] Although all patients were women, there is no other common denominator and the cause of this phenomenon remains obscure. Anesthesia was given in only one case.[68] One aspiration was interrupted when the patient swallowed.[69] Enlargement was rapid, yet transient, with no ecchymoses or airway obstruction. Cold packs were used to effectively reduce gland enlargement within hours. In the third patient, swelling was noticed at least 24 hours postaspiration.[70] Ultrasound examination indicated edema of the prethyroidal soft tissues. Corticosteroids gradually decreased the swelling within 48 hours.

Kobayashi et al.[71] recently reported a phenomenon referred to as postaspiration thyrotoxicosis. Their retrospective 4-year review revealed a total of 5 patients out of 500 who developed transient thyrotoxicosis following FNAB (21- to 23-gauge needles) of thyroid cysts. All of these patients had relatively large cysts. None developed significant symptoms of hyperthyroidism following aspiration. This study was preceded by a brief report by Shulkin[72] who noted the development of a "hot" nodule following FNAB of a thyroid cyst in the same region, suggesting that some follicular disruption or leakage may account for these changes.

Needle tract seeding during a *fine* needle aspiration biopsy of the thyroid has not been documented.[73] In 1990, Hales and Hsu reported implantation of cells from a papillary carcinoma of the thyroid in the cutaneous portion of the needle tract.[74] This patient had undergone three FNABs of the thyroid using 20-, 21-, and finally 25-gauge needles over a 7-year period. The location, amount of fibrosis, and size of the implant suggested that this slow-growing deposit was seeded during one of the first two aspirations. Despite an initial diagnosis of papillary carcinoma, the patient refused surgical excision.

PARATHYROID

Although multiple articles have been written describing the cytomorphology of parathyroid lesions, cytology's usefulness has really been limited to intraoperative scrape or touch imprint diagnoses. This is primarily because the parathyroid glands are located deep within the neck and upper thorax. Even when enlarged, masses within parathyroid glands are rarely encountered during FNAB of head and neck lesions. A typical presentation is an individual with a small, palpable mass assumed to be located within the thyroid. Ultrasound may have already indicated this mass as potentially cystic. The most likely explanation is a nonneoplastic thyroid nodule.

Normal Cytology

Although normal parathyroid cytology differs somewhat from that of the thyroid, even with experience it is difficult to distinguish the two. The two major cell types that compose the parathyroid gland, chief and clear cells, look quite similar on cytologic smears. The cytoplasm of the clear cells tends to be easily disrupted during smear preparation, resulting in numerous naked nuclei (Figure 3.40). The nuclei are somewhat smaller than thyroid follicular cells and tend to form loose, rosettelike structures rather than obvious follicles. Debris, histiocytes, and colloid are usually not present.

Nonfunctioning Cysts

Fortunately, differentiating thyroid nodules, even with prominent cystic degeneration from nonfunctioning parathyroid cysts, is very straightforward. FNAB results in decompression and drainage of water-clear fluid from parathyroid cysts.[75–78] No other cyst in the head and neck region will yield this type of crystal-clear fluid. Chemical analysis of this fluid will reveal an extremely high parathormone level (PTH) in most cases.[79,80] These

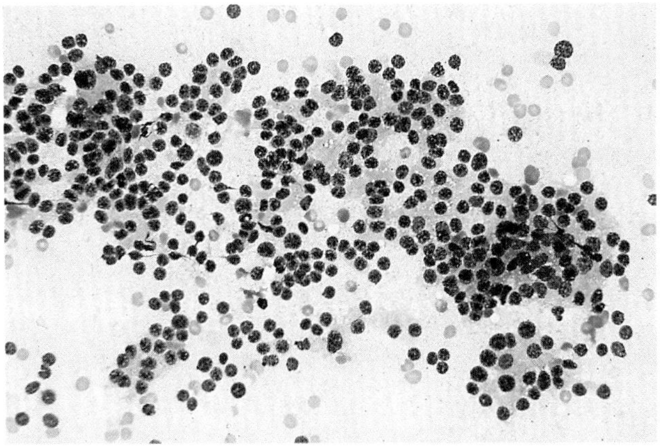

A

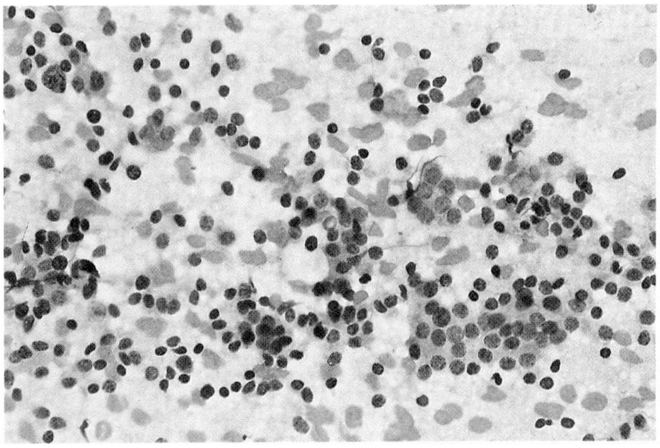

B

FIGURE 3.40 Normal cytology of the parathyroid gland showing small uniform nuclei with minimal cytoplasm. Touch preparation, (A) Diff-Quik® 100×; (B) Papanicolaou 200×.

cysts are likely to reaccumulate over a period of several months; some patients opt to have repeated FNAB for decompression rather than surgery. In the authors' (WJF and CNP) experience of nine cases, only one has recurred after decompression by FNAB.

Hyperplasia versus Adenoma

There are times when ultrasonography may reveal nonpalpable masses in the head and neck that, when placed in clinical context, are presumed to represent either parathyroid adenomas or parathyroid hyperplasia. Although many surgeons still rely on intraoperative diagnoses, the use of ultrasound imaging in conjunction with FNAB to obtain material for a diagnosis has been previously documented.[81–83] The "rules" for differentiating adenoma from hyperplasia are the same regardless of whether the lesion is diagnosed by FNAB cytology or during intraoperative consultation. If only one gland is involved, then *adenoma* is the preferred diagnosis. If multiple glands show enlargement and hypercellularity, then the term *hyperplasia* is chosen. In either case, the cytomorphology is similar: reduced amounts of fibroadipose

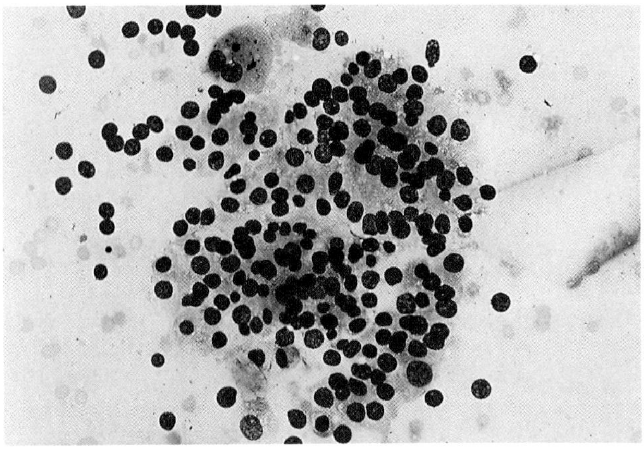

FIGURE 3.41 Parathyroid adenoma. Loosely arranged fragment of parathyroid cells showing anisonucleosis. Diff-Quik® 400×.

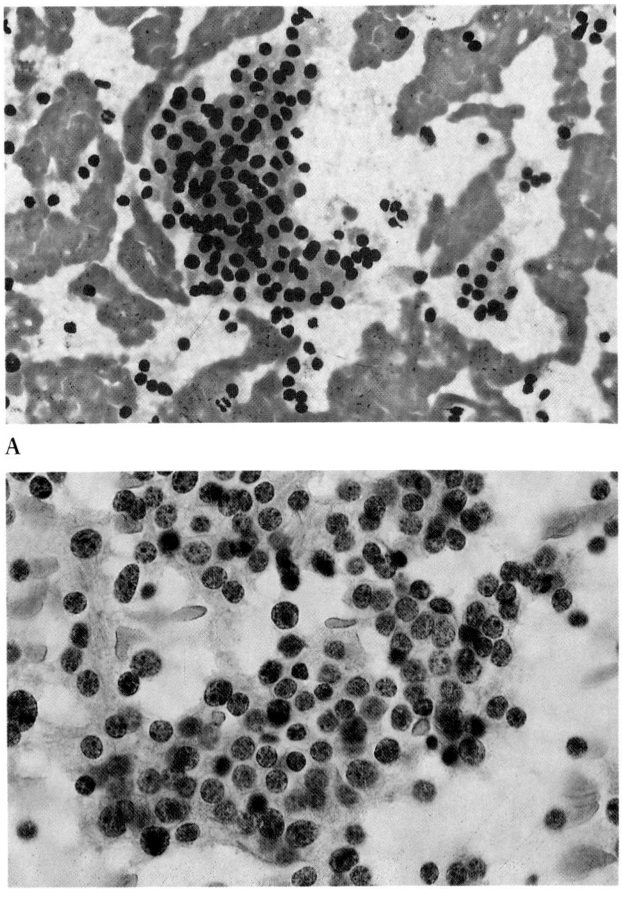

A

B

FIGURE 3.42 Parathyroid hyperplasia. Similar cytomorphology to normal parathyroid cells (see Figure 3.40). Diagnosis based in large measure on increased cellularity and presence of a nodule. Cytologic atypia should not be used to distinguish hyperplasia from a neoplasm. (A) Diff-Quik® 250×; (B) Papanicolaou 400×.

tissue with corresponding increase in parathyroid cells. From a strict cytologic perspective, adenomas demonstrate cells with giant nuclei and anisonucleosis as well as cells with multiple nuclei (morulas) more often than do cases of parathyroid hyperplasia (Figures 3.41 and 3.42). Carcinoma of the parathyroid has to be determined by the surgical pathology features of invasive growth and metastasis and cannot be specifically diagnosed by FNAB except in a metastatic site with prior clinical knowledge that the patient has such a malignancy.

REFERENCES

Thyroid

1. Frable WJ. Thin-needle aspiration biopsy. In Bennington JL (ed.), *Major problems in pathology,* Vol. 14. Philadelphia: W.B. Saunders Co., 1983.

2. Koss LG, Woyke S, Olszewski W. *Aspiration biopsy: Cytologic interpretation and histologic bases.* New York: Igaku-Shoin, 1984.

3. Lowhagen T, Sprenger E. Cytologic presentation of thyroid tumors in aspiration biopsy smears. *Acta Cytol* 1974;18:192–197.

4. Frable MA, Frable WJ. Thin needle aspiration biopsy of the thyroid gland. *Laryngoscope* 1980;90: 1619–1625.

5. Griffies WS, Donegan E, Abel ME. The role of fine needle aspiration in the management of the thyroid nodule. *Laryngoscope* 1985;95:1103–1106.

6. Frable WJ. The treatment of thyroid cancer: The role of fine needle aspiration cytology. *Arch Otolaryngol Head Neck Surg* 1986;112:1200–1203.

7. Kini SR. *Guides to clinical aspiration biopsy: Thyroid.* New York: Igaku-Shoin, 1987.

8. LiVolsi VA. Surgical pathology of the thyroid. In Bennington JL (ed.), *Major problems in pathology,* Vol. 22. Philadelphia: W.B. Saunders Co., 1990.

9. Silverman JF, West RL, Larkin EW, et al. The role of fine-needle aspiration biopsy in the rapid diagnosis and management of thyroid neoplasm. *Cancer* 1986;57:1167–1170.

10. Asp AA, Georgitis W, Waldron EJ, Sims JE, Kidd GS. Fine needle aspiration of the thyroid: Use in an average health-care facility. *Am J Med* 1987; 83:489–493.

11. Caruso D, Mazzaferri EL. Fine needle aspiration biopsy in the management of thyroid nodules. *Endocrinologist* 1991;1:194–202.

12. Hamburger JI, Miller JM, Kini SR. *Clinical-pathological evaluation of thyroid nodules—handbook and atlas.* (Private publication, 1979).

13. Hamburger JI, Husain M. Semiquantitative criteria for fine-needle biopsy diagnosis: Reduced false negative diagnosis. *Diagn Cytopathol* 1988;4:14–17.

14. Hamburger JI, Husain M, Nishiyama R, Nunez C, Solomon D. Increasing the accuracy of fine-

needle biopsy for thyroid nodules. *Arch Pathol Lab Med* 1989;113:1035–1041.

15. Kini SR. Needle aspiration biopsy of the thyroid: Revisited. *Diagn Cytopathol* 1993;9(3):249–251.

16. Ramzy I. *Clinical cytopathology and aspiration biopsy: Fundamental principles and practice.* Norwalk, CT: Appelton and Lange, 1990.

17. Bisi H, de Camargo RYA, Fihlo AL. Role of fine-needle aspiration cytology in the management of thyroid nodules: Review of experience with 1,925 cases. *Diagn Cytopathol* 1992;8:504–510.

18. Gharib H. Fine-needle aspiration biopsy of thyroid nodules: Advantages, limitations and effect. *Mayo Clin Proc* 1994;69:44–49.

19. Szporn AH, Tepper S, Watson CW. Disseminated cryptococcosis presenting as thyroiditis. *Acta Cytol* 1985;29:449–453.

20. Solary E, Rifle G, Chalopin JM. Disseminated aspergillosis revealed by thyroiditis in a renal allograft recipient. *Transplant* 1987;44:839–840.

21. Vaidya KP, Lomvardias S. Cryptococcal thyroiditis: Report of a case diagnosed by fine-needle aspiration cytology. *Diagn Cytopathol* 1991;7:415–416.

22. Guarda LA, Baskin J. Inflammatory and lymphoid lesions of the thyroid gland: Cytopathology by fine needle aspiration. *Am J Clin Pathol* 1987;87:14–22.

23. Tani E, Skoog L. Fine needle aspiration cytology and immunocytochemistry in the diagnosis of lymphoid lesions of the thyroid gland. *Acta Cytol* 1989; 33:48–52.

24. Nilsson G. Marginal vacuoles in fine needle aspiration biopsy smears of toxic goitres. *Acta Pathol Microbiol Scand*(A) 1972;80:289–293.

25. Jayaram G, Singh B, Marwaha RK. Graves' disease: Appearance in cytologic smears from fine needle aspirates of the thyroid gland. *Acta Cytol* 1989; 33:36–40.

26. Frable WJ. Controversies in the pathology and cytology of well-differentiated thyroid carcinoma. *Head Neck* 1990;2:170–175.

27. Suen KC. How does one separate follicular lesions of the thyroid by fine-needle aspiration biopsy? *Diagn Cytopathol* 1988;4:78–81.

28. Ravinsky E, Safneck JR. Fine needle aspirations of follicular lesions of the thyroid gland: The intermediate type smear. *Acta Cytol* 1990;34:813–820.

29. Layfield L. Editorial comments: Fine-needle aspiration evaluation of the solitary thyroid nodule—the imprecision of diagnostic criteria. *Diagn Cytopathol* 1993;9:355–357.

30. Kini SR, Miller JM, Hamburger JI. Cytopathology of Hurthle cell lesions of the thyroid gland by fine needle aspiration. *Acta Cytol* 1981;25:647–652.

31. Gonzalez JL, Wang HH, Ducatman BS. Fine-needle aspiration of Hurthle cell lesions: A cytomorphologic approach to diagnosis. *Am J Clin Pathol* 1993;100:231–235.

32. Kaur A, Jayarm G. Thyroid tumors: Cytomorphology of Hurthle cell tumors, including an uncommon papillary variant. *Diagn Cytopathol* 1993;9:135–137.

33. Kini SR, Miller JM, Hamburger JI, Smith MJ. Cytopathology of papillary carcinoma of the thyroid by fine-needle aspiration. *Acta Cytol* 1980;24:511–512.

34. Miller JM, Hamburger JI, Kini SR. The needle biopsy diagnosis of papillary thyroid carcinoma. *Cancer* 1981;48:989–993.

35. Akhtar M, Ali MA, Huq M, Bakry M. Fine-needle aspiration biopsy of papillary thyroid carcinoma: Cytologic, histologic and ultrastructural correlations. *Diagn Cytopathol* 1991;7:373–379.

36. Gould E, Watzak L, Chamizo W, Albores-Saavedra J. Nuclear grooves in cytologic preparations: A study of the utility of this feature in the diagnosis of papillary carcinoma. *Acta Cytol* 1988;33:16–20.

37. Shurbaji MS, Gupta PK, Frost JK. Nuclear grooves: A useful criterion in the cytopathologic diagnosis of papillary thyroid carcinoma. *Diagn Cytopathol* 1988;4:91–94.

38. Rupp M, Ehya H. Nuclear grooves in the aspiration cytology of papillary carcinoma of the thyroid. *Acta Cytol* 1988;33:21–26.

39. Carcangiu ML, Zampi G, Rosai J. Poorly differentiated ("insular") thyroid carcinoma: A reinterpretation of Langhans' "wuchernde Struma." *Am J Surg Pathol* 1984;8:655–668.

40. Flynn SD, Forman BH, Stewart AF, Kinder BK. Poorly differentiated ("insular") carcinoma of the thyroid gland: An aggressive subset of differentiated thyroid neoplasms. *Surgery* 1988;104:963–970.

41. Pietribiasi F, Sapino A, Papotti M, Bussolati G. Cytologic features of poorly differentiated "insular" carcinoma of the thyroid, as revealed by fine-needle aspiration biopsy. *Am J Clin Pathol* 1990;94:687–692.

42. Sironi M, Collini P, Cantaboni A. Fine needle aspiration cytology of insular thyroid carcinoma: A report of four cases. *Acta Cytol* 1992;36:435–439.

43. Larson RS, Wick MR. Primary mucoepidermoid carcinoma of the thyroid: Diagnosis by fine-needle aspiration biopsy. *Diagn Cytopathol* 1993;9:438–443.

44. Andrion A, Gaglio A, Dogliani N, Bosco E, Mazzucco G. Liposarcoma of the thyroid gland: Fine-needle aspiration cytology, immunohistology and ultrastructure. *Am J Clin Pathol* 1991;95:675–679.

45. Akerman M, Tennvall J, Biorklund A, Martensson H, Moler T. Sensitivity and specificity of fine needle aspiration cytology in the diagnosis of tumors of the thyroid gland. *Acta Cytol* 1985;29:850–855.

46. Bedrossian CWM, Martinez F, Silverberg AB. Fine needle aspiration. In Gnepp DR (ed.), *Pathology of the head and neck.* New York: Churchill Livingstone 1988:pp. 25–99.

47. Suen KC, Quenville NF. Fine needle aspiration of the thyroid gland: A study of 304 cases. *J Clin Pathol* 1983;36:1036–1045.

48. Hsu C, Boey J. Diagnostic pitfalls in fine needle aspiration of thyroid nodules. *Acta Cytol* 1987; 31:699–704.

49. Jayaram G. Fine needle aspiration cytologic study of the solitary thyroid nodule: Profile of 308 cases with histologic correlation. *Acta Cytol* 1985;29: 967–973.

50. Ananthakrishnan N, Rao KM, Narasimhan R, Veliath AJ. Problems and limitations with fine needle aspiration cytology of solitary thyroid nodules. *Aust N Z J Surg* 1990;60:35–39.

51. Harach HR, Zusman SB, Day ES. Nodular goiter: A histo-cytological study with some emphasis on pitfalls of fine-needle aspiration cytology. *Diagn Cytopathol* 1992;8:409–419.

52. LiVolsi VA, Gupta PK. Thyroid fine-needle aspiration: Intranuclear inclusions, nuclear grooves and psammoma bodies—Paraganglioma-like adenoma of the thyroid. *Diagn Cytopathol* 1992;8:82–84.

53. Fiorella RM, Isley W, Miller LK, Kragel PJ. Multinodular goiter of the thyroid mimicking malignancy: Diagnostic pitfalls in fine-needle aspiration biopsy. *Diagn Cytopathol* 1993;9:351–357.

54. Caraway NP, Sneige N, Samaan NA. Diagnostic pitfalls in thyroid fine-needle aspiration: A review of 394 cases. *Diagn Cytopathol* 1993;9(3):345–350.

55. Heinmann A, Gritsman A. Diagnostic problems and pitfalls in aspiration cytology of thyroid nodules. In Schmidt WA (ed.), *Cytopathology annual.* Baltimore: Williams and Wilkins, 1993.

56. Betsill W. Thyroid fine needle aspiration in pregnant women. *Diagn Cytopathol* 1985;1:53–54.

57. Fukuda K, Hachisuga T, Sugimori H, Tsuzuku M. Papillary carcinoma of the thyroid occurring during pregnancy: Report of a case diagnosed by fine needle aspiration cytology. *Acta Cytol* 1991;35: 725–727.

58. LiVolsi VA, Merino MJ. Worrisome histologic alterations following fine needle aspiration of thyroid. *Mod Pathol* 1990;3:59A.

59. Jones JD, Pittman DL, Sanders LR. Necrosis of thyroid nodules after fine needle aspiration. *Acta Cytol* 1985;29:29–32.

60. Kini SR, Miller JM. Infarction of thyroid neoplasms following aspiration biopsy. *Acta Cytol* 1986; 30:591.

61. Jayaram G, Aggarwal S. Infarction of thyroid nodule: A rare complication following fine needle aspiration. *Acta Cytol* 1989;33:940–941.

62. Keyhani-Rofagha S, Kooner DS, Keyhani M, O'Toole RV. Necrosis of a Hurthle cell tumor of the thyroid following fine needle aspiration: Case report and literature review. *Acta Cytol* 1990;34:805–808.

63. Alejo M, Matias-Guiu X, de las Hera Duran P. Infarction of a papillary thyroid carcinoma after fine needle aspiration. *Acta Cytol* 1991;35:478–479.

64. Us-Krasovec M, Golouh R, Auesperg M, Pogacnik A. Tissue damage after fine needle aspiration biopsy. *Acta Cytol* 1992;36:456–457.

65. Bauman A, Strawbridge HTG. Spontaneous disappearance of an atypical Hurthle cell adenoma. *Am J Clin Pathol* 1983;80:399–402.

66. Axiotis CA, Merino MJ, Ain K, Norton JA. Papillary endothelial hyperplasia in the thyroid following fine-needle aspiration. *Arch Pathol Lab Med* 1991; 115:240–242.

67. Tsang K, Duggan MA. Vascular proliferation of the thyroid: A complication of fine-needle aspiration. *Arch Pathol Lab Med* 1992;116:1040–1042.

68. Haas SN. Acute thyroid swelling after needle biopsy of the thyroid. *N Engl J Med* 1982;307:1349.

69. Dal Fabbro S, Barbazza R, Fabris C, Perelli R. Acute thyroid swelling after fine needle aspiration biopsy. *J Endocrinol Invest* 1987;10:105.

70. Velkeniers B, Noppen M, Vanhaelst L. Delayed swelling of prethyroid soft tissue after fine needle aspiration. *J Endocrinol Invest* 1988;11:225.

71. Kobayashi A, Kuma K, Matsuzuka F, Hirai K, Fukata S, Sugawara M. Thyrotoxicosis after needle aspiration of thyroid cyst. *J Clin Endocrinol Metab* 1992;75:21–24.

72. Shulkin BL. Hot nodule after fine needle aspiration. *Clin Nucl Med* 1988;13:131.

73. Powers CN. Fine needle aspiration biopsy: Perspectives on Complications—The reality behind the myth. In Schmidt WA (ed.), *Cytopathology annual 1995.* Baltimore: William and Wilkins, (in press).

74. Hales MS, Hsu FSF. Needle tract implantation of papillary carcinoma of the thyroid following aspiration biopsy. *Acta Cytol* 1990;34:801–804.

Parathyroid

75. Katz AD, Dunkelman D. Needle aspiration of nonfunctional parathyroid cysts. *Arch Surg* 1984; 119:307–308.

76. Pacini F, Antonelli A, Lari R, Gasperini L, Bacheri L, Pinchera A. Unsuspected parathyroid cysts diagnosed by measurement of thyroglobulin and parathyroid hormone concentration in fluid aspiration. *Ann Intern Med* 1985;102:793–794.

77. Silverman JF, Khazanie PG, Norris HT, Fore WW. Parathyroid hormone (PTH) assay of parathyroid cysts examined by fine needle aspiration biopsy. *Am J Clin Pathol* 1986;86:776–780.

78. Oertel YC, Wargotz ES. Diagnosis of parathyroid cysts (letter). *Am J Clin Pathol* 1987;88: 252–253.

79. Prinz RA, Peters JR, Kane JM, Wood J. Needle aspiration of non-functioning parathyroid cysts. *Am Surg* 1990;56:420–422.

80. Layfield LJ. Fine-needle aspiration cytology of cystic parathyroid lesions: A cytomorphologic overlap with cystic lesions of the thyroid. *Acta Cytol* 1991; 35:447–450.

81. Clark OH, Gooding GAW, Ljung BM. Locating a parathyroid adenoma by ultrasonography and aspiration biopsy cytology. *West J Med* 1981;135:154–158.

82. Solbiati L, Montali G, Croce F, Bellotti E, Giangrande A, Ravetto C. Parathyroid tumors detected by fine-needle aspiration biopsy under ultrasound guidance. *Radiology* 1983;148:793–797.

83. DeRaimo AJ, Kane RA, Katz JF, Rolla AP. Parathyroid cysts: Diagnosis by sonography and needle aspiration. *Am J Roentgenol* 1984;14:1227–1228.

CHAPTER

4

Lymph Nodes

In the head and neck, lymph nodes are usually noted rather promptly by the patient or by others. Most commonly, the lymph nodes are enlarged in the cervical area, either anterior or posterior to the sternocleidomastoid muscle, but they may be present in the submaxillary and submental area, the occipital area, adjacent to the thyroid, and both pre- and postauricular in close proximity to the parotid salivary gland. When near or in the same location as another organ such as a salivary gland, there is an immediate differential diagnosis between an actual lymph node enlargement and a process that directly involves the salivary gland or thyroid or even a skin adnexal tumor.[1]

CLINICAL EVALUATION

It is important to learn the circumstances of the lymph node enlargement to obtain a clear clinical picture before performing the aspiration biopsy. For example, a history of ear infections, tonsillitis, or a recent bout of influenza followed by a cervical lymph node enlargement usually points to a reactive process in the node.[2] In the spring and fall, cat-scratch disease is active and can be seen most often in children with a single and sometimes unusual node, such as a submental lymph node, that is enlarged.[3] In contrast, a child or an adult with a very large node but who also has other constitutional symptoms more often suggests a malignant neoplasm, particularly a malignant lymphoma in the pediatric age group.[4] A history of human immunodeficiency virus (HIV) infection or clinical signs of AIDS indicates an immediate list of differential diagnoses including infections, lymphoid hyperplasia, or malignant lymphoma.[5,6] Table 4.1 summarizes some general guidelines in evaluating an enlarged lymph node.

Physical Examination

Remember the following points in palpation of the lymph nodes: size, location with relation to other structures, consistency, and the presence of other nodes in the head and neck area that may be less obviously enlarged (Table 4.2). Metastatic tumors usually present as round, firm and very discrete nodes. Relatively soft and flat nodes of less than 2 centimeters are most often reactive, while enlarged supraclavicular nodes are most frequently the result of metastatic tumors or, in children, are part of the typical presentation of acute lymphoblastic lymphoma. This malignancy may be already confirmed clinically by the presence of a mediastinal mass.[4] In young adults, a very large, firm cervical node, most often in the left cervical area, suggests Hodgkin's disease and the need for a chest film if one is not already available.

It is important to look in the oral cavity, including the floor of the mouth under the tongue and the throat, paying particular attention to the tonsil area. Use a good head light to see these structures clearly. If a metastatic carcinoma from a head and neck primary is suspected, it is also important to palpate within the oral cavity because the neoplasm may be easier to feel as an induration rather than visualize directly.

TECHNICAL CONSIDERATIONS

The technique of aspiration biopsy of lymph nodes is summarized in Table 4.3 and in Chapter 1. Most often, 22-gauge needles will suffice when one suspects metastatic carcinomas. This size needle is usually not contaminated with too much blood in the presence of metastatic carcinoma. Reactive lymph nodes are often

Table 4.1 General Guides to Clinical Evaluation of Lymph Nodes

1. Determine if the patient has a past history of a malignancy or other significant disease process, i.e., collagen vascular disease, immune suppression, etc.
2. Examine the patient carefully for any current clinical evidence of malignancy or other significant disease.
3. Ask about any generalized systemic symptoms, i.e., fever, sweating, chills, weight loss.
4. Inquire how long the lymph nodes have been enlarged. Have the nodes become larger or smaller; if so, how fast? Are there other lymph nodes that have appeared or disappeared?
5. Question the patient about exposure to infectious agents, drugs, or animals.

Table 4.2 General Guides to Physical Examination of Lymph Nodes

1. How extensive is the lymphadenopathy and what node or node groups are enlarged?
2. Is the site of the mass one that may be a structure other than a lymph node, i.e., salivary gland, thyroid, inguinal hernia?
3. How large are the lymph nodes? Are they firm, hard, or soft? Are the enlarged nodes tender? Are they fixed?
4. Is there enlargement of the liver or spleen?
5. Is there evidence for a malignancy in an organ whose lymphatics would drain into the enlarged lymph node or node group?
6. Is there localized evidence of infection in the region of the lymph node or at another site, i.e., ear or oral cavity, specifically a tooth, sore throat, skin, or genital infection?

Table 4.3 General Guides for Aspiration of Lymph Nodes

1. Use standard techniques as described in Chapter 1.
2. Use 22-, 23-, or 25-gauge needles.
3. Try the needle-only method for very small nodes or following an initial aspiration from a small node that is mostly blood.
4. Make smears by the usual horizontal method, particularly if a lymphoproliferative process or malignancy is suspected. The compression smear technique will suffice for other cases that are most often metastatic carcinoma.
5. Stain a few initial air-dried smears by Diff-Quik® to see at least the cellularity and the potential differential diagnosis.
6. Perform additional aspirates as needed for diagnosis and triage for special studies.

bloody so that thinner, higher gauge needles and the use of the needle-only technique may result in a more adequate aspiration biopsy. If there is a group of enlarged lymph nodes, aspirate the largest one.

Aspiration biopsy is the most likely technique to reflect the underlying disease process. If the node is flat and very small, but clinically sufficient to aspirate, it is important to pin it between two fingers and perform the initial aspiration with the needle-only technique for more precise control of the tip of the needle. It is important to avoid traversing the sternocleidomastoid muscle as this will usually make the aspiration painful. Traversing a large muscle often results in a good muscle biopsy but samples nothing from the target lymph node. Roll the muscle out of the way or make an approach with the needle that avoids this large muscle altogether.[7]

Potential Problems

Palpable lymph nodes in the neck may lie in close proximity to the carotid artery, with a pulsation transmitted from that vessel. With this situation, there is also the clinical possibility of a carotid body tumor if the apparently enlarged node is in the midanterior cervical area.[7] Try listening with a stethoscope to detect a bruit. Carotid body tumors have been aspirated successfully but have also produced some complications.[8]

If the mass is suspected to be a carotid artery aneurysm, either forgo the aspiration until that possibility is ruled out by angiographic or other studies or approach the mass cautiously with a 25-gauge needle. Use the needle-only technique. The aspirator should be able to feel the wall of the aneurysm as a rather firm structure; similarly, the wall of the carotid artery itself is also quite firm. If you do puncture this artery, it will be immediately apparent from the blood running relatively rapidly into the syringe. Withdraw the needle quickly and put firm pressure on the puncture site and the artery for a full 10 minutes by the clock. This should take care of the problem.

Preliminary Evaluation

Ensure adequacy of the initial aspiration by immediate evaluation of some of the smears stained by a rapid method, preferably a Romanowsky stain or modification such as Diff-Quik®. It is often possible to make or at least get some idea of the diagnosis from initial evaluation of the stained smears (Table 4.4). The results of this initial study often dictate how subsequent aspirates are partitioned for various special studies as illustrated in the algorithm (Figure 4.1). Smears can be made by any of the methods described in Chapter 1 on techniques. Compression smears suffice for a quick screen and diagnosis of metastatic carcinomas. If one suspects a lymphoproliferative process, it is better to make smears in the more traditional manner as for a bone marrow sample

TABLE 4.4 General Guides for Interpretation of Stains of Lymph Node Aspiration Smears

Features Emphasized by Diff-Quik®	*Features Emphasized by Papanicolaou*
Polymorphism	Nuclear outline
Plasmacytoid features	Chromatin
Lymphoglandular bodies	Nucleoli
Hematopoietic cells	Detail in solid tissue fragments
Bizarre cells	

by separating the slides horizontally (see Figures 1.1 through 1.3). This method has more of a tendency to preserve some semblance of the architecture of the node, which will be helpful in interpretation both for reactive nodes and lymphomas.

It is important to make the microscopic evaluation of a lymph node aspiration systematically (Table 4.5). This is particularly true for examples of lymphoproliferative processes, be they reactive or neoplastic.[9] Diagnoses of metastatic tumors are usually quite obvious after a quick microscopic study of a few or even one smear. The diagnostic range and complexity of lymphoproliferative processes, however, requires the thorough and systematic evaluation of all smears.

The first question is, has a lymph node been aspirated or is the mass an enlarged salivary gland, a cyst of some type of process, a thyroid nodule, a skin adenexal tumor, a paraganglioma, or a soft tissue tumor? The cytopathologist must be familiar with the clinical presentation and the cytologic appearance of these lesions and recognize that they are not lymph nodes, though some have lymphoid tissue.

If it is determined that a lymph node has actually been aspirated, then begin the microscopic evaluation (Table 4.6) at low power. Determine the adequacy of the preparation, cellularity, and any pattern of cell arrangement, specifically isolated cells versus aggregates. Look for any pattern of distribution of aggregates versus isolated cells. Is it uniform or haphazard? (Figures 4.2 and 4.3).

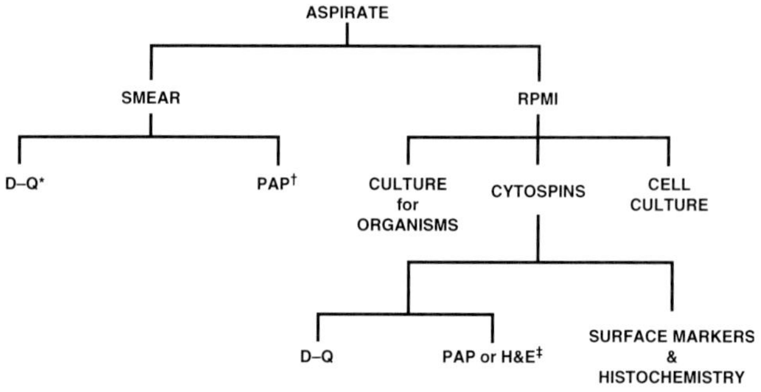

FIGURE 4.1 Algorithm for triage of aspiration biopsy specimen of a lymph node. *Diff-Quik®, †Papanicolaou, ‡Hemahexylin and eosin.

TABLE 4.5 General Guides to Microscopic Evaluation of the Smear

Masses commonly mistaken for lymph nodes include:

1. Cysts—epidermal, sebaceous, branchial cleft, thyroglossal duct, parathyroid.
2. Soft tissue masses—fat, connective tissue, neural, smooth and skeletal muscle, vascular tumors.
3. Skin appendage tumors—sweat gland, sebaceous gland, hair follicle origin.
4. Inflammatory masses—fat necrosis, abscess, granulation tissue or granulomas.
5. Salivary gland masses—sialadenitis, primary and metastatic tumors of the salivary glands.
6. Paragangliomas (carotid body tumor).

TABLE 4.6 Systematic Microscopic Evaluation of the Smear

Low-Power Examination (scanning power 4×)

1. Cellularity of the aspirate—low, moderate, high.
2. Adequacy of the preparation—distribution, staining quality.
3. Pattern of arrangement of cells—aggregates, isolated.

Medium-Power Examination (10× and/or 20×)

1. Presence of bizarre cells, i.e., few carcinoma cells or polyploid cells of Hodgkin's disease or polymorphous T-cell lymphoma.
2. Nature of any small cell aggregates—small lymphocytes, small-round-cell tumors, other.
3. Division of lymphoid cell population into three categories: (a) exclusively or predominantly small cells; (b) mixture of large and small cells; (c) dominance of large cells.
4. Presence of cells with plasmacytoid features, definitive plasma cells and the presence of tingible body macrophages.
5. Prominence of eosinophils or polymorphonuclear leukocytes.
6. Presence of granulomas, granulation tissue fragments.

High-Power Examination (40×)

1. Type of cells in cell aggregates.
2. Identification of bizarre cells.

Oil Immersion (1000×)

1. Nuclear Morphology—cleaves, indentations.
2. Chromatin Distribution—smooth, regular, clumped.
3. Nucleoli—size, shape.

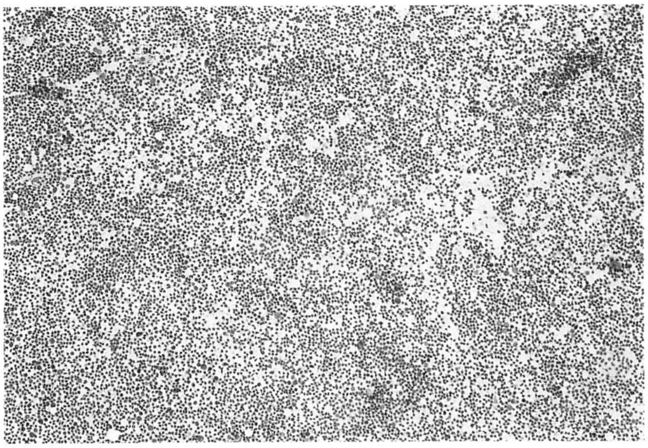

FIGURE 4.2 Aspirate of cervical lymph node. Smear with moderate to high cellularity and minimal aggregates of cells. Looking closely, even at this power, there is no dominant type of cell, large or small, that can be identified. Scattered large cells can be seen. Reactive lymph node. Diff-Quik® 100×.

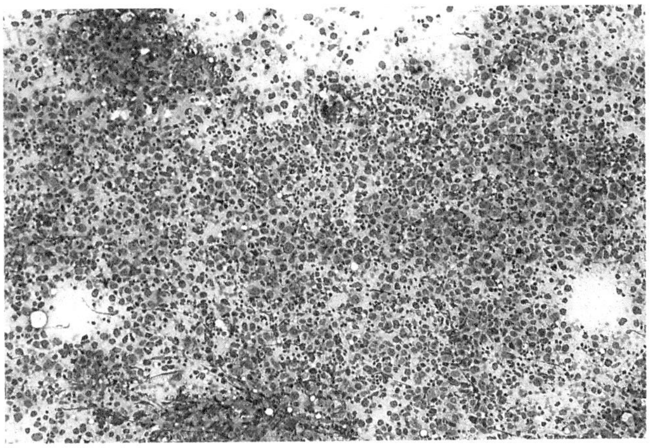

FIGURE 4.3 Aspirate of cervical lymph node. Highly cellular smear with uniform distribution and dominant pattern of large cells. Large cell lymphoma. Diff-Quik® 100×.

Using the medium power of the microscope, look for the presence of bizarre cells; for example, a few carcinoma cells or the polyploid cells of a T-cell lymphoma or Hodgkin's disease (Figure 4.4). Determine what type of cells make up any small-cell aggregates—small lymphocytes or the cells of metastatic small-cell carcinoma from, perhaps, the lung (Figure 4.5). If the smear is composed of a lymphoid cell population, how is it divided? Is it predominantly small cells, predominantly large cells, or a mixture of large and small cells (Figures 4.6 and 4.7)?

Examine the smears for lymphoid cells with plasmacytoid features, the presence of actual plasma cells or large cells that have phagocytosed debris, and tingible body macrophages (Figure 4.8). Tingible body macrophages may be surrounded by lymphocytes. Sometimes these lymphohistiocytic aggregates are only few in number and scattered; in other cases, they are abundant. The

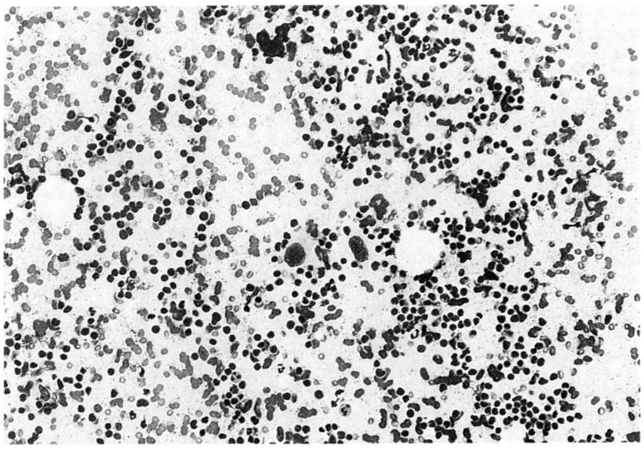

FIGURE 4.4 Aspiration of cervical lymph node. Scattered, large, somewhat bizarre cells from a case of Hodgkin's disease. Diff-Quik® 250×.

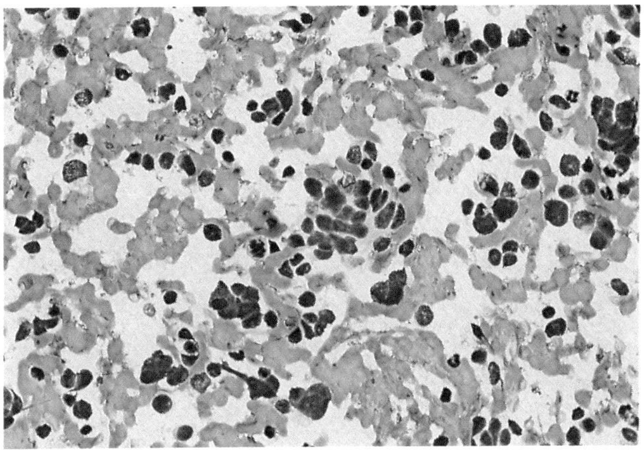

FIGURE 4.5 Aspiration of supraclavicular lymph node. Aggregates of small cells with marked nuclear molding. The smear has a bloody background with scattered smaller cells that are necrotic tumor cells, not lymphocytes. Metastatic small-cell carcinoma of the lung. Diff-Quik® 250×.

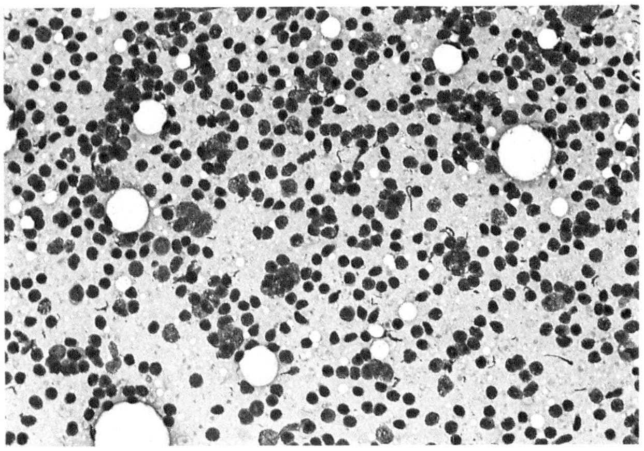

FIGURE 4.6 Aspiration of cervical lymph node. Cellular smear with monotonous pattern of predominantly small cells. Note some uniform small aggregates. Malignant lymphoma, small lymphocytic, poorly differentiated. Diff-Quik® 250×.

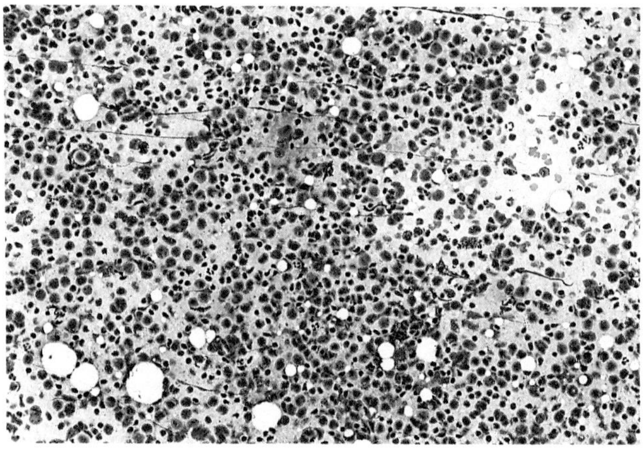

FIGURE 4.7 Aspiration of cervical lymph node. Cellular smear with mixture of small and large cells with no intermediate-sized cells. Mixed small- and large-cell lymphoma. Diff-Quik® 250×.

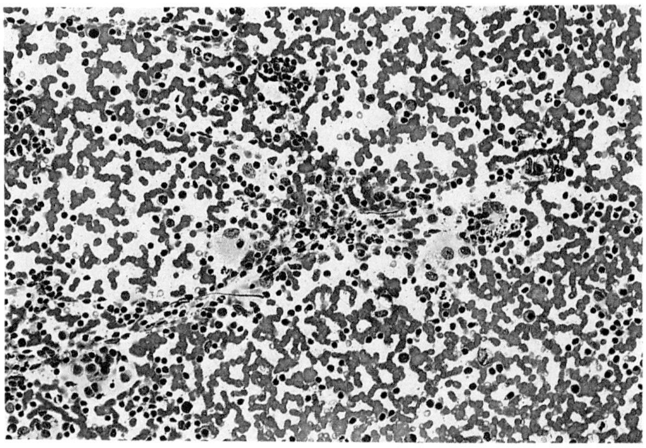

FIGURE 4.9 Aspiration of cervical lymph node. Small sheet of large histiocytic cells surrounded by lymphocytes. This predominant pattern suggests a diagnosis of sinus histiocytosis with massive lymphadenopathy, Rosai-Dorfman disease, histologically confirmed in this case. Diff-Quik® 250×.

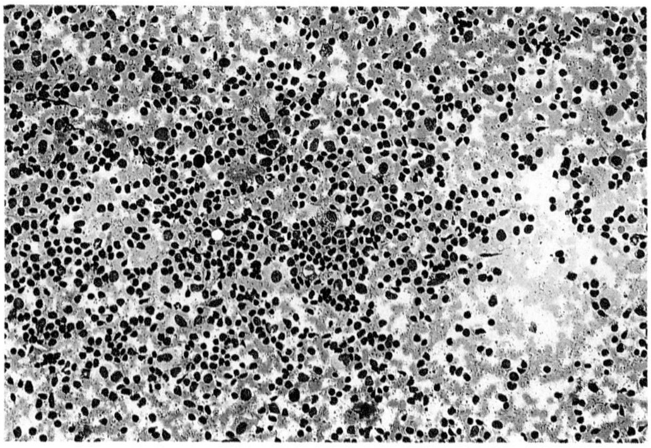

FIGURE 4.8 Aspiration of cervical lymph node. Tingible body macrophages with engulfed nuclear debris. Diff-Quik® 250×.

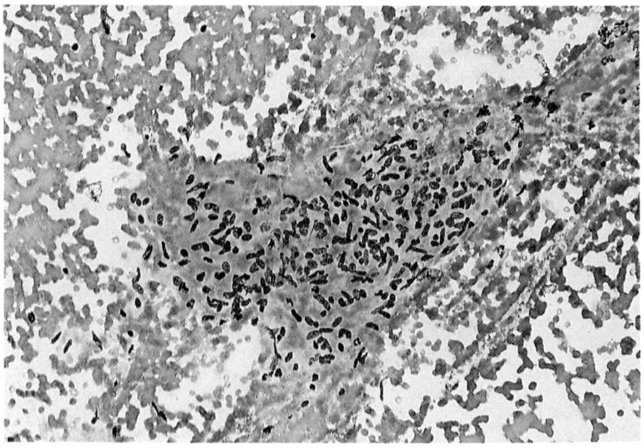

FIGURE 4.10 Aspiration of cervical lymph node. Discrete and cohesive epithelioid cell granulomas found in aspirates of lymph nodes from patients with sarcoid. Diff-Quik® 250×.

application of the lymphocytes to the histiocytes, which may aggregate, can be quite close as in sinus histiocytosis with massive lymphadenopathy, Rosai-Dorfman disease (Figure 4.9).[10,11]

At medium power, also look for the presence of eosinophils or a predominance of polymorphonuclear leukocytes often found with necrosis. This indicates suppuration in the lymph node and the formation of an abscess. Finally, look carefully for granulomas, which in sarcoid are often quite discrete and epithelioid in appearance (Figure 4.10).[12] Sarcoid granulomas contrast with the very loose and poorly structured granulomas with background necrosis found in aspirations from lymph nodes involved with tuberculosis.[13–15]

With any predominantly inflammatory aspiration smear pattern from a lymph node, begin to look for the presence of a specific organism. The refractile capsule of cryptococcus, blastomyces, and coccidiodes can be seen at medium power. The capsule of these organisms can be accentuated in suspected cases by lowering the substage condenser on the microscope to enhance their refractility (Figure 4.11). If an aspiration smear demonstrates a background of necrosis that is very homogeneous but with few cells, look very carefully for the presence of negative images. These are curved, striated thin lines that do not take any stain and thus appear slightly refractile. They are found in patients with AIDS who are infected with atypical mycobacteria that are involving lymph nodes (Figure 4.12).[16]

Many diagnoses in lymph node aspirates are made at medium power, most often metastatic carcinomas. The presence of the foreign malignant cells in the node usually displaces most of the lymphoid elements, making the diagnosis of a metastatic tumor quite easy.

Examining the smears at higher power may help identify the type of cell within cell aggregates. This is true with small lymphocytes versus metastatic small-cell car-

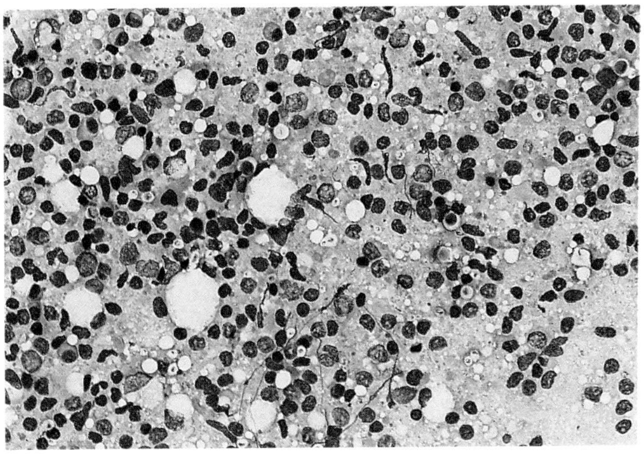

FIGURE 4.11 Aspiration of supraclavicular lymph node. Inflammatory background with refractile structures representing *Cryptococcus neoformans*. Diff-Quik® 400×.

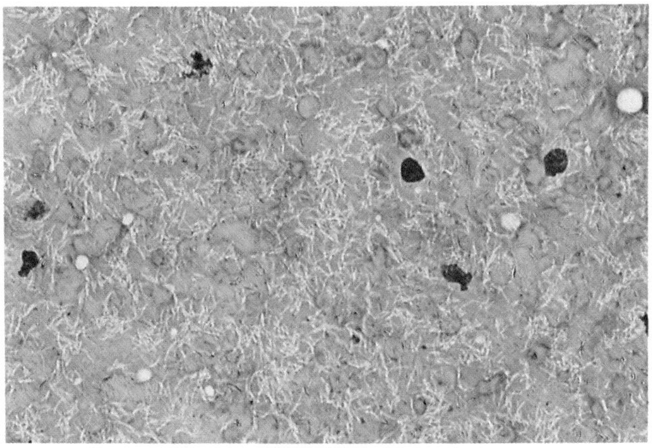

FIGURE 4.12 Aspiration of cervical lymph node. Homogeneous necrotic background with few inflammatory cells. Note the slightly curved, clear linear spaces, which represent infiltration of the node by atypical mycobacteria. Patient with AIDS and disseminated mycobacterial infection. Diff-Quik® 600×.

cinoma and small-round-cell tumors of childhood that have spread to lymph nodes, Ewing's sarcoma, neuroblastoma, and rhabdomyosarcoma (Figures 4.13 and 4.14). The background and cell size, however, are much different in rhabdomyosarcoma when compared to any of the lymphomas (Figure 4.15).[17]

Also at high power, when evaluating the smear, look for the type and details of bizarre cells that may be present, including Reed-Sternberg cells. These cells often have reddish blue nucleoli with Romanowsky stains as opposed to malignant T cells that have many bizarre shapes and features similar to Reed-Sternberg cells but usually have large deep blue nucleoli with Romanowsky stains (Figures 4.16 and 4.17).

Microscopic examination using a very high dry objective or oil immersion may be necessary to visualize cleaves in lymphoid nuclei. Both abnormal chromatin

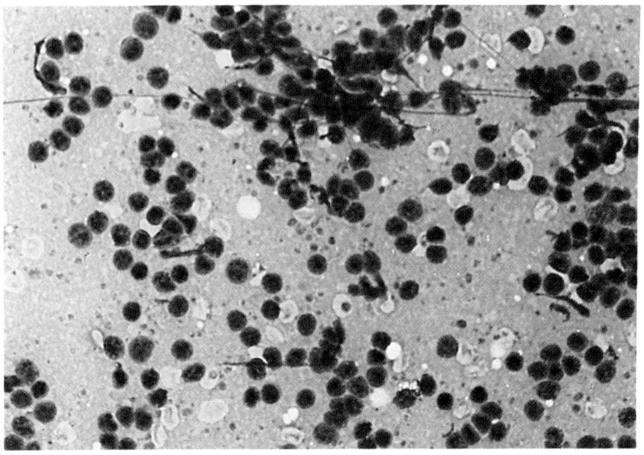

FIGURE 4.13 Aspiration of cervical lymph node. Clusters of small lymphocytes with associated lymphoglandular bodies found in aspirate of small-cell lymphocytic lymphoma, poorly differentiated. Diff-Quik® 400×.

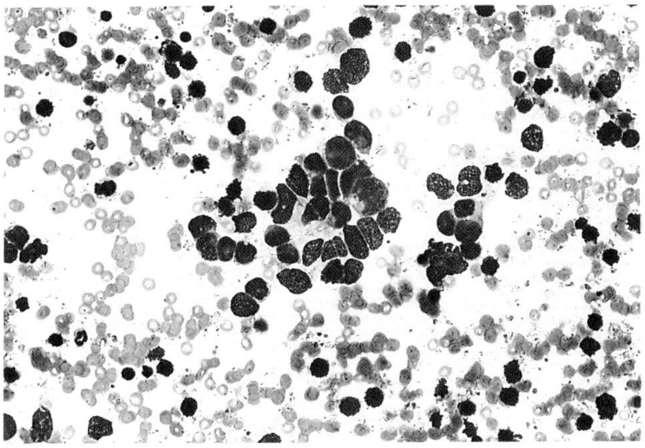

FIGURE 4.14 Aspiration of cervical lymph node. Clusters of small cells not unlike lymphocytes but with much more nuclear molding and more pronounced nuclear irregularities and variation in nuclear size. Metastatic neuroblastoma. Diff-Quik® 400×.

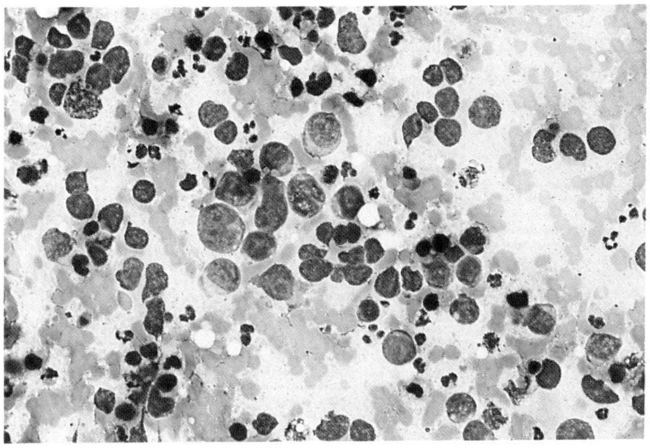

FIGURE 4.15 Aspiration of cervical lymph node. Cellular smear with clustering of tumor cells and great variation in size of nuclei. Lymphoglandular bodies are absent. Metastatic rhabdomyosarcoma. Diff-Quik® 400×.

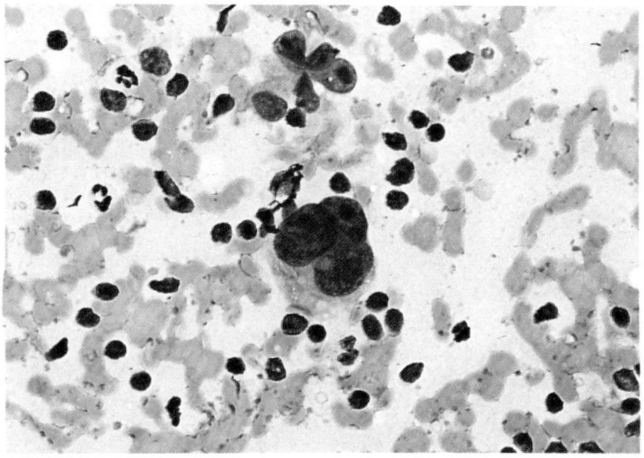

FIGURE 4.16 Aspiration of cervical lymph node. Typical double-nucleated Reed-Sternberg cell. Note the more reddish blue color of the nucleoli. Diff-Quik® 600×.

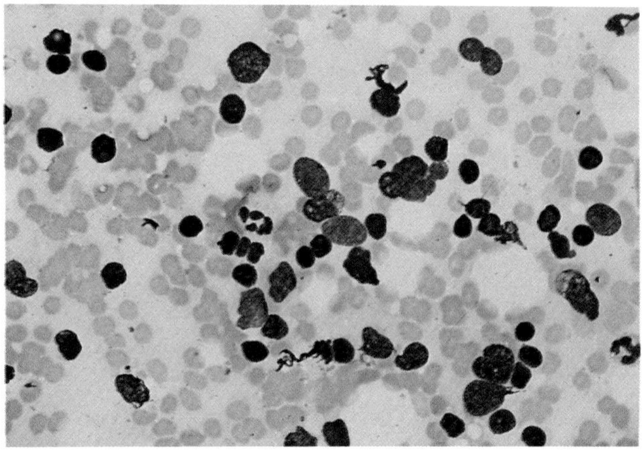

FIGURE 4.17 Aspiration of cervical lymph node. Bizarre large cells of T-cell lymphoma. Note very blue staining of the large nucleoli. Diff-Quik® 600×.

pattern and enlarged misshapen nucleoli can also be confirmed at this very high magnification (Figure 4.18).

INFECTIOUS PROCESSES AND GRANULOMAS

Infectious agents may involve the lymph node directly and can be identified by FNA. More often, there is a region or organ that is infected, with subsequent drainage to a lymph node that induces a secondary, nonspecific reactive response (Table 4.7).[18] The most common infectious agents identified in the lymph node by FNA are mycobacteria and fungi. The incidence of both groups of organisms producing enlarged lymph nodes has substantially increased with the AIDS epidemic.[16,19] The majority of bacteria identified by aspiration are actually derived from abscesses, which clinically can be mistaken for enlarged lymph nodes. The aspirate is composed principally of acute inflammatory exudate with necrosis. The organisms may be present in large numbers

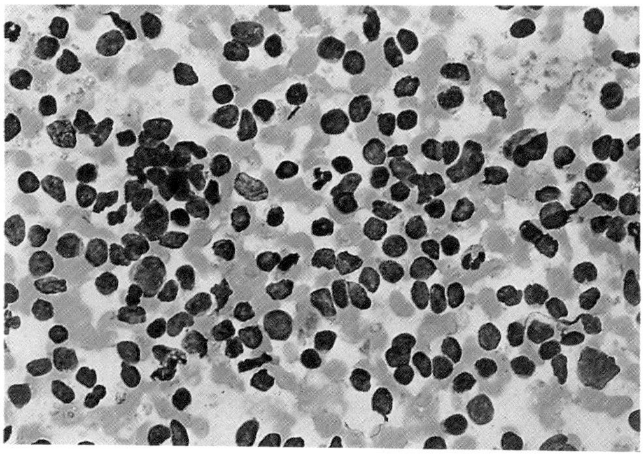

FIGURE 4.18 Aspiration of cervical lymph node. Note irregular shape of nuclei in small-cleaved-cell lymphoma. Actual grooves or lines can also be seen in some nuclei, though they will be more apparent in an alcohol-fixed and Papanicolaou-stained smear. Diff-Quik® 600×.

TABLE 4.7 Cytology of Tuberculosis, Fungal Infections, Sarcoid, and Nonspecific Necrotizing Granulomatous Lymphadenitis

	Tuberculosis and Fungal Infections
1.	The composition of the aspirate varies with the stage of the inflammatory process.
2.	Aspirates may demonstrate only necrosis and accompanying inflammation, necessitating a careful search for a few epithelioid histiocytes (suggestive of granulomas).
3.	Necrosis and granulomas may be abundant.
4.	Later stages with fibrosis/hyalinization of the node make it hard with few cells or none found on biopsy. Rare aggregate of epithelioid cells, giant cells, or a few fibroblasts (nonspecific picture).
	Sarcoidosis
1.	Varying numbers of tightly cohesive (hard) granulomas.
2.	A background of mature lymphocytes and plasma cells.
3.	Necrosis, with rare exception, not a feature.
	Necrotizing Granulomatous Lymphadenitis
1.	Material varies with the stage of the process.
2.	Initial phase lymphoid, follicular hyperplasia pattern.
3.	Isolated epithelioid histiocytes and some in loose, small clusters.
4.	Rare finding of trophozoites (lymphogranuloma) engulfed in histiocytes.
5.	Suppurative pattern with granulomas and necrotic centers in the later phase.

and can be easily seen even without special stains, but some patients may have had antibiotics, rendering the abscess sterile.

Granulomata and necrosis are the most common elements found in aspirates, suggesting that the lymphadenopathy may be secondary to infection.[13] However, not only is a granulomatous response seen in a wide variety of infectious agents, but also it may occur as a result of noninfectious processes, both benign and malignant.[20] The cytologic features should be evaluated to include granulomas, granulomas with necrosis, granulomas in a background of hyperplasia, and granulomas with bizarre cells.

The most common granulomas among our cases are not infectious but are the typical, cohesive epithelioid granulomas of sarcoid. There may be relatively few background lymphocytes in these cases or the granulomas may be few in number (see Figure 4.9). Clinical correlation is important to confirm the diagnosis of sarcoidosis, but surgical biopsy of the node need not be required if there has been a good aspiration biopsy.

Granulomas with necrosis most often have resulted from tuberculosis. The granulomas are loosely formed and may not be readily apparent at first scanning of the aspirate. With the atypical mycobacterial infections seen in AIDS, the background is dominated by a homogeneous necrosis that contains faint, clear, curved lines—so-called "negative images" (see Figure 4.12). Cells present in this type of aspirate from a lymph node will be histiocytes that are packed with these clear lines, giving the cell an appearance similar to the Gaucher cell.[21] Stains for acid-fast organisms will show staining of these clear negative image areas revealing that the Gaucher-like cells are filled with organisms (Figure 4.19).

In conventional tuberculosis, the organism may be quite hard to find, requiring a diligent search of smears that are stained using acid-fast methods. Fungus infections, both primary pathogens—blastomyces, cryptococcus, coccidioides—and saprophytes, of which there are a large variety, produce granulomas with a background of necrosis. In blastomycosis, the organisms may be few in number with very extensive necrosis and few or no identifiable granulomas (Figure 4.20). In lymph node aspirates, blastomycosis is most often secondary to lung involvement, the latter feature producing a radiographic picture that may resemble a primary lung tumor. Both cryptococcus and coccidioides are illustrated in Figures 4.11 and 4.21. These two cases were from patients with AIDS. For that reason, there are a very large number of organisms, necrosis dominates the smear, and there are very few definitive granulomas.

Actinomycosis is illustrated in an aspirate of a neck mass in the area of cervical lymph nodes (Figure 4.22). Clinically, actinomycosis produces a picture of a large, sometimes fixed and very firm cervical mass while the aspirate is most often only necrosis and acute inflammation. The organisms are scattered as ball-like structures

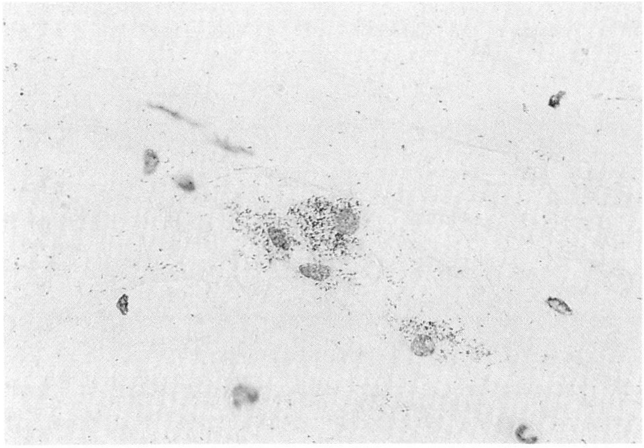

FIGURE 4.19 Aspiration of cervical lymph node. Large histiocytic cells stuffed with acid-fast-staining organisms of atypical mycobacteria. Ziehl-Neilseen stain 600×.

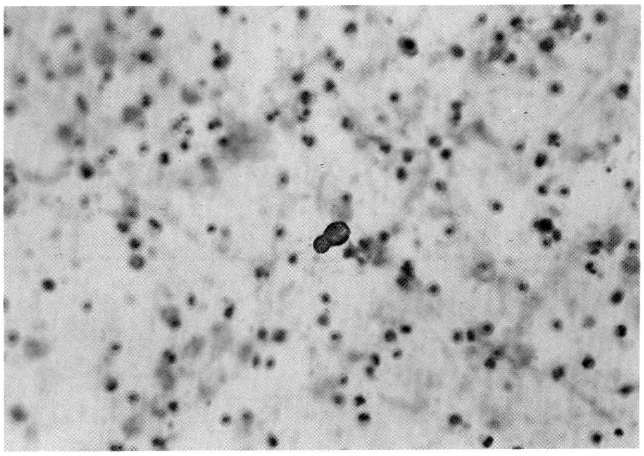

FIGURE 4.20 Aspiration of cervical lymph node. Organisms of blastomycosis detected with silver stain. Gomori methenamine silver 600×.

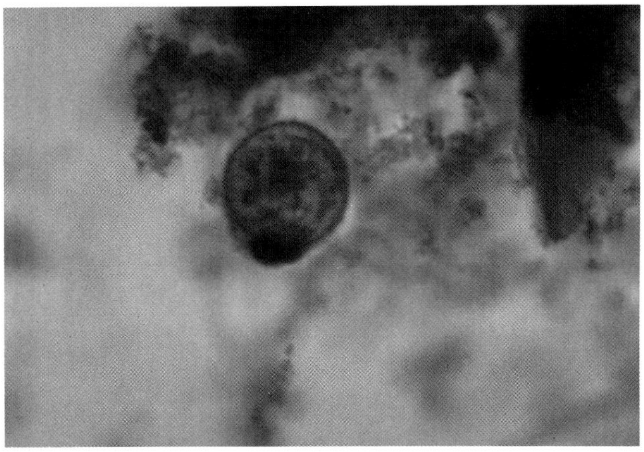

FIGURE 4.21 Aspiration of cervical lymph node. Spherules with organisms of *Coccidioides immitus*. Papanicolaou 1000×

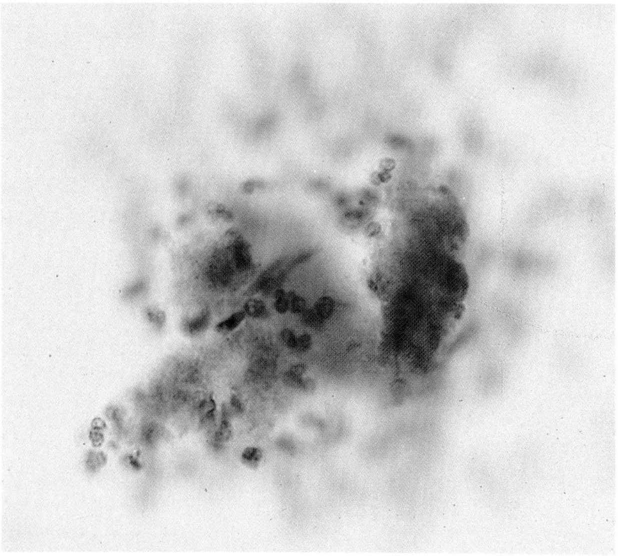

FIGURE 4.22 Aspiration of cervical mass. Filamentous organisms causing actinomycosis (*Actinomyces*) with surrounding acute inflammatory exudate. Papanicolaou 600×.

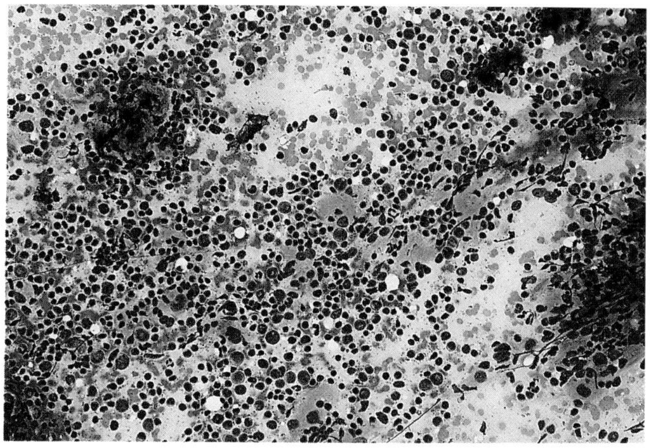

FIGURE 4.23 Aspiration of cervical lymph node. Moderately cellular smear with mixed lymphoid cell population typical of reactive hyperplastic node. This patient was clinically suspected to have cat-scratch disease. The aspiration smear pattern is consistent with that but not specific. Diff-Quik® 250×.

with the clubs protruding from the surface. Although very uncommon, aspergillus may produce a similar clinical picture. This variable group of organisms is identified from its typical treelike branching of hyphal fragments, most often in a background of extensive necrosis. Aspergillus and the *Phycomycetes* may infect the paranasal sinuses producing a mass lesion that can be aspirated for diagnosis.

Necrotizing granulomatous lymphadenitis varies with the stage of the process and is often without a clearcut etiology. Initially, the process is dominated by lymphoid hyperplasia and few or no granulomas are identified (Figure 4.23). Next, the node may suppurate and the smear pattern will show both lymphoid hyperplasia and necrosis. This is followed by granuloma formation that is of the loose epithelioid variety with admixed lymphocytes in various stages of maturation, reflecting the underlying hyperplasia (Figure 4.24).

In the most typical clinical situation a careful history will suggest cat-scratch disease. This disease can produce some remarkably enlarged lymph nodes, particularly in children.[3] These enlarged nodes may be located is less typical places for lymphomas, for example in the submental, post auricular and occipital areas. Cat-scratch disease also seems to be seasonal with a predominance of cases in the spring and fall. When the aspirate demonstrates a cytologic picture as described and there is a reasonable clinical history supporting cat-scratch disease or some other infectious process—a recent influenza, sore throat, tonsillitis, or ear infection—then it is quite acceptable to observe the lymph node over several weeks to see if it regresses. This is usually the case with or without prophylactic antibiotic therapy.

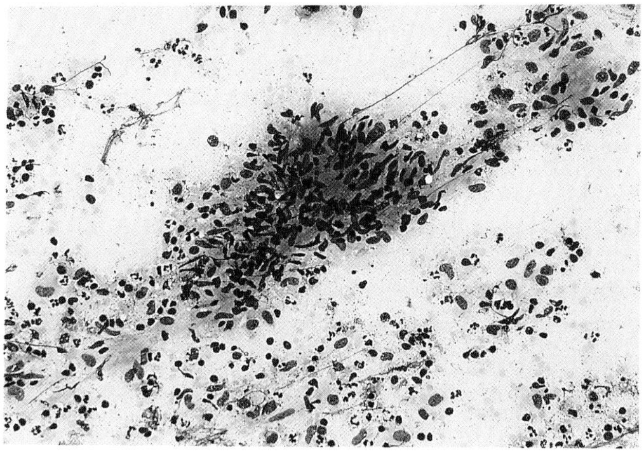

FIGURE 4.24 Aspiration of cervical lymph node. Loose epithelioid granuloma with surrounding mixed population of lymphocytes and macrophages, reflecting reactive hyperplasia. Diff-Quik® 250×.

METASTATIC MALIGNANCY

The detection of metastatic disease is one of the primary indications for aspiration biopsy of a lymph node. The detection of malignancy in an aspiration may be made for recurrent disease, staging, or in uncovering an occult primary.[21–23] Use of ultrasound, computerized tomography (CT), and image-guided fine-needle aspiration biopsy of small, clinically undetected lymph nodes may enhance preoperative staging in carcinomas of the upper aero-digestive tracts.[24–26]

The diagnosis of malignancy in aspiration smears is rarely difficult because, in the majority of cases, abundant cells foreign to the normal lymph node are present. Occasional problem smears are encountered because of extensive necrosis or partial lymph node involvement by the malignant process. When necrotic, the metastatic tumor cells are distorted with indistinct morphology. It then becomes difficult to make either a definitive statement or even a suggestion of the probable primary tumor. Extensive necrosis of a metastatic tumor may give an initial impression on smears of an abscess, but there is a paucity or absence of acute inflammatory cells.

With partial node involvement, the metastatic tumor cells may not be present at all (sampling error) or are present in very small numbers in a background of reactive lymphocytes. Single or very small aggregates of tumor cells surrounded by a few lymphocytes may simulate a granuloma or a reactive, hyperplastic lymphoid follicle. Immunohistochemistry may be helpful if a panel of epithelial markers identifies cells as foreign to the node.[27] It should be remembered that dendritic reticulum cells within a lymph node may stain with cytokeratin and simulate foreign epithelial cells.[28]

A more common problem found with aspiration smears is the distinction of undifferentiated carcinoma from a large-cell lymphoma or the separation of the small-round-cell tumors of childhood and small-cell undifferentiated lymphomas. Careful reviews of cytologic criteria can usually resolve these problems, but special stains, immunohistochemistry, and electron microscopy are sometimes needed for confirmation of a specific diagnosis. The differential cytologic criteria, helpful in this situation, are summarized in Table 4.8. In difficult cases, immunologic determination of carcinoma can usually be made with the application of epithelial markers such as epithelial membrane antigen (EMA) or cytokeratin antibodies using either cytospin preparations or direct smears. Typing of lymphoid cells of a lymphoma can be determined by a variety of lymphocyte markers currently available, flow cytometry, or even molecular diagnostic techniques that are being developed rapidly.

Lymphoglandular bodies are small, round or oval, gray-staining, flat structures of variable size seen in air-dried, Romanowsky-stained smears. They are quite helpful in identifying the accompanying cellular components as lymphoid tissue in aspiration smears (Figure 4.25).[29] Lymphoglandular bodies are quite reliable for this identification but can also be seen in aspirates from small-cell undifferentiated carcinomas or small-round-cell tumors of childhood (Figure 4.26).[30] The following examples illustrate the cytologic features seen in aspirates from some of the common primary tumors metastatic to the lymph nodes.

TABLE 4.8 Cytologic Criteria Differentiating Carcinoma from Lymphoma

Carcinoma	*Lymphoma*
Cells arranged in aggregates	Cells in isolation
Lymphoglandular bodies absent	Lymphoglandular bodies present

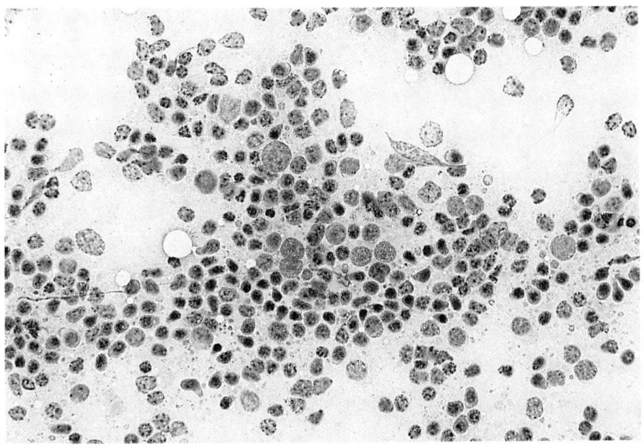

FIGURE 4.25 Aspiration of cervical lymph node. Small, gray bodies of variable size that are pale staining are lymphoglandular bodies representing fragments of cytoplasm of lymphoid cells and are useful in identifying aspirates from lymphoid tissue. Diff-Quik® 400×.

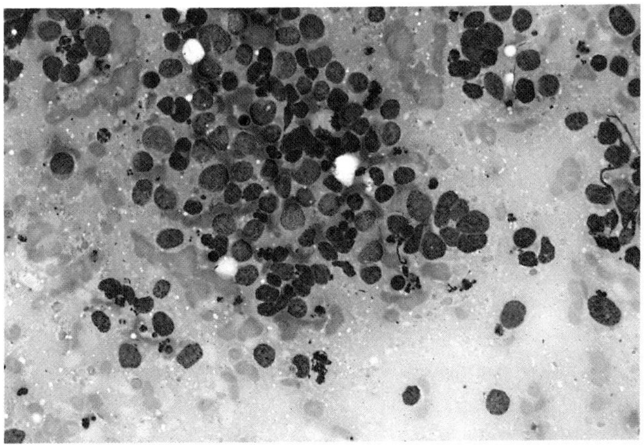

FIGURE 4.26 Aspiration of supraclavicular lymph node. Similar small, gray structures simulating lymphoglandular bodies in the aspirate from metastatic small-round-cell tumor of childhood, in this case neuroblastoma. Diff-Quik® 400×.

Metastatic Squamous Cell Carcinoma

Squamous cell carcinoma is the most frequently detected metastatic malignancy in lymph nodes of the head and neck. The site of origin is usually the oral cavity, pharynx and larynx, or lung. This neoplasm may be well, moderately, or poorly differentiated. Moderately differentiated and poorly differentiated squamous cell carcinomas are easily diagnosed as malignant; however, metastasis from poorly differentiated squamous cell carcinoma may not always be recognizable as squamous in origin. Two features that consistently identify them as squamous cells are dense cytoplasm and well-defined cell

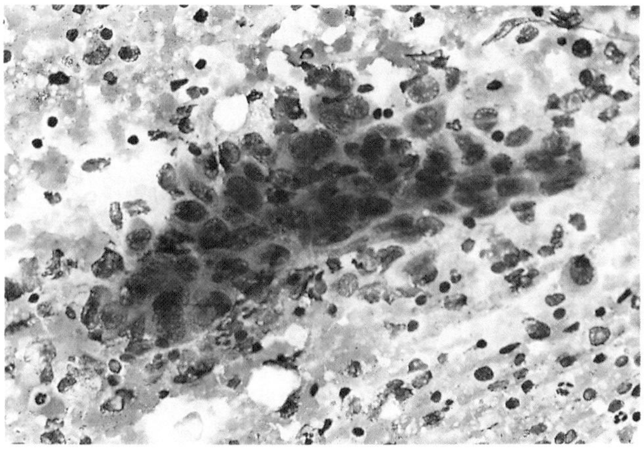

FIGURE 4.27 Aspiration of cervical lymph node. Sheets of poorly differentiated squamous cells with dense cytoplasm, well-defined cell borders and definite but small nucleoli. Chromatin pattern is typically coarse. Diff-Quik® 400×.

boundaries. The nuclear chromatin is coarse and nucleoli are small but quite easily observed (Figure 4.27).

Well-differentiated, heavily keratinized squamous cell carcinoma more commonly arises from the oropharynx, including the tongue, and from the larynx. The degree of dysplasia in aspirates of some keratinizing squamous cell carcinomas may be minimal. Distinction from benign squamous lesions, such as infected branchial cleft cysts or Warthin's tumors with areas of atypical squamous metaplasia, may be difficult in aspiration smears. Usually, in these two benign situations there are relatively few squamous-appearing cells and little or no necrosis.

Small and sometimes occult tonsil primary squamous cell carcinomas may be quite well differentiated and may present first as a cervical mass due to metastatic disease (Figure 4.28). The differential diagnosis is a branchial cleft cyst. Although the cells of metastatic carcinoma are abundant, they are often quite degenerated because this type of metastasis in a lymph node tends to be cystic and extensively necrotic. It is important to remember that with cystic metastases of squamous cell carcinoma there are often many cells with features that are recognizable at the very least as atypical, in contrast to branchial cleft cysts or Warthin's tumor with squamous atypia.

Metastatic Adenocarcinoma

The most common primaries for metastatic adenocarcinoma found on aspiration biopsy of lymph nodes are lung and breast. The supraclavicular nodes are also the most commonly involved when metastasis to the head and neck area occur with these two primary cancers. Other primary sites of carcinoma with metastasis to lymph nodes of the head and neck include the gastrointestinal tract, pancreas, and prostate. The better-differentiated forms of these cancers are characterized by papillary, acinar, or glandular groupings. These cell patterns are expressed in smears as true three-dimensional clusters or cells that overlap each other with poorly defined cell boundaries and relatively transparent cytoplasm (Figure 4.29). Some or a majority of cells of adenocarcinoma viewed in smears often have eccentric nuclei. Cytoplasmic vacuoles may be present. The more poorly differentiated adenocarcinomas from the primaries from the gastrointestinal tract, pancreas, prostate, and including the female genital tract cannot always be determined to be glandular in origin.

In many cases, when carcinoma is detected by lymph node aspiration, the cytologic pattern, while diagnosable as metastatic, lacks distinct enough features to point exclusively to one primary site.[31] Some malignancies do have relatively specific cytologic patterns that

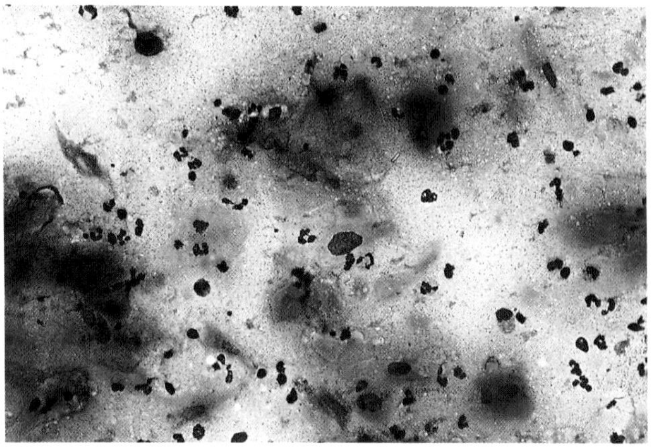

FIGURE 4.28 Aspiration of cervical lymph node. Atypical but scattered keratinized cells from metastatic occult squamous cell carcinoma. Primary found in the tonsil. Diff-Quik® 400×.

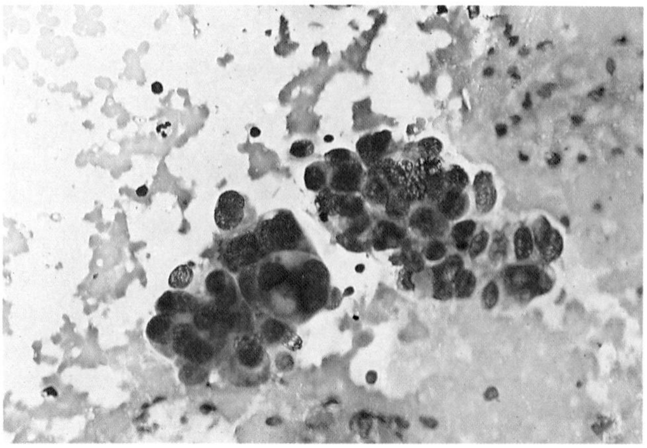

FIGURE 4.29 Aspiration of cervical lymph node. Overlapping and three-dimensional clusters of tumor cells from metastatic papillary carcinoma of the ovary. Diff-Quik® 400×.

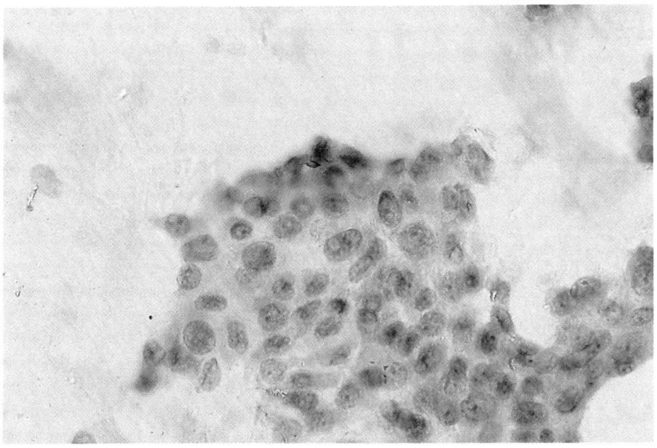

FIGURE 4.30 Aspiration of cervical lymph node. Papillary groups of cells with nuclei demonstrating intranuclear inclusions and nuclear grooves. Diagnosis of metastatic papillary carcinoma of the thyroid. Papanicolaou 600×.

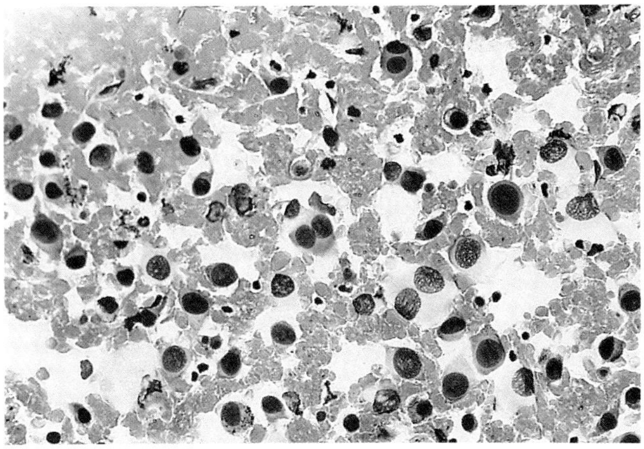

FIGURE 4.31 Metastatic melanoma. Aspiration of cervical lymph node. Cellular aspirate with large, dispersed single cells. Note examples of binucleate tumor cells with mirror-image position of the nuclei. Diff-Quik® 400×.

allow the cytopathologist to at least suggest the primary site (Figure 4.30).

Malignant Melanoma

Malignant melanoma occurs with some frequency from the second decade onward. Usually, though not always, in the presence of metastatic melanoma, there is a history of melanoma or of a pigmented skin lesion. This tumor is more common in fair-skinned individuals and is clearly related to excessive sun exposure. When a head and neck lymph node is involved with metastatic melanoma, the primary is more often in the same area. In aspiration smears, melanoma cells tend to be isolated with some small sheets or aggregates. Binucleate and multinucleate tumor cells are not unusual. In tumor cells that are binucleate examples, the nuclei are usually positioned as mirror images of each other (Figure 4.31).[32,33]

The cells representing the most common histologic pattern, epithelial melanoma, are usually round or oval. If the histologic pattern of the melanoma is spindle cell, then the tumor cells in the aspiration smear of a lymph node or other metastases will likely be spindle shaped. Without a known primary, this spindle cell pattern in an aspiration smear may look like a poorly differentiated spindle cell sarcoma (Figure 4.32). Cells of melanoma often have a moderate amount of cytoplasm that may exhibit a biphasic staining pattern with Romanowsky stains (Figure 4.33).

Macronucleoli are often present in cells of malignant melanoma, and large intranuclear inclusions in some melanomas may be striking. Melanin pigment, when present, is blue-black with Romanowsky stains, but may be visible as a brown dusting or as very coarse, brown cytoplasmic granules in smears stained with the Papanicolaou method (Figure 4.34). If needed, immunohistochemical stains for S-100 protein and HMB 45 are

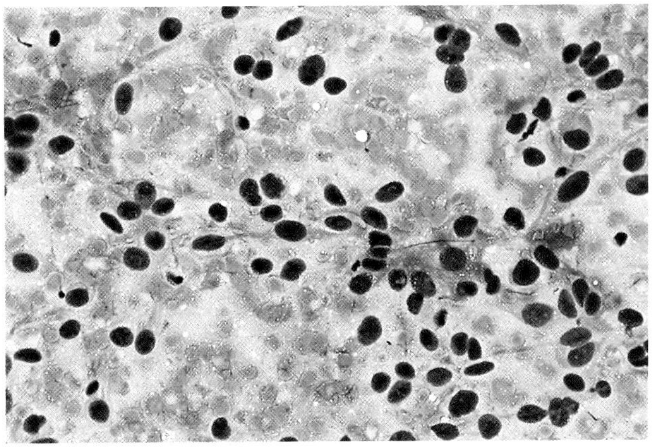

FIGURE 4.32 Aspiration of cervical lymph node. Metastatic melanoma with a predominantly spindle cell pattern. Diff-Quik® 400×.

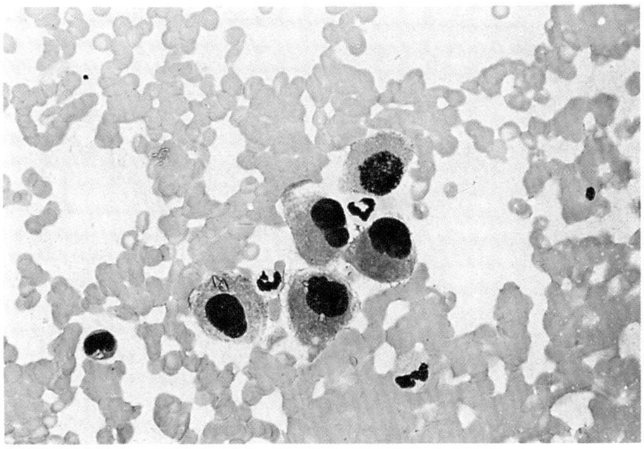

FIGURE 4.33 Aspiration of cervical lymph node. Cells of metastatic melanoma with a biphasic color to the cytoplasm. Diff-Quik® 600×.

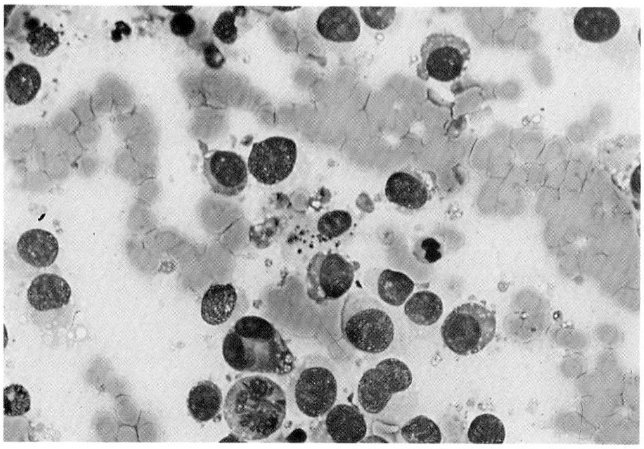

FIGURE 4.34 Aspiration of cervical lymph node. Metastatic melanoma demonstrating tumor cells with blue-black pigment. Diff-Quik® 400×.

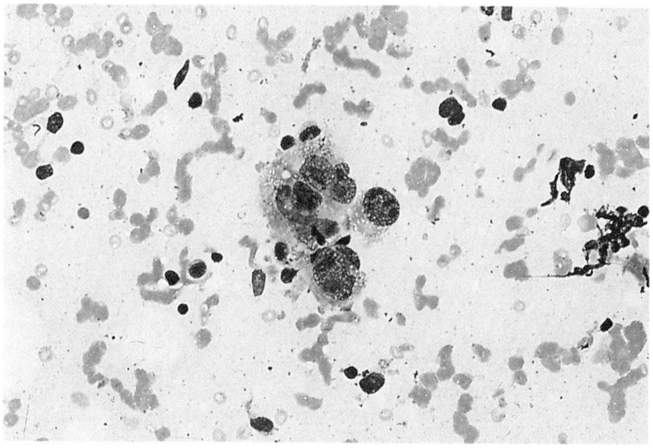

FIGURE 4.35 Aspiration of cervical lymph node. Ki-1 large-cell lymphoma with a very epithelial pattern and individual cells that resemble those found in metastatic malignant melanoma. Diff-Quik® 400×.

positive in nearly all cases. The rare Ki-1 lymphoma may closely simulate malignant melanoma or other epithelial malignancies cytologically (Figure 4.35).[34]

MALIGNANT MELANOMA

Background clean, bloody, or filled with pigmented debris

Monomorphic population of pleomorphic cells**
- **–Large cells with a moderate amount of cytoplasm**
- **–Pigment variable in consistency: fine to coarse**
  - **–Powder blue to cobalt blue on Diff-Quik®**
  - **–Brown to golden on Papanicolaou**
- **–Large nuclei often bi- (mirror image) or multinucleated**
- **–Prominent nucleoli**

****Spindle cell or mixed spindle-epithelioid melanomas can occur**

Lymphoglandular bodies that identify lymphoid tissue can usually be found with the Ki-1 lymphoma. Immunohistochemical studies will also separate this lymphoma from metastatic melanoma or other epithelial tumors.[35]

Small-Cell Undifferentiated Carcinoma

This cancer, most often primary in the lung, is rare in people under the age of 40, and there is usually a history of heavy tobacco use. Clinical or radiologic evidence of a lung neoplasm is frequently present. The aspirate shows a large number of tumor cells that are small and monomorphic. These tumor cells are about twice the size of a mature lymphocyte.[36] While aggregates of these small tumor cells are dominant in most smears, the key to the diagnosis is actually appreciating two populations of malignant cells. Well-preserved cells are larger than the second population of tumor cells, which are necrotic and therefore small, the so-called two-cell population (Figure 4.36). The two-cell pattern, relatively large cells and small cells, is one of the most characteristic features of aspiration smears from small-cell carcinomas, regardless of their primary site.

SMALL-CELL CARCINOMA

Dirty background—cell debris and tingible body macrophages

DNA artifact—nuclear material in long strings
- **–Two-cell population**
- **–Small, hyperchromatic—pyknotic cells (nonviable)**
- **–Slightly larger, viable cells**
  - **–Scant cytoplasm**
  - **–Round to oval nuclei**
  - **–Finely granular, smudgy chromatin**
  - **–Indistinct/absent nucleoli**

Smears of small-cell undifferentiated carcinoma also have a necrotic background with strings of nuclear DNA streaked across the slide due to the very fragile nature of the tumor cells. Malignant lymphomas or lymphoproliferative processes seldom show this marked DNA artifact unless excessive pressure is used in preparing the smears. In some cases of metastatic small-cell carcinoma, neuron-specific enolase may be positive, but this marker is quite nonspecific. Chromogranin positivity is also found in some small-cell undifferentiated carcinomas.

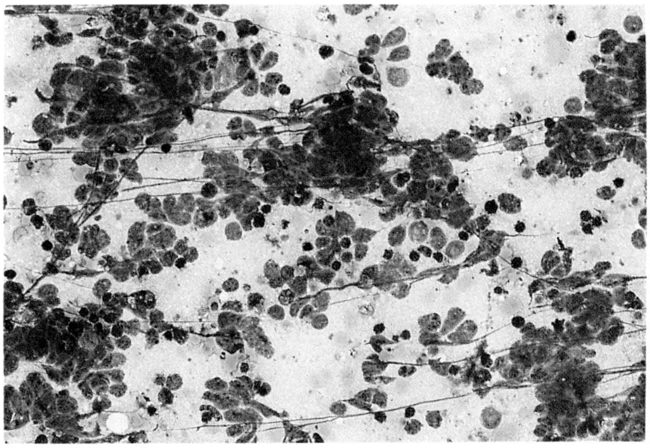

FIGURE 4.36 Aspiration of supraclavicular lymph node. Metastatic small-cell undifferentiated carcinoma of the lung. Note the population of both large, well-preserved cells and small, necrotic tumor cells. The latter look like lymphocytes. Diff-Quik® 400×.

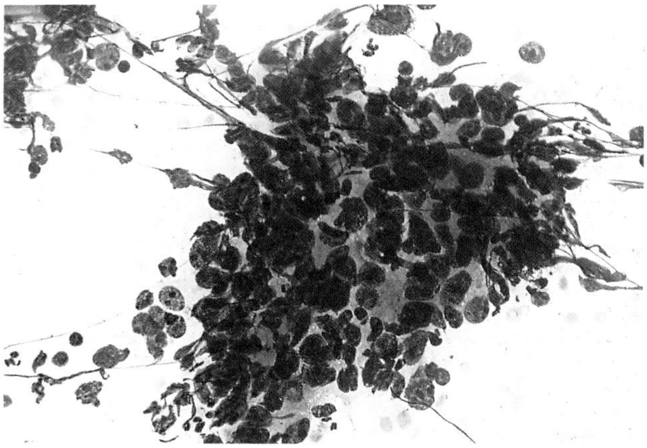

FIGURE 4.37 Lymphoepithelioma. Aspiration of cervical lymph node. Large, undifferentiated tumor cells in a loose grouping. Note coarse chromatin and prominent nucleoli. These tumor cells in a predominantly single-cell pattern may simulate large-cell lymphoma. Diff-Quik® 400×.

Lymphoepithelioma

This tumor is seen in both young patients and again as a second peak incidence in the sixth decade. Lymphoepithelioma arises in the nasopharynx where the primary may remain small and often undetected until the patient presents with cervical lymph node metastases. Some patients have symptoms attributable to the nasopharyngeal primary, such as postnasal drip, nasal stuffiness, or obstruction.[36]

The cells of metastatic lymphoepithelioma are large to medium sized with a very coarse and irregular chromatin pattern but a relatively clear cytoplasm (Figure 4.37). The prominent central nucleolus stands out in the background of this coarse or pale chromatin.[37] The cells of metastatic lymphoepithelioma may occur in sheets and may be dispersed as single cells in air-dried smears. They are usually only seen in aggregates following fixation and staining with Papanicolaou.

LYMPHOEPITHELIOMA

Variable cellularity

Biphasic population
- **Large to medium size epithelial cells**
- **Moderate amount of clear cytoplasm**
- **Large nuclei with coarse chromatin**
- **Prominent central nucleoli**

Lymphocytes
- **Intermingled with epithelial cells or**
- **Scattered around the periphery of nests of epithelial cells**

The lymph nodes involved by metastatic lymphoepithelioma are often large and dominated by a lymphoid proliferation that may hide a relatively few tumor cells (Figure 4.38). The tumor cells of lymphoepithelioma may also look like hyperplastic follicular center cells within this dominant lymphoid background. This feature is accentuated by the fact that the tumor cells may also have a very bland appearance. The presence of metastatic lymphoepithelioma may also induce a granulomatous reaction that can incorporate the tumor cells and make their identification quite difficult (Figure 4.39).

The use of immunohistochemical stains, epithelial membrane antigen (EMA), and cytokeratin on either a direct smear or a cytospin preparation is quite helpful in finding a few tumor cells of metastatic lymphoepithelioma in a very hyperplastic or granulomatous background. Epstein-Barr virus has been detected using

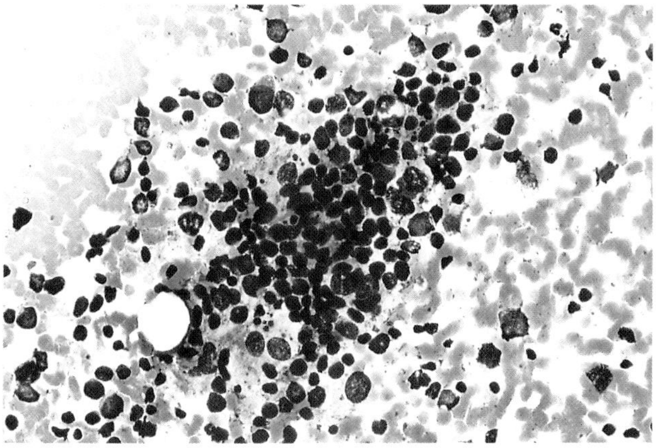

FIGURE 4.38 Lymphoepithelioma. Aspiration of cervical lymph node. A few large tumor cells found in a background of abundant lymphocytes. With only a few tumor cells present, they may be overlooked in the hyperplastic lymphoid background. Diff-Quik® 400×.

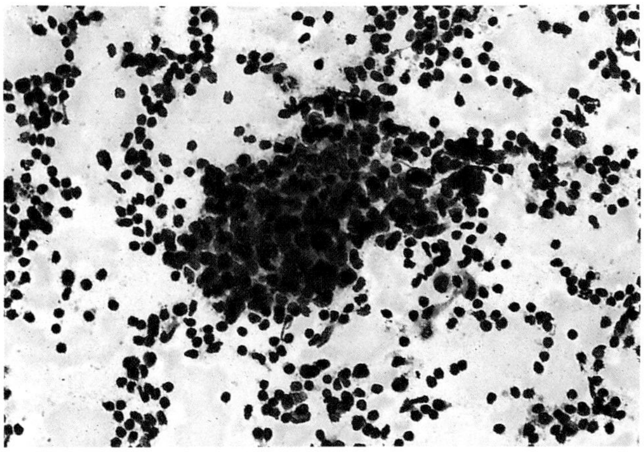

FIGURE 4.39 Aspiration of cervical lymph node. Granulomatous pattern found in aspirate from metastatic lymphoepithelioma. Tumor cells may be quite difficult to detect in the presence of a granulomatous reaction. If found, they may suggest the diagnosis of Hodgkin's disease. Diff-Quik® 400×.

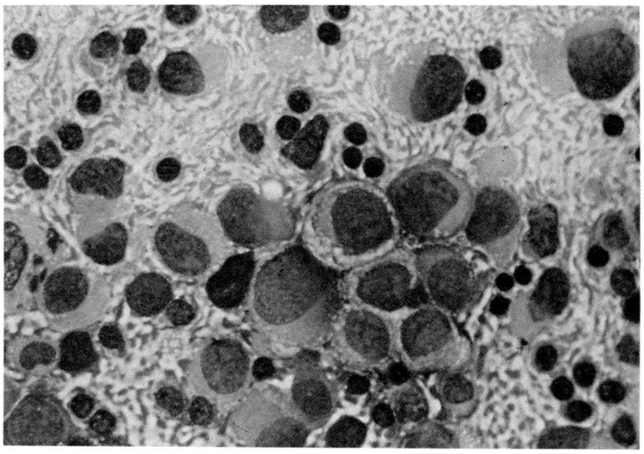

FIGURE 4.40 Metastatic seminoma. Aspiration of cervical lymph node. Large, undifferentiated tumor cells seen in a background of striations or strips of dispersed cytoplasm, "tigroid" background. This is a very useful feature in identifying metastatic seminoma. Diff-Quik® 400×.

polymerase chain reaction on aspirates from a majority of lymphoepithelioma-type nasopharyngeal carcinoma.[38] This tumor may also be quite difficult to diagnose by FNA if there is only partial lymph node involvement by metastasis.[36]

Seminoma

Seminoma is not commonly found metastatic to lymph nodes of the head and neck area, but the author has seen examples of metastasis from this neoplasm to supraclavicular, occipital, and cervical nodes as the first indication of the spread of seminoma. Mediastinal nodes are often involved at the same time, though they may not be readily apparent with conventional radiographs. The cytologic features of seminoma in aspiration smears demonstrate large cells with abundant but fragile cytoplasm, relatively pale but coarse nuclear chromatin, and a prominent central red or red-blue nucleolus. The tumor cells are isolated or in sheets but will form small aggregates with fixation of the smears and staining with Papanicolaou.

The background of the smear in metastatic seminoma is one of the most characteristic features because it has a striped appearance due to spreading and dislocation of the fragile cytoplasm. This is accentuated on Romanowsky-stained preparations and has been referred to as a "tigroid" background (Figure 4.40).[39] This feature is quite reliable for seminoma, but it has been seen in cases of embryonal rhabdomyosarcoma.[17] Without careful preparation of the aspiration smears, this unusual cytologic feature may be lost.

SEMINOMA

High cellularity

"Tigroid" background on Diff-Quik® (cytoplasmic dislocation)

Birmorphic population
- **–Large "epithelioid" cells**
  - **–Moderate amount of fragile cytoplasm**
  - **–Large nuclei with pale, coarse chromatin**
  - **–Prominent nucleolus**
- **–Small, mature lymphocytes**

As in the histopathology of its primary, seminoma may also have both variable numbers of lymphocytes and plasma cells, and granulomatous features. The tumor cells usually dominate the smears with lymphocytes and plasma cells present, but a marked granulomatous pattern may obscure the presence of recognizable tumor cells in the aspiration smear. Usually there is a history of prior primary testicular seminoma or germ-cell tumor, which is a helpful clinical finding when faced with the granulomatous aspiration smear pattern of metastatic seminoma.

Prostate Adenocarcinoma

Mortality from carcinoma of the prostate has shown a steady increase in the last decade. This tumor occurs in men, usually over the age of 50. Screening with prostatic specific antigen (PSA) has dramatically raised the detection of low-grade and low-stage prostatic carcinoma and led to a resurgence of radical prostatectomy as the major treatment. Prostate cancer is infrequently

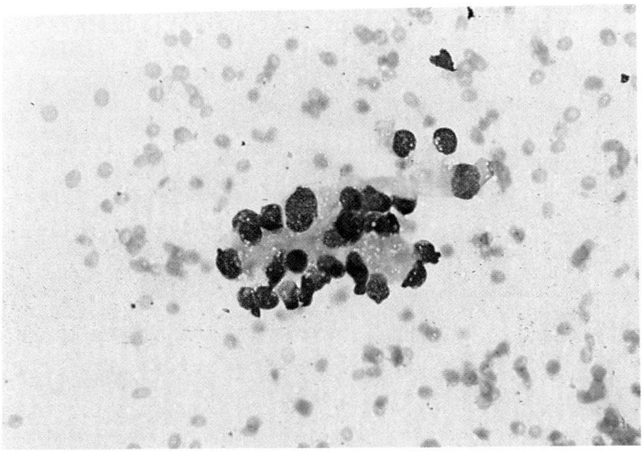

FIGURE 4.41 Aspiration of supraclavicular lymph node. Malignant well-differentiated tumor cells in a microacinar arrangement. The very uniform nature of the microacini simulates the same pattern in well- to moderately differentiated prostatic adenocarcinomas and is a feature that suggests that diagnosis in aspirates from metastatic sites. Diff-Quik® 400×.

found metastatic to lymph nodes in the head and neck area. Occasionally, patients with prostate cancer will first present with an enlarged lymph node. Because of the drainage system of the urogenital tract, the enlarged lymph node is often in the left supraclavicular space. Better-differentiated adenocarcinomas of the prostate have a pattern suggestive of primary prostatic carcinoma with well-formed microacinar arrangements of tumor cells (Figure 4.41).

METASTATIC PROSTATIC CARCINOMA

High cellularity

Monomorphic population of small to medium sized cells

Uniform, microacinar pattern

Moderate amount of clear cytoplasm

Uniform nuclei

Single, central, prominent nucleolus

Most poorly differentiated carcinomas metastatic from the prostate cannot be distinguished cytologically from other metastatic poorly differentiated carcinomas. Similar to the histologic features of well- and moderately well-differentiated prostatic carcinoma, the tumor cells are relatively uniform, have a clear cytoplasm, little variation in nuclear size and shape, and most of them have a central, single, and prominent nucleolus. Staining of direct smears or cytospin preparations with PSA and/or prostatic specific acid phosphatase (PSAP) will show positivity in essentially all differentiated prostatic carcinomas and in many of the undifferentiated prostate carcinomas (Figure 4.42).[2] There may be high background staining in aspiration smears but because PSA and PSAP are terminally differentiated proteins, granular staining of the tumor cells can still be considered positive.

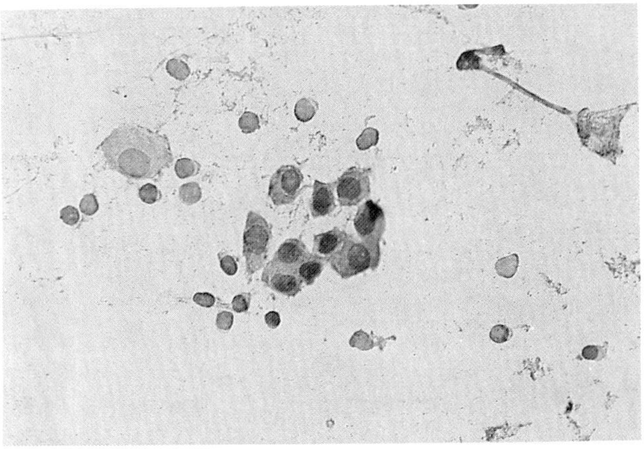

FIGURE 4.42 Aspiration of supraclavicular lymph node. Aspirate demonstrating positive staining of tumor cells with PSAP. Avidin-biotin complex method 600×.

Renal Cell Carcinoma

Renal cell carcinoma (hypernephroma) may initially present with metastases to lymph nodes, including those in the head and neck, but the route of spread of this malignancy is usually hematogenous. Lung, brain, bone, skin, and soft tissue are more common sites of metastases and may occur some years after the primary tumor has been treated. Renal cell carcinoma may be quite pleomorphic and look frankly sarcomatous both in the aspiration of primary renal tumors or metastatic sites (Figure 4.43.)[40] This pattern of spindle and pleomorphic tumor cells can be quite confusing for a diagnosis of metastatic renal cell carcinoma because it resembles poorly differentiated pleomorphic sarcomas, including malignant fibrous histiocytoma.

METASTATIC RENAL CELL CARCINOMA

High cellularity, often bloody

Monomorphic population of bland cells
–Moderate amount of clear to granular cytoplasm
–Round, uniform nuclei
–Small, distinct nucleoli

****Sarcomatoid variant may be encountered**

More often, renal cell carcinoma has large cells with clear or granular cytoplasm. Both types of cyto-

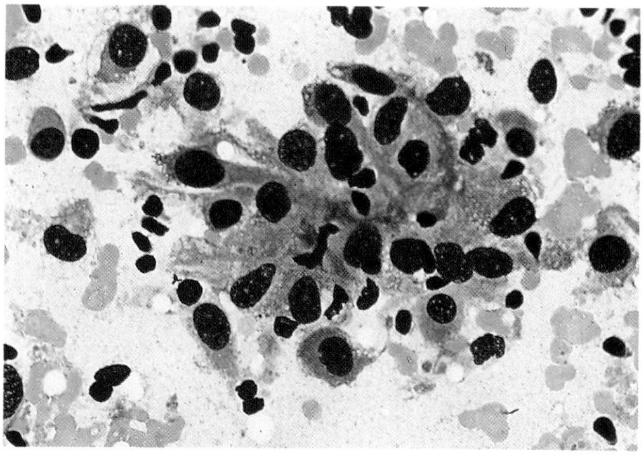

FIGURE 4.43 Aspiration of cervical lymph node. Pleomorphic and predominantly spindle-shaped tumor cells found in metastatic renal cell carcinoma with a sarcomatoid pattern. Tumor cells do not look epithelial, making the exact diagnosis quite difficult without comparison to the original primary tumor. Diff-Quik® 400×.

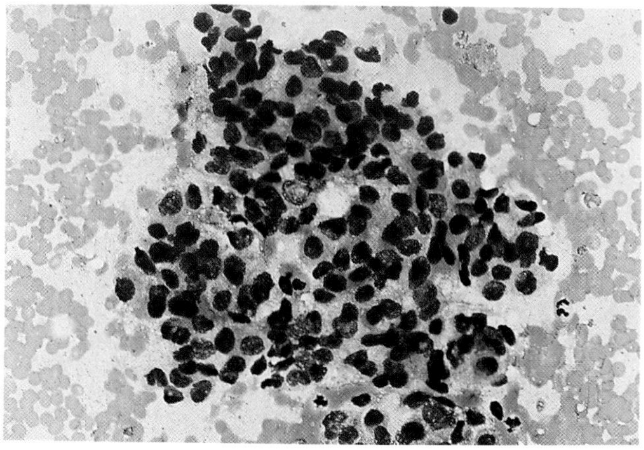

FIGURE 4.45 Aspiration of supraclavicular lymph node. Relatively small and uniform tumor cells with consistently eccentric position of the nucleus. This pattern suggests a metastatic signet-cell carcinoma, of which stomach or other parts of the gastrointestinal tract are the most likely primary sites. Diff-Quik® 400×.

plasm may be seen in tumor cells within the same aspirate. Nucleoli are prominent while the nuclear chromatin can vary from homogeneous, but usually hyperchromatic, in well-differentiated tumors to coarse in less-differentiated renal cell carcinomas. The tumor cells occur both in sheets and loose aggregates, the latter may be bounded by visible portions of a capillary blood vessel that recapitulates closely the tissue pattern of this tumor (Figure 4.44).

Gastric Carcinoma

As in histologic patterns, the cytology of gastric cancer varies from the intestinal type with tall columnar

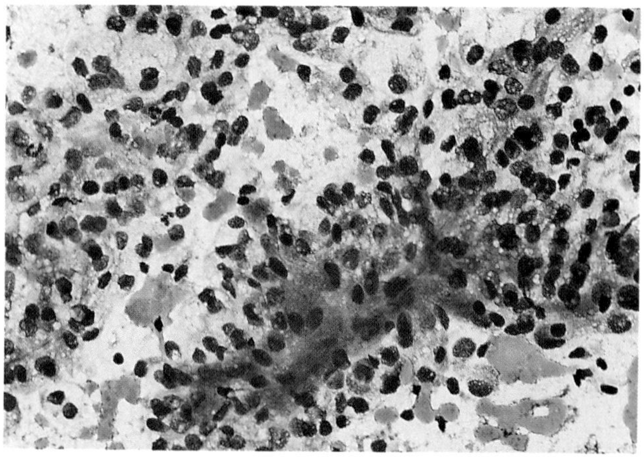

FIGURE 4.44 Aspiration of supraclavicular lymph node. Aggregates of cells with both clear and granular cytoplasm surrounded in part by a thin capillary blood vessel. In the aspiration smear, this recapitulates the pattern of a typical renal cell carcinoma. Diff-Quik® 400×.

cells to the superficial, spreading diffuse type with small cuboidal and very uniform signet-ring cells. In aspiration smears, signet-ring cells occur in predominantly cohesive aggregates. The background of the smear is often quite clean. The nucleus of these tumor cells consistently appears eccentric but is not dramatically flattened against the cell boundary as is observed with the cells of signet-cell carcinoma in histopathology (Figure 4.45).

METASTATIC GASTRIC CARCINOMA

High cellularity

Clean background

Variable cytology—columnar, cuboidal or signet-ring cells
- **–Variable amounts of cytoplasm, may be vacuolated**
- **–Nuclei eccentric (compressed in signet-ring cells)**

Signet-ring cells may be seen in other adenocarcinomas, notably breast. They may be present in aspirates from pancreatic carcinomas, cholangiocarcinomas, and rarely, primary carcinomas of the large intestine. Very rarely a signet-cell aspiration and histologic pattern may be found in lymphoma.[2,41] The conventional duct types of adenocarcinomas of the pancreas and bile ducts are not cytologically distinctive. They both may produce abundant colloid, which gives a very metachromatic background to the smear, but this occurs also with some carcinomas of the large intestine (Figure 4.46).

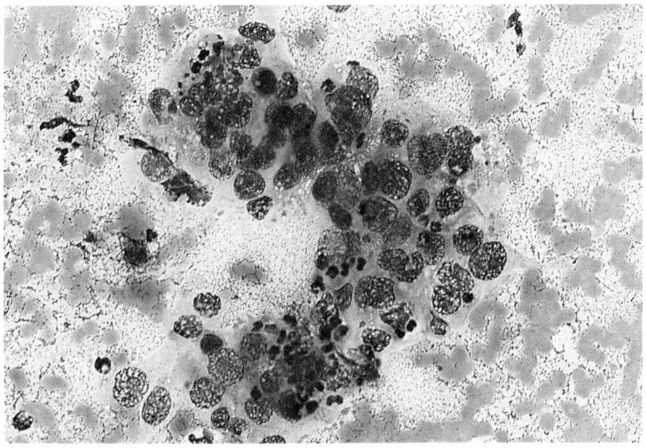

FIGURE 4.46 Aspiration of cervical lymph node. Columnar-shaped tumor cells in a background of metachromatic mucinous material. Metastatic adenocarcinoma from the pancreas. Diff-Quik® 400×.

Colonic Carcinoma

Adenocarcinoma of the colon can metastasize via the perivertebral lymphatics and present as an enlarged supraclavicular or cervical lymph node. There is usually a strikingly necrotic background. If the tumor is predominantly of colloid type, a very metachromatic background may be seen in smears stained by Romanowsky methods. The tumor cells are distinctly columnar and occur predominantly in sheets. The tumor cells within these sheets may form some recognizable acinar structures (Figure 4.47).

Because of degeneration and necrosis, the cells of colonic adenocarcinomas may appear smaller than one would expect but they still retain their columnar shape. The nuclei are also elongated and, in well-preserved tumor cells, the nuclei have coarse chromatin and prominent nucleoli. In large sheets of tumor cells, long serpiginous glands may be detected with a careful examination of the smear. This pattern seems to occur more often in carcinoma of the colon than in differentiated adenocarcinomas of pancreatic ducts.

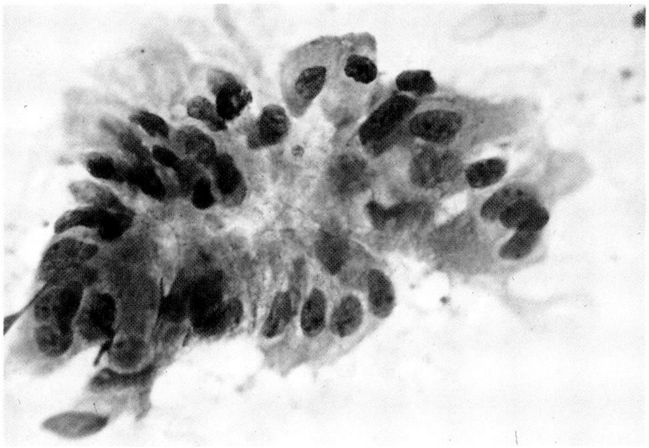

FIGURE 4.47 Aspiration of supraclavicular lymph node. Distinctly columnar-shaped tumor cells in a necrotic background. This is the most common aspiration smear pattern of metastatic colonic carcinoma. Diff-Quik® 400×.

METASTATIC COLONIC ADENOCARCINOMA

High cellularity

Scattered foci of necrosis

Clusters, linear and acinar arrangements of epithelial cells
- **–Columnar, with moderate amount of finely vacuolated cytoplasm**
- **–Basally oriented elongated nucleus**
- **–Granular chromatin**
- **–Central (luminal) necrosis**

Sarcomas

Rhabdomyosarcoma is the most frequent soft tissue sarcoma to involve lymph nodes, particularly in the head and neck area. Synovial sarcomas will also be found metastasizing to lymph nodes.[42] Other types of sarcomas usually metastasize hematogenously. The cytologic features of rhabdomyosarcomas are usually cellular smears with predominantly single cells, oval to spindle in shape and with occasionally larger cells with proportional enlargement of the nucleus. The nucleus is frequently eccentrically placed in the cell with a cytoplasmic tag to one side that mimics the tissue pattern of this tumor, most commonly the embryonal variant (Figure 4.48).

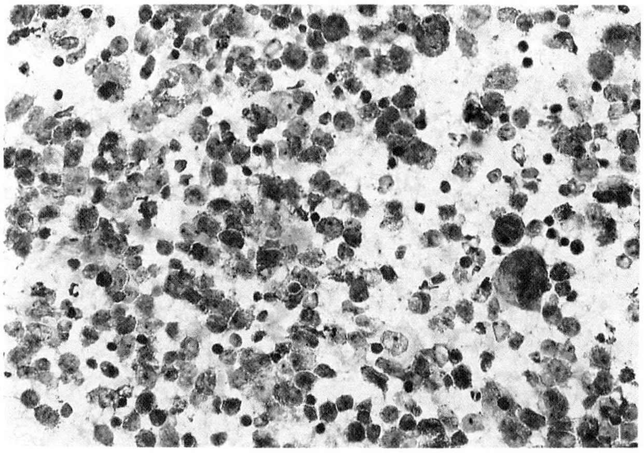

FIGURE 4.48 Aspiration of cervical lymph node. Sheets and many single tumor cells with very undifferentiated features. Note variation in nuclear size, including a few giant nuclei. There is often a small cytoplasmic tag to one side of the nucleus, a feature often found with rhabdomyosarcoma. Diff-Quik® 400×.

The cytoplasm of rhabdomyosarcoma, while somewhat fragile, is dense. The rather delicate nature of the cytoplasm may create a tigroid background, in some cases identical to the smears from metastatic seminoma. This is apparent in 3 of 18 examples in a recently reported series.[17] Cytoplasmic fragments detached from cells of rhabdomyosarcoma may also simulate lymphoglandular bodies. With the embryonal variant, there may be cells in clusters surrounded by a faint metachromatic stroma. Desmin and myoglobin immunohistochemical stains are useful when positive as additional confirmation of the diagnosis.

LYMPHOPROLIFERATIVE DISEASE

There is a very great spectrum of pathologic processes that can involve lymph nodes when dealing with lymphoproliferative disease. It is therefore very important to have a systematic approach to interpretation of needle aspirations when trying to diagnose this diverse group of entities. The aim of such an approach is to reduce the number of diagnostic possibilities for any given case. A convenient starting point is to subdivide the lymphoproliferative processes into three groups based on the predominant cell size: small cells, mixed small and large cells, or large cells. The diagnostic possibilities can then be further narrowed down by looking at chiefly background elements to arrive at a working differential diagnosis. This approach is followed in outline form below:[9,37]

Predominance of Small Lymphocytes in the Aspiration

Benign	*Malignant*
mild hyperplasia	lymphoma, small-cell (well-differentiated lymphocytic, WDL)
medullary cord expansion	lymphoma, small-cleaved-cell (poorly differentiated lymphocytic, PDL)
dermatopathic lymphadenopathy	lymphoma, lymphoblastic
	Castleman's disease
	lymphoma, small-non-cleaved-cell (intermediate size)(Burkitt's)
	Hodgkin's disease lymphocyte-predominant plasma cell tumors, small blue cell tumors of childhood

With the exception of Hodgkin's disease, the cellularity of a malignant lymphoma and a small-cell dominant pattern will be much greater and much more obviously monotonous than in the benign reactive processes listed above. Hodgkin's disease, while it may

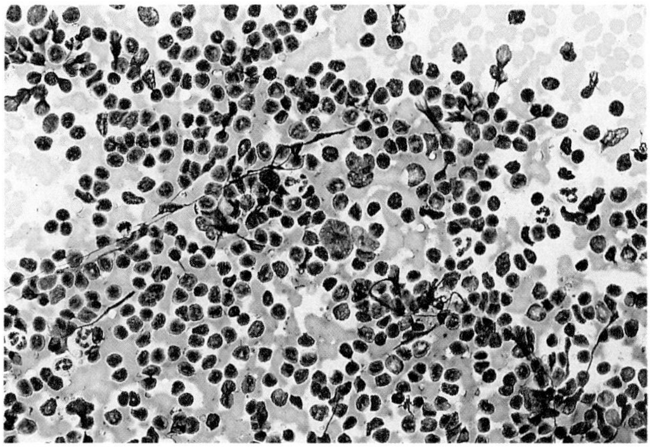

FIGURE 4.49 Hodgkins's disease. Aspiration of cervical lymph node. Scattered large polymorphous cells in a background otherwise dominated by small lymphocytes. Essentially no cells of intermediate size are present. Diff-Quik® 250×.

have a small-cell dominant pattern and low cellularity, must demonstrate some typical large Reed-Sternberg cells to be diagnosed from an aspiration biopsy. Though acceptable examples of Reed-Sternberg cells may be quite sparse in the aspiration smear from some cases of Hodgkin's disease, the size differential between them and the small lymphocytes is quite striking during initial scanning of the smears (Figure 4.49).[43] This dichotomy of cell size is often the first and major clue to the diagnosis of lymphocyte-predominant Hodgkin's disease from aspiration biopsy smears.

Mixture of Large and Small Cells in the Aspiration

Benign	*Malignant*
moderate hyperplasia—follicular	lymphoma, mixed large- and small-cell, follicular center-cell lymphoma, mixed large- and small-cell, T-cell lymphoma, polymorphous plasmacytoid
	Hodgkin's disease, nodular sclerotic (NS) and mixed cellularity lymphoma with partial node involvement

With aspiration smears that have a mixture of large and small cells, the clue to the diagnosis of malignant lymphoma is that there is little or no transition in cell sizes. Two distinct cell populations are seen in reviewing the smears, with no or very few intermediate sized cells. This pattern of two cell populations based on size will be most marked with Hodgkin's disease of the nodular sclerotic type or mixed cellularity, but this pattern is also seen with mixed small- and large-cell lymphomas. Reed-

Sternberg cells, in nodular sclerotic and mixed cellularity Hodgkin's disease, will be relatively easy to find.

Granuloma-like collections of cells may be present in both Hodgkin's disease and T-cell lymphomas. The polymorphism of T cells, variable patterns of the smear, and a wide range in cellularity of smears from T-cell lymphomas make them the most difficult to distinguish from Hodgkin's disease or to diagnose as malignant lymphoma in some cases.[44,45] With polymorphous T-cell lymphomas, the largest cells have prominent nucleoli that are very deep blue in color when observed in Romanowsky-stained smears while the nucleoli of Reed-Sternberg cells have red to blue-red nucleoli. This observation has been found useful in bone marrow smears to separate these two lymphomas. Molecular diagnostic techniques have also been used to identify these difficult lymphomas and to recognize more common lymphomas both in aspiration biopsy and sometimes in histologic sections (Figure 4.50).[46–51]

The mixed large- and small-cell lymphomas with plasmacytoid features may be confused with the relatively rare occurrence of a myeloma involving a lymph node.[52] Clinical features of bone involvement with true myeloma helps in making this separation, while frankly malignant features of the lymphoid cells found in smears from this type of malignant lymphoma and the rather striking polymorphism of the tumor cells also helps to establish the diagnosis (Figure 4.51).

The most confusing aspiration smear patterns will occur when a mixed small- and large-cell lymphoma has partially involved a node. The distinctly different two-cell population of this mixed lymphoma will be masked by portions of the smear that demonstrate the uninvolved node—a spectrum of cell sizes from large to small accompanied by some lymphohistiocytic aggregates.[53] This same feature of partial node involvement results in aspiration smears that are very difficult to interpret with any type of lymphoma and

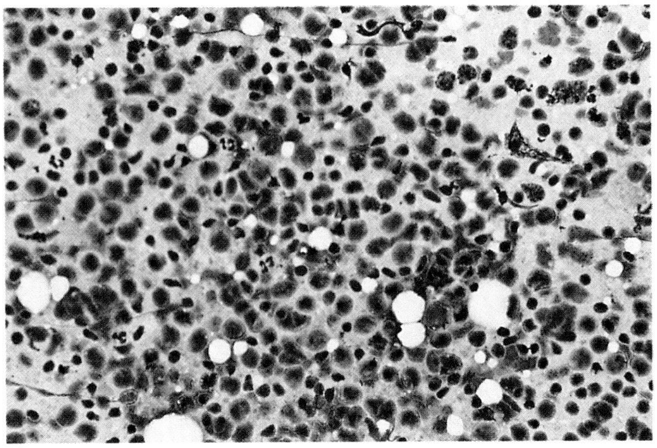

FIGURE 4.50 Aspiration of cervical lymph node. Large polymorphous cells with deep-blue nucleoli. Polymorphous T-cell lymphoma. Diff-Quik® 600×.

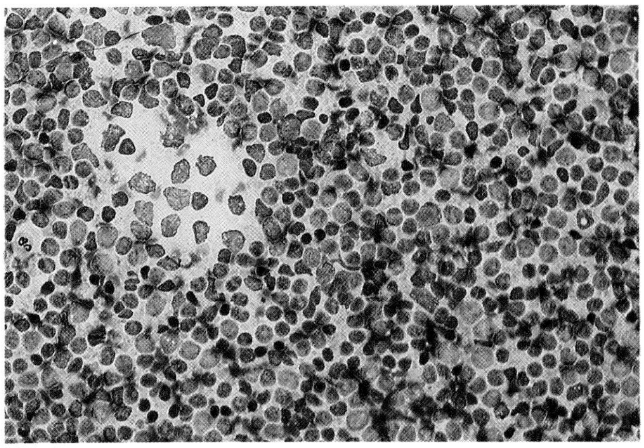

FIGURE 4.51 Aspiration of cervical lymph node. Cellular smear with mixed large and small cells. Some smaller lymphocytes have plasmacytoid features. Mixed small- and large-cell lymphoma. Diff-Quik® 400×.

this is often nondiagnostic with the small-cell lymphomas. If the nodes are large and there are other clinical features suggesting a lymphoma, it is wise to report these smears as at least suspicious for a malignant lymphoproliferative process and proceed with an excisional biopsy of the node aspirated and/or adjacent nodes.

Predominance of Large Cells

Benign	*Malignant*
marked hyperplasia—follicular infectious mononucleosis	lymphoma, large-cell immunoblastic
	Hodgkin's disease, lymphocyte depleted and nodular sclerosis
	granulocytic sarcoma
	carcinoma, undifferentiated
	sarcomas, undifferentiated
	melanoma

The aspiration smears with a predominance of large cells are nearly always malignant, but they can include not only large-cell lymphomas and lymphocyte-depleted Hodgkin's disease but metastatic carcinomas, sarcomas, and melanomas. In aspiration smears, Ki-1 lymphomas may also appear to be quite similar to melanomas, other epithelial malignant tumors metastatic to lymph nodes, and even some poorly differentiated sarcomas (Figure 4.52).[52,54]

With its dominance of single large cells and few aggregates or sheets, metastatic melanoma particularly may closely mimic some large-cell lymphomas, particularly Ki-1 as noted above.[35,54] Immunohistochemistry is quite helpful in these problem cases. Antibody panels to

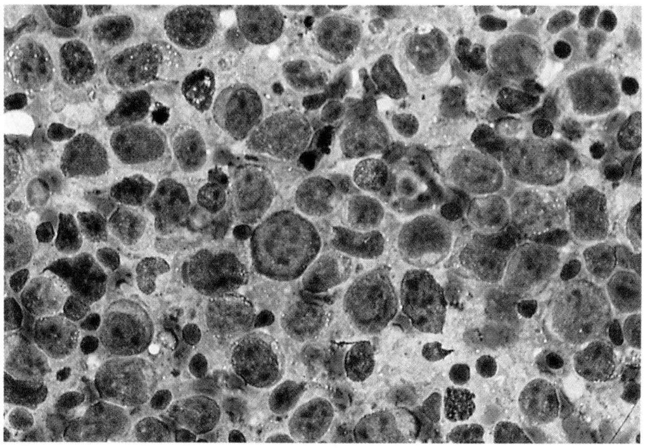

Figure 4.52 Ki-1 lymphoma. Aspiration of cervical lymph node. Large malignant cells with some clustering and an epithelial appearance. There are very few lymphoglandular bodies in the background of the smear. Diff-Quik® 400×.

help in making these differential diagnoses are listed in Table 4.9.

The only proliferative process in which the FNAB smears are dramatically dominated by large cells is infectious mononucleosis. Clinical features of this disease usually point to the correct diagnosis. A positive heterophil antibody may not be present at the time of the lymph node enlargement. While the smears may at first examination appear to be dominated by large cells, there is usually a spectrum of cell sizes from large to small and

Table 4.9 Markers to Distinguish Undifferentiated Neoplasms

Antibodies	*Results*	*Interpretation*
Cytokeratin	+	Carcinoma or other Epithelial Tumor—Panel I
EMA*	+	
S-100	–	
CD45†	–	
Cytokeratin	–	Melanoma, Neurogenic Tumors—Panel II
EMA	–	
S-100	+	
CD45	–	
Cytokeratin	–	Lymphoma—Panel III
EMA	–	
S-100	–	
CD45	+	
Cytokeratin	–	Granulocytic Sarcoma, Histiocytic Tumors, Germ-Cell Tumors—Panel IV
EMA	–	
S-100	–	
CD45	–	

*EMA—Epithelial Membrane Antigen

†CD45—Common Leukocyte Antigen

an organization of small and intermediate lymphoid cells around collections of large cells. This pattern on the aspiration smears reflects the marked follicular hyperplasia observed histologically with infectious mononucleosis (Figure 4.53).[55]

INFECTIOUS MONONUCLEOSIS

Relatively clean background

Heterogeneous population but dominated by
- **Large atypical cells**
- **Thin rim of basophilic cytoplasm**
- **Uniform nucleus with bland chromatin**
- **Prominent nucleoli**

****Clinical data imperative**

The features described cytologically with the marked hyperplasia of infectious mononucleosis reflect the actual enlarged lymphoid follicles. With poor smear technique, this important finding can be disturbed or destroyed. Careful examination of the nuclear chromatin pattern of these large cells from hyperplastic lymphoid follicles and those of a large-cell lymphoma reveal that they are quite different (Figure 4.54). The reactive follicular center cells have a bland nuclear chromatin with round uniform nucleoli while the cells of large-cell lymphoma have nuclei with a coarse and distinct chromatin pattern and red, large and sometimes irregular and often multiple nucleoli. The cells of large-cell lymphoma occur both singly and in sheets with no pretense to follicle formation even if that pattern is present histologically in the node itself.

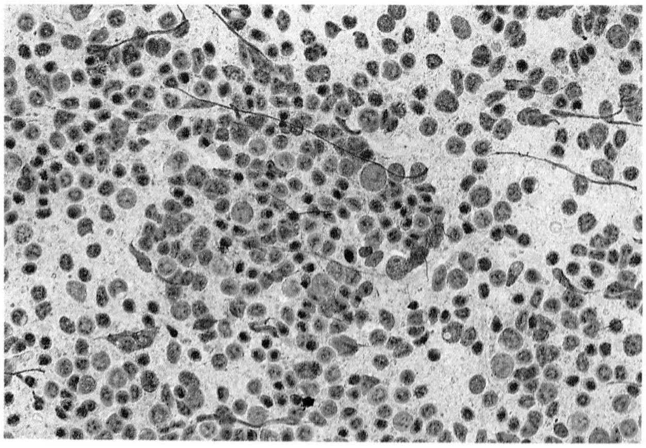

Figure 4.53 Aspiration of cervical lymph node. Very cellular smear with apparent dominance of large cells. These cells are not all similar as some have the dense cytoplasmic rim of immunoblasts. They do not have an abnormal chromatin pattern to the nucleus or multiple large nucleoli found with large-cell lymphoma. Hyperplastic node found in infectious mononucleosis. Diff-Quik® 400×.

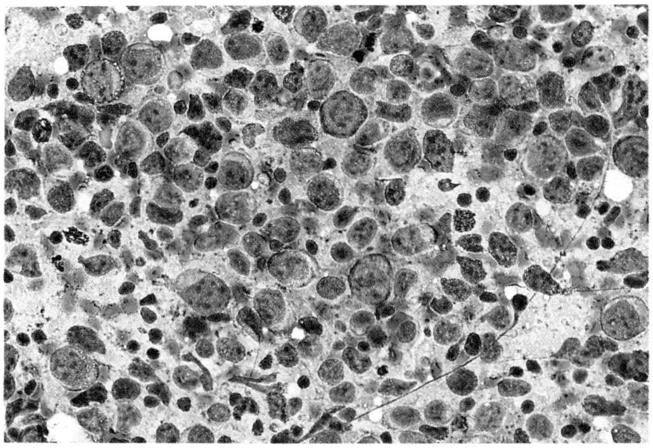

FIGURE 4.54 Aspiration of cervical lymph node. Large undifferentiated cells from large-cell lymphoma. Compare features of nuclear chromatin and nucleoli with the severe hyperplasia of infectious mononucleosis illustrated in Figure 4.53. Diff-Quik® 400×.

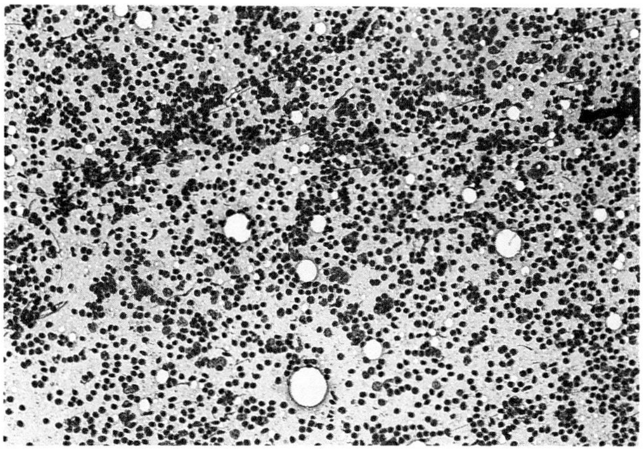

FIGURE 4.55 Aspiration of cervical lymph node. Uniform clumping of small lymphocytes from small-cleaved-cell lymphoma. Diff-Quik® 250×.

Background Elements

When the predominant population of lymphocytes is determined and diagnostic possibilities are reduced, background elements occurring in the aspiration smear can be used to arrive at a more specific diagnosis (Table 4.10). Background elements include cell aggregates, granulomas, necrosis, tingible body macrophages, plasma cells, cells with plasmacytoid features, eosinophils, and individual or collections of bizarre cells. Any one or several of these background elements may be present. It is important to review the smears for the dominant element or elements.[37] For example, cell aggregates are most common in metastatic carcinomas. They are important in differentiating metastatic small-round-cell tumors from small-cell lymphomas, particular lymphoblastic lymphomas, and Burkitt's lymphoma in children. Small-cell lymphoma that is poorly differentiated with cleaved cells is likely to show uniform clumping of the lymphoid cells (Figure 4.55).[56] The presence of lymphoglandular bodies and the uniform distribution and size of the small-cell clumps points toward the correct diagnosis.

Among malignant processes, on aspiration smears, T-cell lymphomas and Hodgkin's disease are the most likely to have background granulomas. The granulomas may actually be the element that is found first in the smears from either Hodgkin's disease or T-cell lymphomas.[43,57,58] Unlike infectious granulomas, with the exception of sarcoid, the granulomas that are a part of some malignant lymphomas are quite cellular and there is considerable pleomorphism among the individual cells making up the granuloma (Figure 4.56).

Necrosis is a prominent feature of both infectious disease and some poorly differentiated carcinomas. It may also occur with metastatic well-differentiated squamous cell carcinoma, producing a cystic metastasis in a cervical lymph node. The cellularity is still relatively high and some cells are usually well enough preserved to clearly indicate a malignant process. One benign reactive lymphoid proliferation rarely seen in the United States is Kikuchi's disease. The background in these aspirates is dominated by necrosis with a reactive pattern of lymphoid elements showing a great deal of degeneration.[59,60] This necrosis may produce a pattern of relatively large and small cells that can suggest metastatic small-cell carcinoma. Usually extensive DNA artifact is lacking in these cases. Immunostains may not be helpful with aspirates from lymph nodes showing necrosis because that feature may produce artifactual background staining that can be carried into the cells making interpretation difficult. Use of cytospin preparation will eliminate all or most of this problem.[61]

Tingible body macrophages usually point to a reactive lymph node most often when associated with sur-

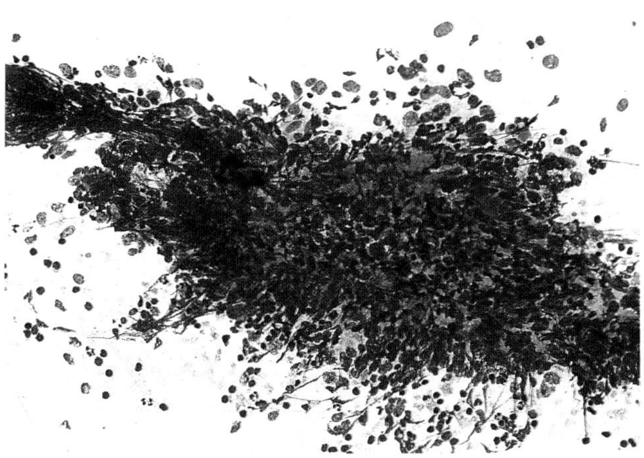

FIGURE 4.56 Aspiration of cervical lymph node. Cellular granuloma seen in aspiration smear of Hodgkin's disease. Pleomorphism of individual cells within the granuloma is important to the diagnosis, prompting a search for typical Reed-Sternberg cells. Diff-Quik® 400×.

TABLE 4.10 Background Elements in the Differential Diagnosis of Lymphoproliferative Processes

Cell Aggregates	
Benign	*Malignant*
follicular center-cell fragments	carcinoma
sinus histiocytosis	lymphoma (small-cleaved-cell)
granulomas	Hodgkin's disease
Granulomas	
Benign	*Malignant*
caseating processes, TB, fungi	lymphoma, T-cell, Hodgkin's disease
sarcoidosis	follicular lymphoma (rare)
acute necrotizing granuloma	seminoma
cat-scratch disease	thymoma
brucellosis	
syphilis	
foreign body reactions	
Necrosis	
Benign	*Malignant*
granulomatous processes	lymphoma, lymphoblastic
abscess; i.e., bacterial infection	lymphoma, small-noncleaved-cell
spontaneous infarction	lymphoma, immunoblastic
Kakuchi's disease	lymphoma, small-cleaved-cell (rare) Hodgkin's disease carcinoma
Tingible Body Macrophages	
Benign	*Malignant*
reactive hyperplasia	lymphoma, lymphoblastic
	lymphoma, small noncleaved
	lymphoma, large-cell
	malignancy with partially involved node

rounding lymphocytes, lymphohistiocytic aggregates that mimic the reactive follicular centers (Figure 4.57).[62,63] They may be associated with a variety of malignant neoplasms in aspiration biopsies but often in this situation stand alone without any organized pattern (Figure 4.58). They are most confusing when seen in an aspirate from a partially involved node by a malignant process because they look like—and are in fact representative of—the reaction within the node.[37]

Plasma cells, plasmacytoid cells, and eosinophils are relatively nonspecific in a differential diagnosis of benign and malignant lymphoid process and are rarely part of carcinoma metastatic to a lymph node. The only exception with respect to plasma cells, plasmacytoid cells, and mature lymphocytes is metastatic lymphoepithelioma from the nasopharynx.[37,38] If plasmacytoid cells are a very dominant element and have enlarged nuclei with variation in size and prominent nucleoli, then a plasma-cell neoplasm, myeloma, is a strong possibility (Figure 4.59). While myeloma is a disease of bone, it can occur in lymph nodes but only as a secondary in advanced disease. The author has also seen myeloma involve soft tissue of the head and neck. Primary plasma-cell tumors may also occur in the head and neck, particularly in the oral cavity where they are accessible to aspiration biopsy.

Bizarre cells, which are usually quite large, point immediately to a malignant process, particularly T-cell lymphomas and Hodgkin's disease. These cells are often so strikingly atypical and large that they are out of place with any of the other lymphoid or other types of cells present. (Figure 4.60). Reactive lymph nodes may have occasional histiocytes or immunoblastic cells that are somewhat bizarre. Histiocytes can be recognized by the

TABLE 4.10 Continued

Benign	Malignant
Plasma Cells	
Benign	*Malignant*
nonspecific reactive process	lymphoma—T-cell
infectious process; i.e., TB, syphilis	Hodgkin's disease, mixed cellularity, NS
collagen vascular diseases	carcinoma
angiofollicular hyperplasia	
Plasmacytoid Cells	
Benign	*Malignant*
nonspecific reactive process	plasmacytoid lymphomas
infectious processes; viral bacterial	small-cell-type polymorphous
drug-induced reactions	B-cell lymphoma
postvaccination hyperplasia	immunoblastic lymphoma
	plasma-cell tumors
Eosinophils	
Benign	*Malignant*
nonspecific reactive processes	lymphoma T-cell
infectious processes; i.e., protozoal	Hodgkin's disease, mixed cellularity and NS
lymphogranuloma	myelogenous leukemia
eosinophilic lymphadenitis	histiocytosis X
Bizarre Cells	
Benign	*Malignant*
	histiocytosis (occasionally non-Hodgkin's lymphomas (some) immunoblasts)
	Hodgkin's disease
	carcinoma
	sarcoma

blandness of their chromatin, inconspicuous nucleoli, abundant cytoplasm, and the frequent presence of a slightly indented nucleus. Immunoblasts have characteristic very deep blue cytoplasm and are accompanied by a range of plasmacytoid cells (Figure 4.61).

The most difficult challenge with aspiration biopsy of lymph nodes and lymphoproliferative processes has been the recognition of T-cell lymphoma and Hodgkin's disease.[45,64] The cytologic features from a number of cases are summarized in Table 4.11. The T-cell lymphomas in particular, in concert with their histologic features, can provide a wealth of different smear patterns that can mimic reactive, granulomatous processes as well as metastatic neoplasms—both carcinomas and sarcomas. Finding large, bizarre individual cells in the smear should alert one to the possibility of a T-cell lymphoma (Figure 4.62). Clinical correlation is important. These patients often have fever and weight loss and the nodes or node is large. From the cytologic features listed in Table 4.11, the overlap with Hodgkin's disease is obvious. Classic double-nucleated Reed-Sternberg cells must be found for a diagnosis of Hodgkin's disease on aspiration biopsy. Reed-Sternberg cells tend to have large nucleoli, and these nucleoli are distinctly red when smears are stained with Romanowsky methods (Figure 4.63).

IMMUNOLOGIC STUDIES IN FINE NEEDLE ASPIRATION OF LYMPH NODES

A wide variety of antibodies are available that have relative specificity in the identification of epithelial, mesenchymal, hematopoietic, and lymphoreticular cells.[65,66] These antibodies can be employed with im-

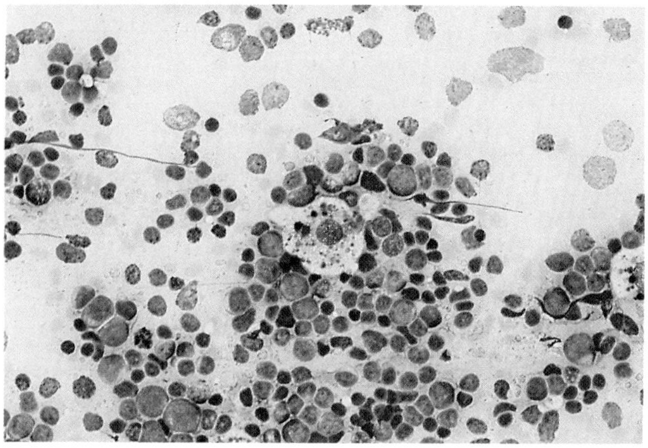

FIGURE 4.57 Aspiration of cervical lymph node. Reactive follicular center with tingible body macrophage, seen in reactive hyperplastic lymphadenitis. Diff-Quik® 400×.

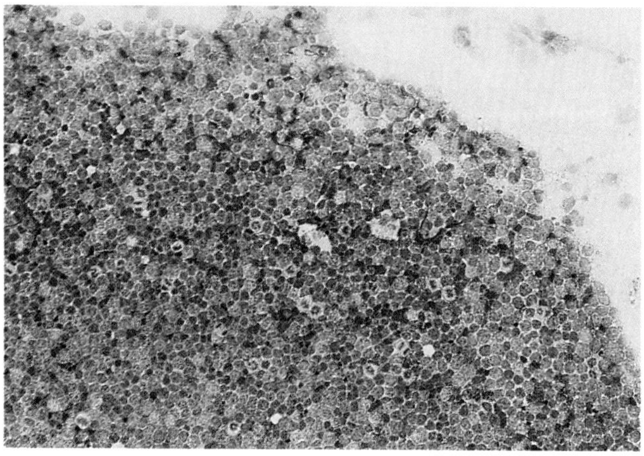

FIGURE 4.58 Aspiration of cervical lymph node. Highly cellular smear with diffuse individual malignant lymphoid cells and scattered tingible body macrophages. This pattern is typical of Burkitt's lymphoma. Diff-Quik® 250×.

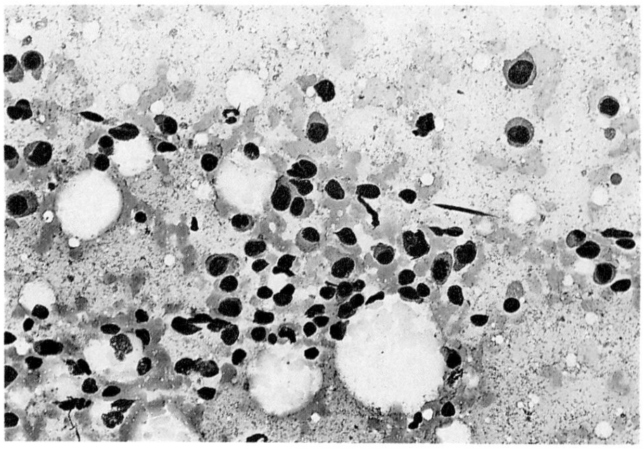

FIGURE 4.59 Multiple myeloma. Aspiration of cervical lymph node. Smear with large numbers of plasma cells that vary in size and shape. Diff-Quik® 400×.

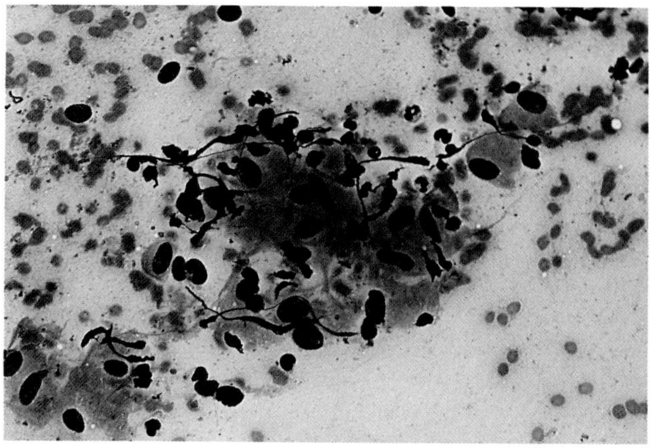

FIGURE 4.60 Aspiration of cervical lymph node. Large bizarre cells found in T-cell lymphoma. Diff-Quik® 400×.

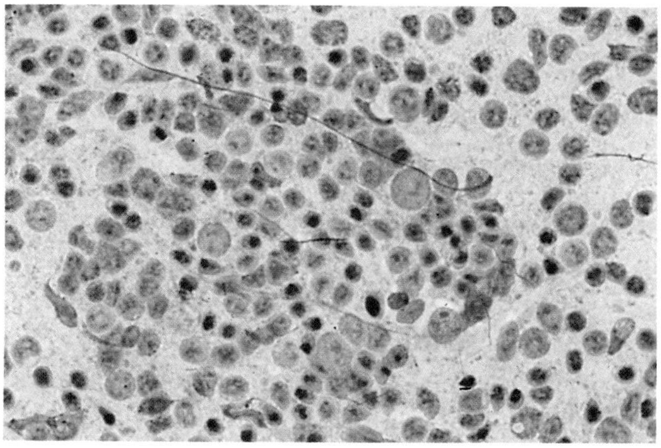

FIGURE 4.61 Aspiration of cervical lymph node. Aspiration smear with large immunoblasts from a very reactive node. Note deep-blue and dense rim of cytoplasm. Diff-Quik® 600×.

TABLE 4.11 Cytologic Features of T-Cell Lymphomas and Hodgkin's Disease

	Lymphoma—Peripheral T-Cell
1.	A mixture of large and small cells present.
2.	Granulomas may be abundant.
3.	Granulomas are highly cellular.
4.	Bizarre cells present individually and within granulomas.
5.	Bizarre cells have large blue nucleoli.
6.	Eosinophils and plasma cells are often present.
	Hodgkin's Disease
1.	Granulomas frequent.
2.	Granulomas are cellular.
3.	Large polyploid cells, mononuclear and binuclear Reed-Sternberg cells.
4.	Eosinophils and plasma cells frequently present.
5.	Necrosis present.
6.	Reed-Sternberg cells have red nucleoli.

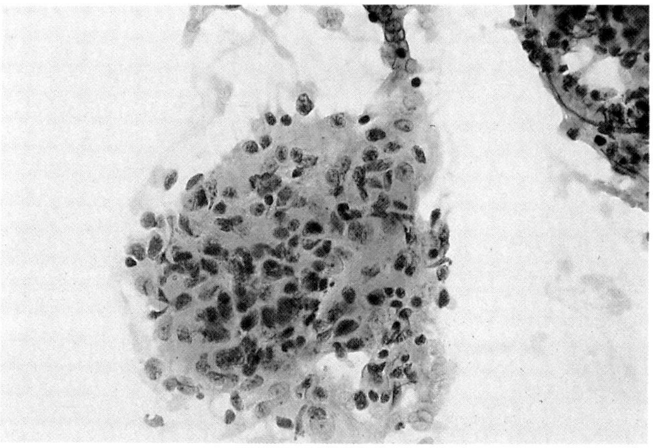

FIGURE 4.62 Aspiration of cervical lymph node. One of the patterns of T-cell lymphoma with granuloma-like aggregates and large bizarre cells. Diff-Quik® 250×.

munohistologic techniques to assist in determining the lineage of a neoplasm and in some cases in differentiating benign processes from malignant ones. However, just as aspiration cytology of lymph nodes complements rather than replaces surgical biopsy, immunologic studies complement but do not replace the cytologic interpretation of an aspirate.

In spite of the utility of immunologic studies, there are problems with this technique. These problems include the following:

1. They limit the cost effectiveness of FNA when used routinely;
2. Sometimes adequate material cannot be obtained to run the necessary panel of markers;
3. Antibodies are only relatively specific to cell antigens and may cross-react with a variety of cell types within and outside a particular cell lineage;

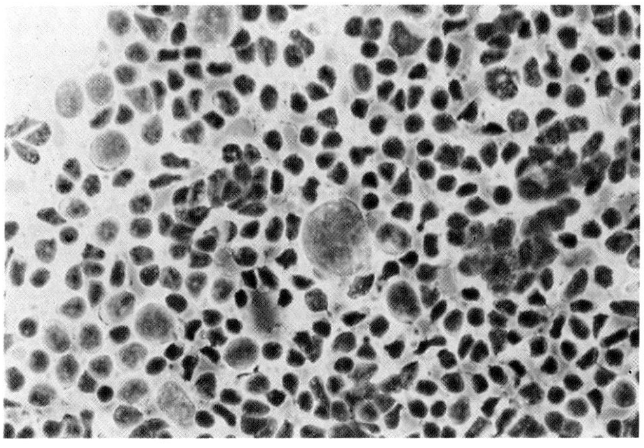

FIGURE 4.63 Aspiration of cervical lymph node. Reed-Sternberg cells from Hodgkin's disease with large, reddish blue nucleoli. Diff-Quik® 600×.

4. Neoplastic cells do not always express the surface antigens found on analogous normal cells; and
5. Peripheral T-cell lymphomas have a heterogeneous immunologic pattern without a marker that is specific for malignancy.

In spite of these handicaps, in selected situations immunologic study of cells obtained by FNAB may be extremely useful.[53,67–69] Some common applications of FNAB from lymph nodes include:

1. Differentiating carcinoma from lymphoma;
2. Distinguishing reactive lymphoid processes from monoclonal B-cell lymphomas;
3. Differentiating hematogenous from lymphoreticular malignancies; and
4. Aiding in the subtyping of lymphomas, namely lymphoblastic lymphoma, and small-cell lymphoma.

Aspirate material may be studied immunologically in several different ways, including examination of direct smears, cytospin preparations from cell suspensions, or by flow cytometry of cell suspensions.[44,70] Immunologic studies utilizing direct smears are of limited use because only a small quantity of slides can be prepared and multiple aspirates are required to make these preparations. In direct smears from lymph nodes, there is often a dense plasmalike background that causes high nonspecific staining that may be carried over into cell cytoplasm. This makes interpretation quite difficult.

Flow cytometry is of limited use because expensive equipment to run this test may not be available. A relatively large number of cells is required for the determination of any single marker, which, in turn, limits the number of panels that can be run on the aspiration biopsy. Finally, the morphology of the cells that stain positively or negatively in flow cytometry cannot be determined.[68]

The author has found that cytospin preparations are the most useful method for immunologic characterization of lymph node aspirates. Advantages include:

1. A large number of slides can be prepared, therefore large panels can be run;
2. Nonspecific staining is not a problem because the background is clean; and
3. Utilizing immunoperoxidase techniques, the morphology of the cells that are reacting with the antibody can be determined.

By actual count, as many as 13×10^6 cells have been obtained from a single aspiration of a lymph node harboring a malignant, poorly differentiated lymphocytic lymphoma. Although reactive nodes most often provide far fewer cells, there are sufficient numbers in most cases to run immunologic markers when there is difficulty interpreting routinely stained smears. Often the most difficult differential diagnoses is that of a very reactive atypical node versus a malignant lymphoma where the cellularity of the aspiration is usually high and the lymph node clinically large.

Preparation of Slides for Immunologic Studies

1. Cell suspensions are prepared by placing the cells obtained by FNA into a small tube containing 5.0 milliliters of RPMI 1640 with 10 percent fetal calf serum (RPMI/FCS). Enough cellular aspirate material should be obtained to make the solution slightly cloudy (about 105 to 106 cells/mL).
2. Two to five drops of cell suspension are placed in the cytospin chamber of the cytocentrifuge. Two additional drops of RPMI/FCS are then added to the chamber. No fixatives are added. Short, low-speed centrifugation is employed, namely, 500 RPM for 3 to 4 minutes, to avoid damage to the cells. Slides are removed immediately after centrifugation and allowed to air-dry as quickly as possible. Slides may be stored in a dessicator at room temperature for up to a week prior to use. For the immunohistochemical method, consult Chapter 1.

Protocols for Marker Studies

The choice of markers to aid in the diagnosis of a neoplasm is based on a variety of factors including clinical history, laboratory and radiographic findings, and the morphologic appearance of the neoplastic cells. There is no optimal panel of markers for studying lymphoid and nonlymphoid neoplasms. Varying sets of circumstances dictate the need for panels composed of different antibodies. Panels of antibodies should be utilized to resolve the questions raised by clinical and cytologic findings.

The panels listed in Tables 4.12–4.15 are expected to serve as general guides but should not be considered preemptive. New antibodies are constantly becoming available. Panels need to be revised regularly as these new antibodies become available, additional information about existing antibodies is published, and experience increases with repeated use of antibodies.[37] Remember that the morphologic diagnosis is the single most important factor in deciding what antibody studies should be performed and this must be reflected in the decision process.

TABLE 4.12 Lymphoid Process Versus Nonlymphoid Process (see Table 4.9)

Morphology Favors Lymphoid Process
Panel II and Panel III
Morphology Favors Nonlymphoid Process
Panel IV
Morphology Cannot Tell If Lymphoid or Nonlymphoid
Panel I

UTILITY OF ASPIRATION BIOPSY OF LYMPH NODES

Aspiration biopsy of lymph nodes for the diagnosis of metastatic neoplasms is well established. It is the quickest, safest and most cost-effective test for confirming metastases in lymph nodes. The application and utility for diagnosing lymphoproliferative disease is now gaining some acceptance. Objections to FNAB for the diagnosis of lymphoproliferative disease have been[37]

1. many hematopathologists are not knowledgeable or comfortable with aspiration cytology,
2. many cytopathologists are not familiar with lymphoreticular pathology,
3. the spectrum of pathologic processes involving lymph nodes is both large and complex,
4. many standard cytologic criteria for individual cells do not apply to interpretation of aspirations of lymph nodes, and
5. there is some degree of overlap in the appearance cytologically of some lymphoproliferative processes, making FNA diagnosis less precise and accurate than in other organ systems.

Despite the difficulties enumerated above, FNAB of lymph nodes can be a valuable tool in patient management. It provides a rapid, simple means of directly sampling the mass in question as a guide to clinical management. In some cases, FNAB will serve as an extension of the physical examination with surgical biopsy as the next possible step. FNAB may substitute for surgical biopsy in some cases, particularly with metastatic disease, and therapy can be started or the patient can be followed clinically.[71,72] In a small percentage of cases, the results of FNAB of lymph nodes will be inconclusive or even misleading. These inconclusive findings do not invalidate the procedure. As in any other diagnostic procedure, care and common sense must be used in the interpretation and application of the results of lymph node aspiration biopsy.[2]

The authors' experience with FNAB of lymph nodes confirms that metastatic disease can be diagnosed with confidence and appropriate management instituted. When aspiration is coupled with special stains and cultures, infectious lesions can also often be effectively diagnosed by FNA. Reactive, hyperplastic lymphadenopathy, in most cases, can be diagnosed with enough confidence that the patient can be followed clinically. If the enlarged lymph nodes continue to be worrisome, surgical biopsy must then be performed. Diagnosis by FNAB

TABLE 4.13 Initial Panel for Lymphoma Typing

Antibodies	*Cells Identified*	*Detects*
CD 3	T Lymphocytes	T-Cell Lymphomas and Leukemias
CD 5	T Lymphocytes	T-Cell Lymphomas, B-Cell SCL/CLL
Anti-HLADR	B Lymphocytes	B-Cell Lymphomas monocytes; myeloid cells; some T-Cell Lymphomas cells; activated T cells, Granulocytic Sarcoma cells; histiocytes
CD 20	B Lymphocytes	B-Cell Lymphomas
Anti-kappa & lambda	B Lymphocytes	B-Cell Lymphomas
Anti-mu	B Lymphocytes	B-Cell Lymphomas
CD 10	Pre-B Lymphocytes	Lymphoblastic lymphoma
		Pre-T Lymphocytes and Leukemia
		Follicular Center-Cell Lymphomas (some)

TABLE 4.14 Extended Lymphocytes Marker Panel for Lymphoma

Antibodies	*Cells Identified*	*Detects*
CD 1	Thymic Lymphocytes	Lymphoblastic Lymphoma and Leukemia, T-cell; Thymoma (lymphoid component); Histiocytosis X
CD 7	Pan T-cell	Lymphoblastic Lymphoma, T-cell; T-ALL; other T-cell Lymphomas
CD 8	Suppressor T-cells	T-cell Lymphomas (some)
CD 4	Helper T-cells	T-cell Lymphomas (some) Mycosis fungoides
CD 13, CD 33	Myeloid/monocytic	AML/Granulocytic Sarcoma
CD 15, CD 14		series cells AML, M4, M5
CD 14	Monocytic cells	AML, M4, M5
Anti-Tdt	Pre T and Thymic lymphocytes:	Lymphoblastic Lymphoma and Leukemia: AML (rarely)
	Pre-B-Lymphocytes	

of a *de novo* lymphoma should, in most instances, be followed by surgical biopsy for confirmation and subtyping. However, the use of immunohistochemical stains for lymphoid markers can subtype many of these cases from adequate FNAB biopsy samples.[9] When the patient is a poor surgical risk, if the aspiration diagnosis is unequivocal, therapy of a lymphoproliferative process may be based on the FNAB diagnosis alone.

Advantages of Lymph Node Fine Needle Aspiration Biopsy[37]

1. Is safe, simple, rapid.
2. Is cost effective.
3. Expedites and directs patient management.
4. Allows the lymph node to remain as a marker for therapy.
5. Does not violate the surgical field for subsequent surgical procedures.

Disadvantages of Lymph Node Fine Needle Aspiration Biopsy[37]

1. Overlap of cytologic patterns in some benign and malignant processes.
2. Inability to differentiate diffuse and nodular patterns of lymphoma.
3. Difficulty in adequately sampling lymph nodes with partial involvement, extensive fibrosis, or necrosis.

TABLE 4.15 Identification of Nonlymphoid Neoplasms

Neoplasm	*Antibodies*	
Neuroendocrine	Neuron-Specific Enolase S-100 Chromogranin	
Endocrine	Insulin Glucagon Somatostatin Thyroglobulin	Calcitonin Gastrin Prolactin ACTH
Sarcoma	Actin Desmin Factor 8	Myoglobin S-100 Ulex
Germ Cell	AFP HCG Alkaline Phosphatase Placental Lactogen	Cytokeratin
Pediatric Round Blue Cell Tumors	CD45 (LCA) NSE Chromogranin	Desmin Myoglobin
Prostate Carcinoma	Prostatic Specific Antigen (PSA) Prostatic Specific Acid Phosphatase (PSAP)	
Breast Carcinoma	Estrogen Receptor Progesterone Receptor Gross Cystic Disease Fluid Protein (GCDFP15)	

Reporting of Lymph Node Fine Needle Aspiration Biopsy Results

The following scheme is recommended for reporting the results of aspiration biopsies of lymph nodes.

1. Lesion not lymphoreticular, that is, mixed tumor of salivary gland, branchial cleft cysts.
2. Metastatic malignancy—consistent with primary if known (if unknown, try to determine the primary).
3. Evidence suggestive of infectious process—recommend confirmation with culture.
4. Hyperplastic lymph node—clinical follow-up recommended.
5. Evidence suggestive of lymphoma—recommend biopsy confirmation.
6. FNAB results inconclusive—recommend biopsy if clinically indicated.

Contraindications and Complications

There are no contraindications to lymph node aspiration biopsy in the head and neck or in any other areas.[2] However, it may be contraindicated to aspirate a carotid body tumor that could be mistaken clinically for a lymph node, but aspiration of this neoplasm has been accomplished successfully.[8]

Several complications from aspiration biopsy of lymph nodes have been reported. Davies and Webb published one of the first reports to causally associate FNAB with tissue damage.[73] They noted a segmental infarction of an axillary lymph node in the area sampled by aspiration biopsy, apparently secondary to venous thrombosis. Although spontaneous infarction of lymph nodes has been documented, it is usually not a localized phenomenon. Shortly after the report of Davies and Webb, a study by Behm et al. addressed the degree of disruption that FNAB may have on lymph node architecture.[74] Twenty-eight benign lymph nodes, excised intact within 4 weeks following FNAB, were accepted into their study. Fifty-seven percent of cases showed no evidence of the previous FNAB. Minimal disruption, usually not exceeding 5 percent of the cross-sectional area examined, was found in 12 cases (43 percent), indicating that FNAB will not compromise histologic assessment in the vast majority of cases. More recently, studies by Dekmezian et al. and Tsang and Chan have confirmed that morphologic changes such as segmental necrosis or hemorrhage can occur but typically do not interfere with histologic assessment.[75,76] Lymph nodes that have been vigorously aspirated or that are involved with malignant lymphoma appear more susceptible to these changes.

REFERENCES

1. Linsk JA, Franzen S. *Clinical aspiration cytology,* 2nd ed. New York: J.B. Lippincott Co., 1989, pp. 39–47.

2. Frable WJ. Thin-needle aspiration biopsy. In Bennington JL (ed.), *Major problems in pathology,* Vol 14. Philadelphia, W.B. Saunders Co., 1983, pp.75, 87, 91, 92.

3. Stastny JF, Wakely PE Jr., Frable WJ. The cytologic features of necrotizing granulomatous disease consistent with cat scratch disease (abstract). *Acta Cytol* 1994;38:868.

4. Wakely PE Jr., Kardos TF, Frable WJ. Application of fine needle aspiration biopsy to pediatrics. *Hum Pathol* 1988;19:1383–1386.

5. Martin-Bates E, Tanner A, Suvarna SK, Glazer G, Coleman DV. Use of fine needle aspiration cytology for investigating lymphadenopathy in HIV positive patients. *J Clin Pathol* 1993;46:564–566.

6. Tao L, Gullane PJ. HIV infection-associated lymphoepithelial lesions of the parotid gland: Aspiration biopsy cytology, histology, and pathogenesis. *Diagn Cytopathol* 1991;7:158–162.

7. Stanley MW, Lowhagen T. *Fine needle aspiration of palpable masses.* Boston: Butterworth-Heinemann, 1993.

8. Engzel U, Franzen S, Zijicek J. Aspiration biopsy of tumors of the neck; II, Cytologic findings in 13 cases of carotid body tumor. *Acta Cytol* 1971;15:25–30.

9. Frable WJ, Kardos TF. Fine needle aspiration biopsy. Applications in the diagnosis of lymphoproliferative disease. *Am J Surg Pathol* 1988;12(Suppl.I):62–72.

10. Chang YW. Sinus histiocytosis with massive lymphadenopathy. Report of a case with fine needle aspiration cytology. *Acta Cytol* 1993;37:186–190.

11. Trautman BC, Stanley MW, Goding GS, et al. Sinus histiocytosis with massive lymphadenopathy (Rosai-Dorfman disease): Diagnosis by fine-needle aspiration. *Diagn Cytopathol* 1991;7:513–516.

12. Wakely PE Jr., Silverman JF, Holbrook CT, et al. Fine needle aspiration biopsy cytology as an adjunct in the diagnosis of childhood sarcoidosis. *Pediatr Pulmonol* 1992;13:117–120.

13. Gupta SK, Chugh TD, Sheikh ZA, Al-Rubah NAR. Cytodiagnosis of tuberculous lymphadenitis: A correlative study with microbiologic examination. *Acta Cytol* 1993;37:329–332.

14. Lau SK, Wei WI, Dwan S, Yew WW. Combined use of fine-needle aspiration cytologic examination and tuberculin skin test in the diagnosis of cervical tuberculous lymphadenitis. A prospective study. *Arch Otolaryngol Head Neck Surg* 1991;117:87–90.

15. Singh UR, Bhatia, A, Gadre DV, Talwar V. Cytologic diagnosis of tuberculous lymphadenitis in children by fine needle aspiration. *Indian J Pediatr* 1992; 59:115–118.

16. Ang GA, Janda WM, Novak RM, Gerardo L. Negative images of mycobacteria in aspiration biopsy smears from the lymph node of a patient with acquired immunodeficiency syndrome (AIDS). Report of a case and a review of the literature (review). *Diagn Cytopathol* 1993;9:325–328.

17. Almeida M, Stastny JF, Wakely PE Jr., et al. Fine-needle aspiration biopsy of childhood rhabdomyosarcoma: Reevaluation of the cytologic criteria for diagnosis. *Diagn Cytopathol* 1994;11:231–236.

18. Gupta AK, Nayar M, Chandra M. Reliability and limitations of fine-needle aspiration cytology of lymphadenopathies. An analysis of 1,261 cases. *Acta Cytol* 1991;35:777–783.

19. Pithie AD, Chicksen B. Fine-needle extrathoracic lymph-node aspiration in HIV-associated sputum-negative tuberculosis. *Lancet* 1992;340:1504–1505.

20. Drut R. Fine-needle aspiration cytology in a case with features of chronic granulomatous disease. *Diagn Cytopathol* 1991;7:57–59.

21. Lee RE, Valaitis J, Kalis O, Sophian A, Schultz E. Lymph node examination by fine needle aspiration in patients with known or suspected malignancy. *Acta Cytol* 1987;31:563–572.

22. Guarda LA. Simultaneous fine-needle aspiration of thyroid lesions and regional cervical lymph nodes: Clinicopathologic implications *Diagn cytopathol* 1992;8:377–379.

23. Matsuda M, Nagumo S, Koyama H, et al. Occult thyroid cancer discovered by fine-needle aspiration cytology of cervical lymph node: A report of three cases. *Diagn Cytopathol* 1991;7:299–303.

24. Baatenburg de Jong RJ, Rongen RJ, Verwoerd CD, et al. Ultrasound-guided fine-needle aspiration biopsy of neck nodes. *Arch Otolaryngol Head Neck Surg* 1991;117:402–404.

25. van den Brekel MW, Castelijns JA, Stel HV, et al. Occult metastatic neck disease: Detection with US and US-guided fine-needle aspiration cytology. *Radiology* 1991;180:457–461.

26. van den Brekel MW, Stel HV, Castelijns JA, Croll GJ, Snow GB. Lymph node staging in patients with clinically negative neck examinations by ultrasound and ultrasound-guided aspiration cytology. *Am J Surg* 1991;162:362–366.

27. Gherardi G, Marveggio C. Immunocytochemistry in head and neck aspirates: Diagnostic applications on direct smears in 16 problematic cases. *Acta Cytol* 1992;36:687–696.

28. Domagala W, Bedner E, Chosia M, et al. Keratin-positive reticulum cells in fine needle aspirates and touch imprints of hyperplastic lymph nodes. A possible pitfall in the immunocytochemical diagnosis of metastatic carcinoma. *Acta Cytol* 1992;36: 241–245.

29. Soderstrom N. The free cytoplasmic fragments of lymphoglandular tissue (lymphoglandular bodies):

A preliminary presentation. *Scand J Haematd* 1968; 5:138–152.

30. Flanders E, Kornstein MJ, Wakely PE Jr., Kardos TF, Frable WJ. Lymphoglandular bodies in fine-needle aspiration cytology smears. *Am J Clin Pathol* 1993;99:566–599.

31. Pilotti S, DiPalma S, Alasio L, Bartoli C, Rilke F. Diagnostic assessment of enlarged superficial lymph nodes by fine needle aspiration. *Acta Cytol* 1993; 37:853–866.

32. Friedman M, Forgione H, Shanbhag V. Needle aspiration of metastatic melanoma. *Acta Cytol* 1980; 24:7–15.

33. Qizilbash AH, Young JEM. *Guides to clinical aspiration biopsy. Head and neck.* New York: Igaku-Shoin, 1988, pp. 190–195.

34. Duesenbery D, Jones DB, Sapp KW, Lemons FM. Cytologic findings in the sarcomatoid variant of large cell anaplastic (Ki-1) lymphoma. A case report. *Acta Cytol* 1993;37:508–514.

35. Tani E, Lowhagen T, Nasiell K, Ost A, et al. Fine needle aspiration cytology and immunocytochemistry of large cell lymphomas expressing the Ki-1 antigen. *Acta Cytol* 1989;33:359–362.

36. Feldman PS, Covell JL, Kardos TF. *Fine needle aspiration cytology. Lymph node, thyroid, and salivary gland.* Chicago: ASCP Press, 1989, pp. 17,29,30.

37. Koss LG, Woyke S, Olszewski W. *Aspiration biopsy. Cytologic interpretation and histologic basis,* 2nd ed. New York: Igaku-Shoin, 1992, p. 247.

38. Grenko RT, Shabb WS. Metastatic nasopharyngeal carcinoma: Cytologic features of 16 cases. *Diagn Cytopathol* 1991;7:562–566.

39. Lopes-Cardozo P. *Atlas of clinical cytology.* Philadelphia: J.B. Lippincott Co., 1976, pp. 512,516.

40. Suen KC. *Guides to clinical aspiration biopsy. Retroperitoneum and intestine,* 2nd ed. New York: Igaku-Shoin, 1994, p. 253,260.

41. Limjoco JMT, Brooks JJ, Alavi JB. Signet-ring cell lymphoma. Report of a case diagnosed by fine needle aspiration cytology. *Acta Cytol* 1991;35:281–284.

42. Enzinger FM, Weiss SW. *Soft tissue tumors.* St. Louis; C.V. Mosby Co., 1995, pp. 572,781.

43. Kardos TF, Vinson JH, Behm FG, et al. Hodgkin's disease: Diagnosis by fine-needle aspiration biopsy. Analysis of cytologic criteria from a selected series. *Am J Clin Pathol* 1986;86:286–291.

44. Chernoff WG, Lampe HB, Cramer H, Banerjee D. The potential clinical impact of the fine needle aspiration/flow cytometric diagnosis of malignant lymphoma. *J Otolaryngol* 1992;1:1–15.

45. Oertel J, Oertel B, Lobeck H, Huhn D. Cytologic and immunocytologic studies of peripheral T-cell lymphomas. *Acta Cytol* 1991;35:285–293.

46. Katz RL, Hirsch-Ginsberg C, Childs C, Dekmezian R, Fanning T, Ordonez N, Cabanillas F, Sneige N. The role of gene rearrangements for antigen receptors in the diagnosis of lymphoma obtained by fine-needle aspiration: A study of 63 cases with concomitant immunophenotyping. *Am J Clin Path* 1991;96:479–490.

47. Lubinski J, Chosia M, Huebner K. Molecular genetic analysis in the diagnosis of lymphoma in fine needle aspiration biopsies: I, Lymphomas versus benign lymphoproliferative disorders. *Acta Cytol* 1988;10: 391–398.

48. Lubinski J, Chosia M, Huebner K. Molecular genetic analysis in the diagnosis of lymphoma in fine needle aspiration biopsies: II, Lymphomas versus non-lymphoid malignant tumors. *Acta Cytol* 1988;10: 399–404.

49. Lubinski J, Chosia M, Kotanska K, Huebner K. Genotypic analysis of DNA isolated from fine needle aspiration biopsies. *Acta Cytol* 1988;10:383–390.

50. Shabb N, Katz R, Ordonez N, Goodacre A, Hirsch-Ginsberg C, El-Naggar A. Fine-needle aspiration evaluation of lymphoproliferative lesions in human immunodeficiency virus-positive patients: A multiparameter approach. *Cancer* 1991;67:1008–1018.

51. Williams ME, Frierson HR Jr., Tabbarah S, et al. Fine-needle aspiration of non-Hodgkin's lymphoma. Southern blot analysis for antigen receptor, *bcl-2,* and *cmyc* gene rearrangements. *Am J Clin Pathol* 1990;93:754–759.

52. Carter TR, Feldman PS, Innes DJ Jr., et al. The role of fine needle aspiration cytology in the diagnosis of lymphoma. *Acta Cytol* 1988;32:848–853.

53. Sneige N, Dekmezian RH, Kat RL, et al. Morphologic and immunocytochemical evaluation of 220 fine needle aspirates of malignant lymphoma and lymphoid hyperplasia. *Acta Cytol* 1990;34:311–322.

54. Cartagena N, Katz RL, Hirsch-Ginsberg C, et al. Accuracy of diagnosis of malignant lymphoma by combining fine-needle aspiration cytomorphology with immunocytochemistry and in selected cases, Southern blotting of aspiration cells: A tissue-controlled study of 86 patients. *Diagn Cytopathol* 1992;8:456–464.

55. Kardos TF, Kornstein MJ, Frable WJ. Cytology and immunocytology of infectious mononucleosis in fine needle aspirates of lymph nodes. *Acta Cytol* 1988;32:722–726.

56. Das DK, Gupta SK, Pathak IC, et al. Burkitt-type lymphoma. Diagnosis by fine needle aspiration cytology. *Acta Cytol* 1987;31:1–7.

57. Das DK, Gupta SK, Datta BN, et al. Diagnosis of Hodgkin's disease and its subtypes. Scope and limitations of fine needle aspiration cytology. *Acta Cytol* 1990;34:329–336.

58. Friedman M, Kim U, Shimaoka K, et al. Appraisal of aspiration cytology in management of Hodgkin's disease. *Cancer* 1980;45:1653–1663.

59. Greenberg ML, Cartwright L, McDonald DA. Histiocytic necrotizing lymphadenitis (Kikuchi's disease): Cytologic diagnosis by fine-needle biopsy. *Diagn Cytopathol* 1993;9:444–447.

60. Hsueh E-J, Ko W-S, Hwang W-S, Yam LT. Fine-needle aspiration of histiocytic necrotizing lymphadenitis (Kikuchi's disease). *Diagn Cytopathol* 1993; 9:448–452.

61. Tani EM, Christensson B, Porwit A, Skoog L. Immunocytochemical analysis and cytomorphologic diagnosis on fine needle aspirates of lymphoproliferative disease. *Acta Cytol* 1988;32:209–215.

62. O'Dowd GJ, Frable WJ, Behm FG. Fine needle aspiration biopsy of lymph node hyperplasia. Diagnostic significance of lymphohistiocytic aggregates. *Acta Cytol* 1985;29:554–558.

63. Stani J. Cytologic diagnosis of reactive lymphadenopathy in fine needle aspiration biopsy specimens. *Acta Cytol* 1987;31:8–13.

64. Oshima K, Tani E, Masuda Y, Skoog L, Kikuchi M. Fine needle aspiration cytology of high grade T-cell lymphomas in human T-lymphotrophic virus type 1 carriers. *Cytopathology* 1992;3:365–372.

65. True L (ed.). *Atlas of diagnostic immunohistopathology.* Philadelphia: J.B. Lippincott Co., 1990.

66. Katz RL. Cytologic diagnosis of leukemia and lymphoma. Values and limitations. *Clin Lab Med* 1991; 11:469–499.

67. Oertel J, Oertel B, Kastner M, Lobeck H, Huhn D. The value of immunocytochemical staining of lymph node aspirates in diagnostic cytology. *Brit J Haematol* 1988;79:307–316.

68. Moriarty AT, Wiersema L, Snyder W, Kotylo PK, McCloskey DW. Immunophenotyping of cytologic specimens by flow cytometry. *Diagn Cytopathol* 1993; 9:252–258.

69. Levitt S, Cheng L, DuPuis MH, Layfield LJ. Fine needle aspiration diagnosis of malignant lymphoma with confirmation by immunoperoxidase staining. *Am J Clin Pathol* 1985;29:895–902.

70. Vick WW, Tello JW, Wikstrand CJ, et al. Application of a panel of antiganglioside monoclonal antibodies to cytologic specimens. *Acta Cytol* 1992; 36:697–705.

71. Patt BS, Schaefer SD, Vuitch F. Role of fine-needle aspiration in the evaluation of neck masses (review). *Med Clin North Am* 1993;77:611–623.

72. Ramzy I, Rone R, Schultenover SJ, Buhaug J. Lymph node aspiration biopsy: Diagnostic reliability and limitations—an analysis of 350 cases. *Diagn Cytopathol* 1985;1:39–45.

73. Davies JD, Webb AJ. Segmental lymph-node infarction after fine-needle aspiration. *J Clin Pathol* 1982;35:855–857.

74. Behm FG, O'Dowd GJ, Frable WJ. Fine-needle aspiration effects on benign lymph node histology *Am J Clin Pathol* 1984;82:195–198.

75. Dekmezian RH, Sneige N, Katz RL. The effect of fine needle aspiration on lymph node morphology in lymphoproliferative disorders. *Acta Cytol* 1989; 33:732–733.

76. Tsang WYW, Chan JKC. Spectrum of morphologic changes in lymph nodes attributable to fine needle aspiration. *Hum Pathol* 1992;23:562–565.

Chapter

5

Skin and Soft Tissue

This chapter discusses not only superficial skin nodules but also palpable tumors of the deep dermis and subcutaneous tissue. FNAB is an obvious choice as a diagnostic procedure for masses of the skin and soft tissue, especially of the head and neck. Many of these are benign neoplasms whose diagnosis is relatively straightforward on aspiration cytology. Yet FNAB is underutilized as an accurate diagnostic procedure for superficial dermal masses. Reasons for the limited use of FNAB include: (1) patients with these lesions often present to dermatologists who are trained in punch- and shave-biopsy techniques rather than FNAB; (2) many of these diagnoses require histologic assessment for definitive identification; and (3) excisional biopsy of skin nodules requires only a small amount of anesthesia and has minimal complications.

TECHNIQUE

FNAB of skin and subcutaneous nodules is similar to FNAB of other body sites. For the very superficial lesions, the fine needle biopsy without aspiration technique, reviewed in Chapter 1, may be more suitable than the use of the somewhat cumbersome aspiration syringe and holder. For well-demarcated, raised skin nodules, it may also be useful to bend the needle tip slightly, so that it can enter the nodule parallel or oblique to the skin surface (Figure 5.1). This allows sampling of the mass without excessive bleeding or penetration of the underlying normal structures, which can obscure the diagnosis. An important parameter to consider prior to aspiration is the selection of proper needle gauge. Superficial nodules are often effortlessly sampled using 23-gauge and 25-gauge needles. While less pain or discomfort and bleeding occur when these smaller gauge needles are used, the needles may not easily penetrate thick skin or scar tissue. For this reason, 22-gauge needles, which have more rigid walls, should be considered for hard or sclerotic masses. Palpation of the nodule prior to aspiration will usually provide sufficient information to select the appropriate needle gauge.

SUPERFICIAL LESIONS

Few would argue that FNAB is not particularly useful in diagnosis of melanocytic, inflammatory, and other dermatologic diseases that require the pattern of histo-architecture for accurate diagnosis. However, FNAB can be very useful in the evaluation of superficial nodules in patients with a history of malignancy.

Although the incidence of dermal metastases from internal malignancies is small (0.7% to 4.4%), the presence of dermal nodules in patients with known cancer is worrisome for the presence of advanced disease.[1–5] Lung and squamous cell carcinoma of the oral cavity in men and breast and ovary in women represent the most common primaries that will metastasize to the skin and subcutaneous region. Other primaries common to both men and women include colon carcinoma, malignant melanoma, and malignant lymphoma. FNAB of these superficial dermal nodules represents a rapid and accurate method for the detection of metastatic disease. The head and neck region followed by anterior chest wall and abdomen are frequent sites for cutaneous metastases. In the majority of cases, patients will be older, at least in their fifth decade, and have a history of a previous primary malignancy. Nodules may be firm, fixed or mobile, single or multiple. They will rarely show signs of inflammation or ulceration.[5] Aspiration cytology will reveal cells that meet the criteria for malignancy. Often

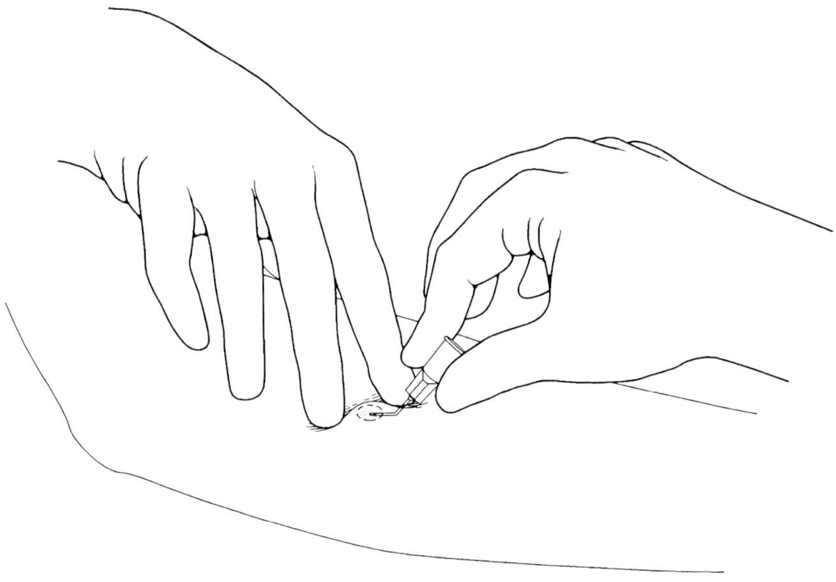

FIGURE 5.1 "Bent tip" technique for FNAB of skin nodules. The needle should enter the skin in a horizontal plane.

these cells will have the same cytomorphology as the primary. If previous histopathology of the original primary is available, it can be reviewed concurrently with the aspiration cytology. In most cases, FNAB is used as confirmation of the spread of disease and in many cases no further biopsy/surgical intervention need be attempted.

Dissemination of malignant cells can occur by hematogenous, lymphatic, or direct spread following interventional procedures (Table 5.1). It is beyond the scope of this book to discuss the cytomorphology of all the cancers that have been documented to metastasize to the skin and subcutaneous tissue.

There are many examples of primary cutaneous lesions, both nonneoplastic and neoplastic, that have been encountered with FNAB. Several of the comprehensive aspiration cytology texts contain short discussions of FNAB of cutaneous, epidermal, and dermal masses, ranging from cysts and adenexal lesions to basal and squamous carcinomas.[6–9] The primary difficulty in FNAB diagnosis of cutaneous lesions is due to (1) the tremendous overlap of cytologic features and (2) the need for architecture for specific diagnosis. Basaloid and squamous cells represent the primary cell type in the vast majority of primary dermal lesions sampled by FNAB. The difficulty in diagnosis of these lesions can be illustrated by a list of the differential diagnoses of squamous-basal cell processes (Table 5.2). This cytologic overlap results in cautious, often nonspecific, diagnoses or lists of differential diagnoses. This is surprising because studies have shown that benign and malignant lesions can be accurately categorized and often specific diagnoses made using FNAB, especially if careful attention is paid to clinical data and physical examination.[10]

TABLE 5.1 Metastatic Tumor Nodules: Route of Dissemination

Direct spread
Invasion of skin from underlying tumor
Extra nodal extension of tumor
Postoperative implantation of tumor in incisions
Tumor implantation in drainage or paracentesis wounds
Tumor implantation in needle (large bore only) biopsy tracts
Hematologic and Lymphatic spread
Dermal lymphatic spread of breast, lung carcinomas
Lymphoma, disseminated
Hematologic spread from distant primaries (renal, GI)
Leukemic infiltrates (chloromas)

TABLE 5.2 Differential Diagnoses: Primary Cutaneous Lesions

Basaloid/Squamous Lesions
Epithelial inclusion cyst
Pilomatrixoma
Tricholemmal cyst
Branchial cleft cyst
Adenexal tumors
Merkel-cell carcinoma
Basal cell carcinoma ± squamous features
Squamous cell carcinoma ± basaloid features
Salivary gland tumors monomorphic adenoma adenoid cystic carcinoma

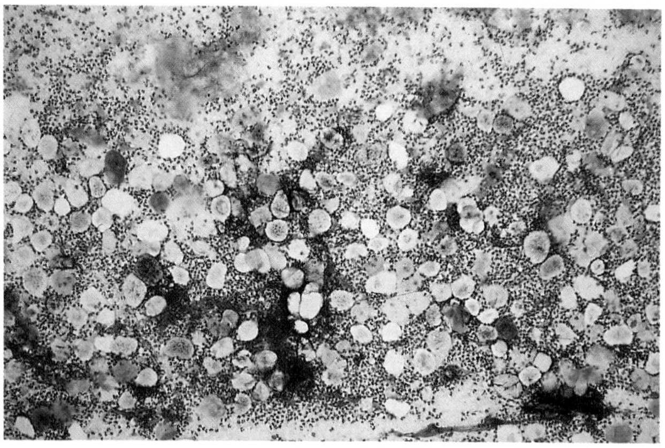

A

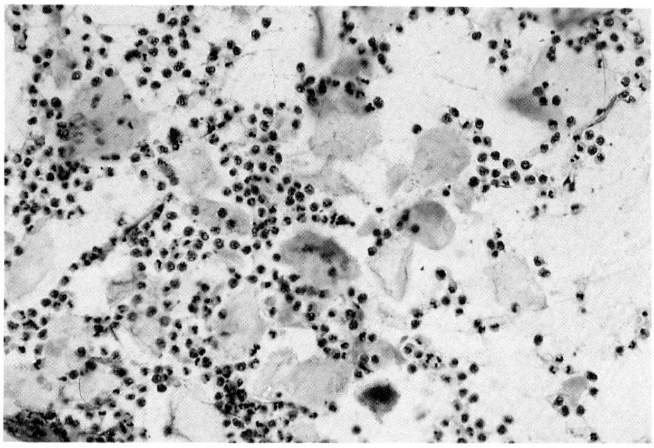

B

FIGURE 5.2 Epidermal inclusion cyst. Numerous benign squamous cells, many of which are anucleate (ghost) cells. Acute inflammatory cells are scattered throughout. (A) The Diff-Quik® stain accentuates ghost or anucleate squamous cells. Diff-Quik® 200×. (B) Varying degrees of orangeophilia indicate the squamous origin of this cyst. Papanicolaou 400×.

CYSTS

Epidermal Inclusion and Sebaceous Cysts

The epidermal inclusion cyst (EIC) followed closely by the sebaceous cyst represent two of the most common nonneoplastic dermal nodules sampled. The aspirated material from both lesions, when expressed from the needle, has a characteristic foul smell and cheesy-white appearance. This thick material is often difficult to smear and may result in very thick, unreadable smears. This may be avoided by expelling all of the aspirated material on one slide and then apportioning very small, manageable portions of this sample to clean slides for smearing. Smears from EIC reveal numerous anucleate and obviously benign squamous cells with scattered acute inflammatory cells (Figure 5.2). While a rapid diagnosis of EIC is usually made, rupture of the EIC results in an intense inflammatory response. In addition to the influx of acute inflammatory cells, predominantly neutrophils, epithelial repair and a foreign body giant-cell reaction may occur. The resultant squamous cell nuclear atypia may make it difficult to differentiate this lesion from squamous cell carcinoma (Figure 5.3).[11] Key cytologic differences include a relatively normal or slightly increased nuclear to cytoplasmic ratio and less nuclear hyperchromasia in the EIC.

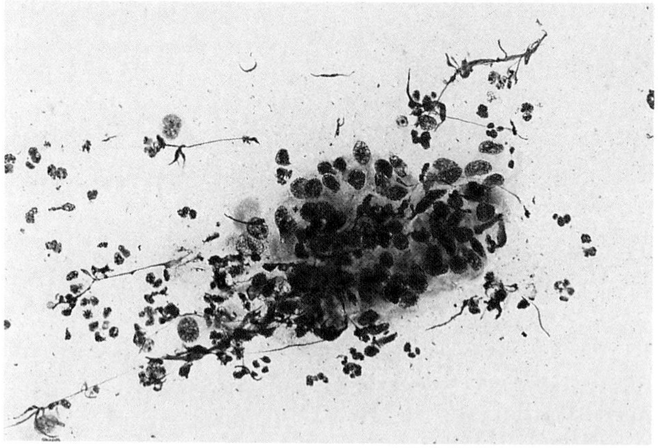

FIGURE 5.3 Epidermal inclusion cyst. An aggregate of immature squamous cells showing some variation in nuclear size and shape. The cells are surrounded by acute inflammatory exudate, which was heavily represented in other portions of the smear and accompanied large numbers of mature squamous cells. Diff-Quik® 400×.

EPIDERMAL INCLUSION CYST (EPIDERMOID CYST)—CYTOLOGIC FEATURES

High cellularity and abundant material

Anucleated squamous cells
- **–Ghost cells**
- **–Orangeophilic (Pap)/dense purple (DQ)**

Nucleate squamous cells
- **–Pyknotic nuclei**

Keratin debris

Acute inflammatory cells

Evidence of epithelial repair
- **–**If EIC is ruptured, then increased numbers of acute inflammatory cells and multinucleated giant cells with engulfed keratin debris are seen.**

SEBACEOUS CYST—CYTOLOGIC FEATURES

High cellularity and abundant material

Sebaceous cells
- **–Large cells**
- **–Vacuolated (foamy) cytoplasm**
  - **–Histiocytic appearance**

Acute inflammatory cells

Pilomatrixoma

Pilomatrixoma (pilomatricoma or calcifying epithelioma of Malherbe) often presents as a slow-growing, palpable, firm mass in the deep dermis or subcutaneous region of the face, neck, or upper extremities. The overlying skin may be normal in appearance or pigmented. Although more common in young people, it may also present as an incidental finding in the workup of patients with head and neck carcinoma. Several articles have delineated the cytologic criteria necessary for diagnosis: basaloid cells, ghost cells, foreign body giant-cell response, and calcific debris (Figures. 5.4 and 5.5).[12–16] Aspiration of these firm masses is sometimes difficult due to the presence of this calcific debris. Thin, flexible 25-gauge needles may obtain limited if any material; indeed, this gauge needle has been bent during FNAB of pilomatrixoma. The "larger" fine needles, that is, 22-gauge, will usually be able to obtain an adequate sample. As difficult as it can be to obtain a specimen from this tumor, it is equally difficult at times to produce quality smears. In addition to very thick smears, crystalline debris will not smoothly compress and results in long streaks/scratches during smearing.

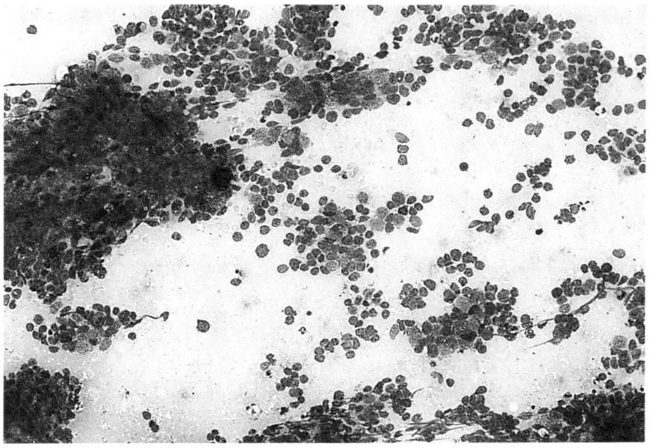

FIGURE 5.4 Pilomatrixoma. Cellular aspirate with sheets of small, round anaplastic-looking cells. The immediate reaction to a smear with this pattern is metastatic small-cell carcinoma or a small-round-cell tumor of childhood, depending on clinical history. Diff-Quik® 250×.

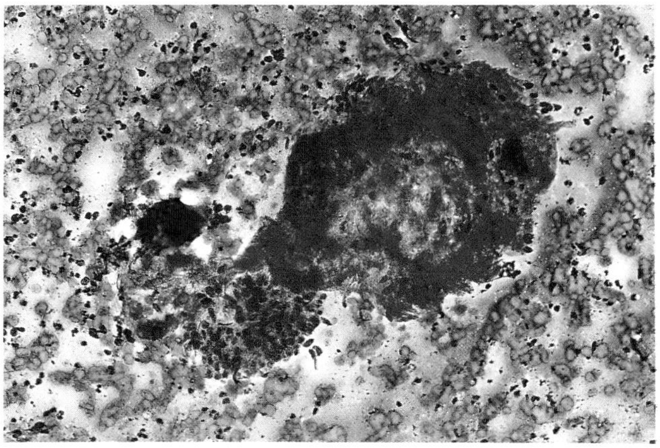

FIGURE 5.5 Pilomatrixoma. Another field from the case above demonstrating the more differentiated squamous cells of the hair matrix. These cells are necrotic and appear as ghosts in a necrotic background. Also present are the small, undifferentiated-appearing round cells, both singly and in groups. Diff-Quik® 250×.

PILOMATRIXOMA—CYTOLOGIC FEATURES

High cellularity and abundant material

Small basaloid cells
- **–Sheets, clusters, and fragments**
- **–Scant cytoplasm**
- **–Uniform, hyperchromatic nuclei**
- **–Finely granular chromatin**
- **–Distinct nucleoli**

Squamous cells
- **–Anucleate and nucleate with pyknotic nuclei**
- **–Ghost cells: pale eosinophilic anucleate squames (Papanicolaou)**

Calcific debris
- **–Glassy blue (DQ)**
- **–Orangeophilic (Pap)**

Multinucleated foreign body giant cells

Epidermal Appendage and Adenexal Tumors

The classification of tumors from the various adenexal structures is difficult even when one is confronted with an excisional biopsy of the complete lesion. As discussed above, the criteria for accurate cytodiagnosis of pilomatrixoma have been described; however, there are only scattered case reports in the literature that illustrate the cytologic features of other cutaneous adenexal tumors. Entities that have been diagnosed by FNAB include chondroid syringoma, syringocystadenoma papilliferum,[17–19] and malignant spiradenoma.[20] The chondroid syringoma has the same cytologic features as benign mixed tumor of salivary glands.

Basal Cell Carcinoma

Basal cell carcinoma (BCC) is the most frequently occurring carcinoma of the skin, occurring on sun-exposed surfaces, especially the face and extremities. Nodules may appear waxy with demarcated, raised borders. They can also be ulcerated and are rarely pigmented. Because of the excellent prognosis if BCC is completely excised, patients with BCC are frequently diagnosed and treated with shave or

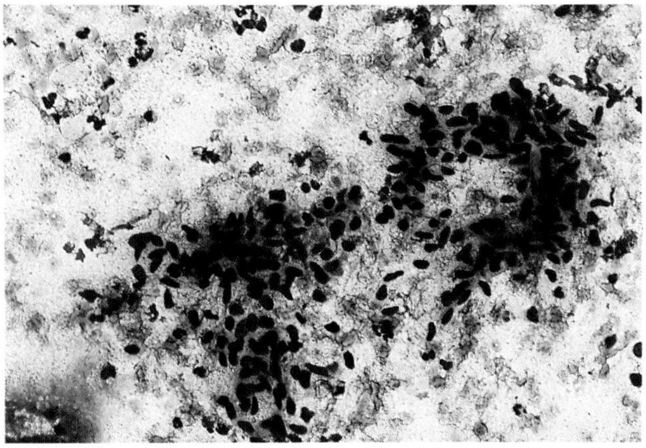

FIGURE 5.6 Basal cell carcinoma. Clusters of small dark cells with smooth peripheral border and some peripheral palisading. Nuclear edges are smooth and there is evidence of peripheral palisading. Some branching of these tight cell fragments is seen reflecting the irregular infiltrative pattern of some basal cell carcinomas. Diff-Quik® 400×.

excisional biopsies by dermatologists and plastic surgeons. The characteristic appearance of BCC and the inclination for histologic confirmation of tumor-free margins make FNAB a less practical option for many. However, FNAB can be used successfully to demonstrate multifocal and recurrent BCC. As with the more common skin nodules, the criteria for diagnosis have been identified and center around the cytomorphology of the basaloid cell.[9,10,21,22]

Cytologically, the most common type of BCC is composed predominantly of fragments of small basal cells that palisade at the edge of the fragments (Figures 5.6 and 5.7). Centrally, there is a somewhat haphazard arrangement of these cells with nuclear crowding and overlapping. Other subtypes of BCC can show focal squamous differentiation (keratotic) that includes keratin formation and vesicular nuclei with prominent nucleoli. This variation of BCC can result in a reluctance to classify the tumor as BCC and reliance on a more nonspecific diagnosis that suggests the possibility of BCC, basosquamous carcinoma, or squamous carcinoma with basaloid features. Rarely, pigmented BCC can occur. Coarse melanin granules are found within the cytoplasm of the neoplastic cells or melanophages. Because of this, malignant melanoma might be a consideration. History and immunocytochemistry can be useful adjuncts in the differential diagnosis. Adenoid BCC is also a rare variant. Small foci of larger cells arranged in glandular structures are seen on aspiration cytology.

BASAL CELL CARCINOMA—CYTOLOGIC FEATURES

Moderate cellularity

Basal cells
- **–Tight clusters and fragments**
- **–Dispersed, single cells**
- **–Peripheral palisading and central overlapping/crowding**
- **–Oval, hyperchromatic nuclei**
- **–Finely granular chromatin**
- **–Absent nucleoli**

***Keratinization and foci of squamoid differentiation (keratotic variant)**

***Melanin pigment and melanophages (rare variant)**

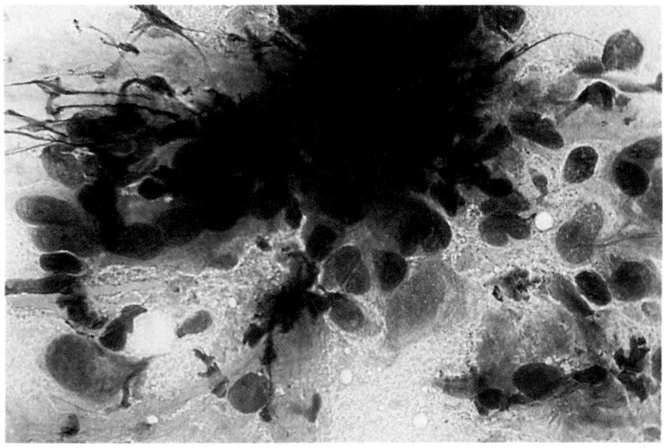

FIGURE 5.7 Basal cell carcinoma. Fragment of BCC with small basaloid cells with high nuclear to cytoplasmic ratio, bland chromatin, and smooth nuclear membranes. Diff-Quik® 1000×.

Merkel-Cell Carcinoma (Primary Neuroendocrine Carcinoma of the Skin)

Merkel-cell carcinoma (MCC), primarily a dermal tumor in older individuals, can resemble BCC. Because its origin is neuroendocrine, there are subtle cytologic clues.[23–28] FNAB smears show dispersed, discohesive, small, hyperchromatic, uniform cells that may line up in a single file ("Indian" filing) and may show pseudorosettes and/or microacinar formations. Nuclei tend to be larger and have granular chromatin compared to those found in BCC (Figure 5.8). Nuclear molding and mitoses can also be seen. As in small-cell carcinoma of the lung, the cytoplasm of the Merkel cells tends to be very fragile and easily stripped during smearing. This results in a background of cytoplasmic contents resembling granular necrotic debris.[23] Scattered naked nuclei are easily identified.

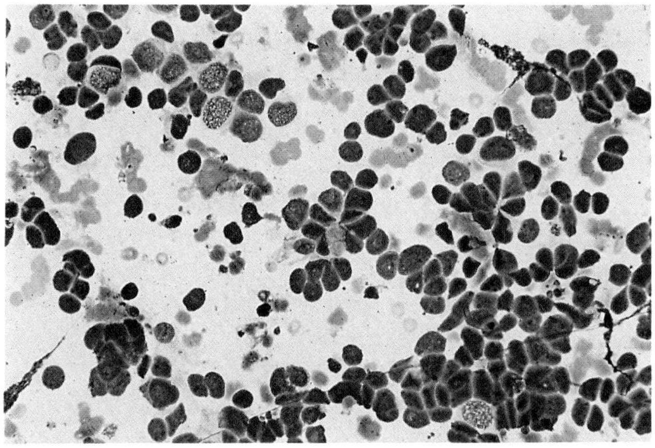

FIGURE 5.8 Merkel-cell carcinoma. Cellular aspirate with irregular sheets and dissociated small cells. Note striking nuclear molding and formation of pseudorosettes (center of the illustration). Necrosis can produce the two-cell pattern of very small and relatively larger cells as seen with metastatic small-cell carcinoma of the lung. The nuclear chromatin appears very powdery rather than smudged as in small-cell carcinomas of the lung. Nucleoli are inconspicuous. Note small metachromatic button (intermediate filaments) in the center of the figure. Diff-Quik® 400×.

MERKEL–CELL CARCINOMA—CYTOLOGIC FEATURES

High cellularity

Discohesive, monomorphic cells
- **–Indian filing, pseudorosette, microacinar formations**
- **–Uniform, round to oval**
- **–Scant cytoplasm**
- **–Medium sized, hyperchromatic nuclei**
- **–Nuclear molding**

Background debris and naked nuclei

Mitoses

Unfortunately, the differential diagnosis for MCC is extensive and includes not only BCC but metastatic small-cell carcinomas and carcinoids, poorly differentiated carcinomas, adenexal skin carcinomas, melanomas, and high-grade lymphomas. Immunocytochemistry can differentiate neuroendocrine carcinomas from BCC, melanoma, and lymphoproliferative lesions (Table 5.3). Cytokeratin, chromogranin, and neuron-specific endase (NSE) positivity are typical of neuroendocrine tumors, both primary and metastatic. Cytokeratin positivity in Merkel-cell carcinoma has been reported to have a distinctive paranuclear dotlike staining pattern. Domgala demonstrated these spherical, eosinophilic, perinuclear cytoplasmic inclusions to be intermediate filaments, termed *IF buttons* (Figure 5.9).[26,27] Because of the similarity among neuroendocrine

TABLE 5.3 Immunocytochemistry in the Differential Diagnosis of Small (Basal)-Cell Tumors

Tumor	*CK*	*VIM*	*LCA*	*S-100*	*HMB 45*	*NSE*	*CG*
SCC	+	–	–	–	–	–	–
BCC	+	–	–	–	–	+	+
Melanoma	±	+	–	+	+	–	–
NHL	–	±*	+	–	–	–	–
MCC	+†	–	–	–	–	+	+
SmCC	+	±	–	–	–	+	+
Carcinoid	+	–	–	–	–	±	±

Immunochemistry: CK, cytokeratin; VIM, vimentin; LCA, leukocyte common antigen; S-100 and HMB 45 neural/melanoma markers; NSE, neuron-specific enolase; CG, chromogranin tumors: SCC, squamous cell carcinoma; BCC, basal cell carcinoma; NHL, non-Hodgkin's lymphoma, MCC, Merkel-cell carcinoma; SmCC, Small-cell carcinoma, lung

*rare positivity in Burkitt's lymphoma

† IF buttons

carcinomas, differentiating primary cutaneous tumors from metastatic neoplasms is difficult and is based on clinical data and physical examination.

Squamous Cell Carcinoma

The differentiation between primary cutaneous squamous cell and metastatic squamous cell carcinoma (SCC) is sometimes very difficult on FNAB cytology alone. Obviously, history of a head and neck primary, especially of the oral cavity, is critical information. Although epidermal nodules do occur in primary SCC, the majority of these tumors are ulcerated with raised borders, therefore clinically obvious primaries. Generally, primary SCC will be well to

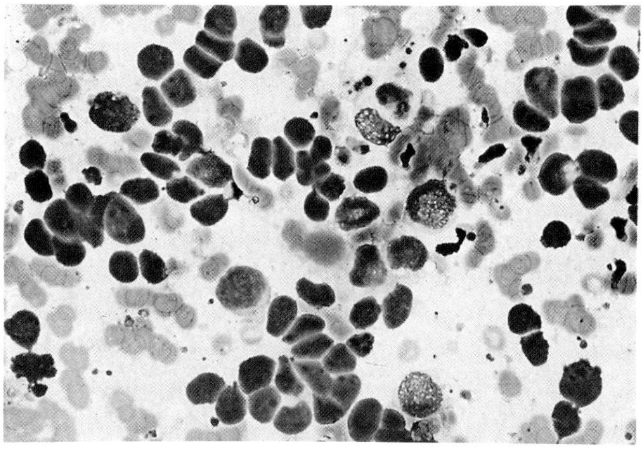

FIGURE 5.9 Merkel-cell carcinoma. Higher magnification to demonstrate two metachromatic IF buttons surrounded by small, undifferentiated tumor cells. Diff-Quik® 600×.

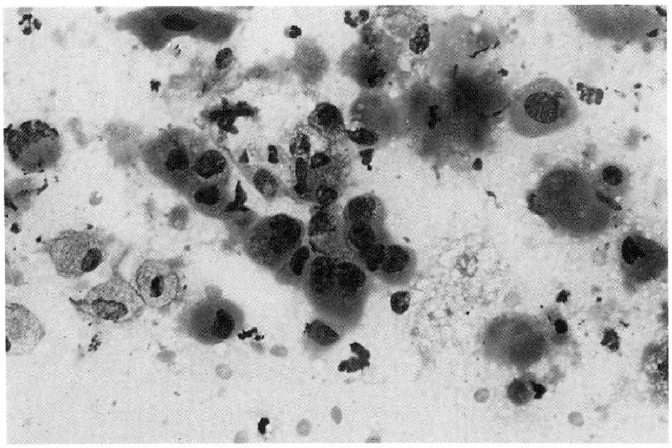

A

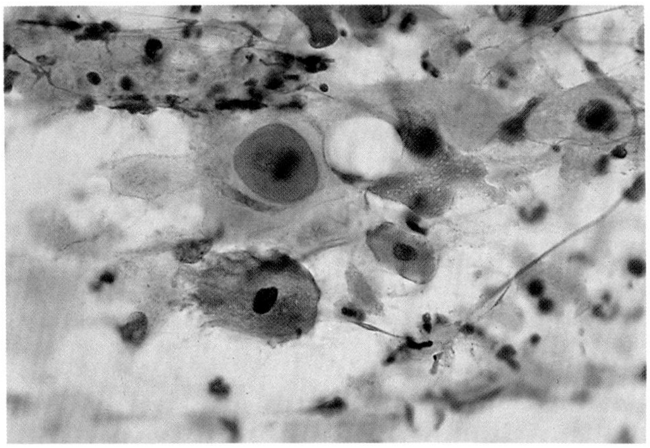

B

FIGURE 5.10 Well-differentiated squamous cell carcinoma. Squamous cells with high nuclear to cytoplasmic ratio in a background of cellular debris. (A) Dense, slate-blue cytoplasm that is characteristic of keratin on Diff-Quik® stain. Diff-Quik® 1000×. (B) Neoplastic keratinized squamous cells with pyknotic nuclei and orangeophilic cytoplasm. Papanicolaou stain 400×.

moderately differentiated, while metastatic tumors will be less differentiated. Metastatic SCC will more often be located in the deeper dermis or lymph nodes and be associated with necrosis. In either case, the neoplastic squamous cells have abundant cytoplasm, vesicular nuclei, and prominent nucleoli. While the detection of keratinization is facilitated using the Papanicolaou stain due to the intense orangeophilia, it can also be identified on Diff-Quik® as dense, slate-blue cytoplasm (Figure 5.10). FNAB smears of well-differentiated SCC show anucleate squames, squamous cells with pyknotic nuclei, pieces of keratinized cytoplasm, and cellular debris. Single bizarre cells are scattered throughout the smears, while smaller tumor cells tend to occur as irregular fragments. These fragments tend to be flat sheets showing a cobblestone pattern accentuated by dense cytoplasmic borders and intracellular bridges (Figure 5.11).

CUTANEOUS SQUAMOUS CELL CARCINOMA—CYTOLOGIC FEATURES

High Cellularity

Squamous cells
- **–Sheets and irregular fragments, single cells**
- **–Atypical/dyskeratotic cells**
- **–Keratinization ("pearls" and debris)**
- **–Vesicular nuclei**
- **–Prominent nucleoli**

Mitoses

Sebaceous Carcinoma

Sebaceous carcinoma, a fairly low-grade tumor except when it occurs in the ocular adenexa (Meibomian gland carcinoma), is infrequently encountered on FNAB. As its name implies, the predominant feature of

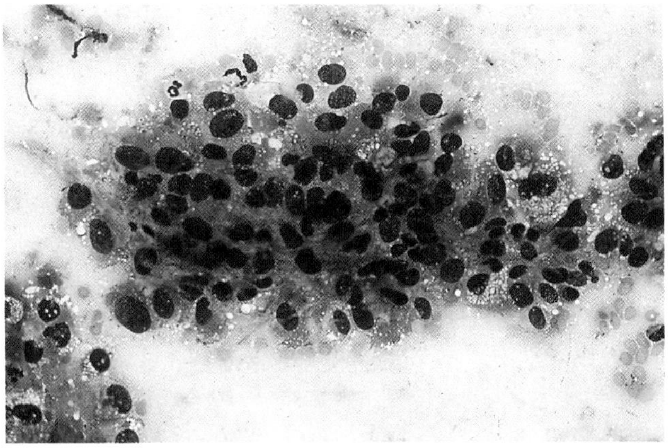

A

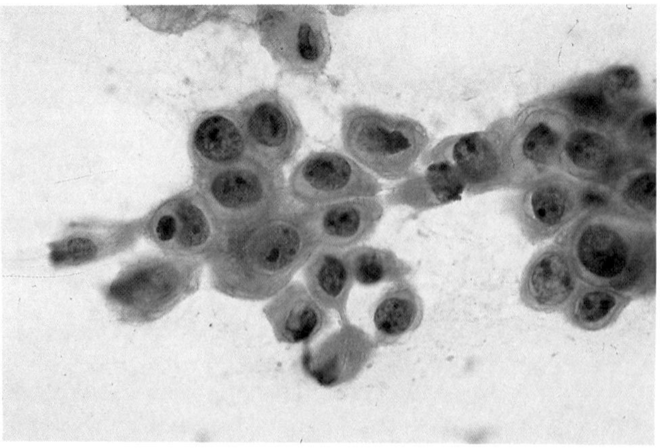

B

FIGURE 5.11 Moderately differentiated squamous cell carcinoma. (A) Flat sheet of carcinoma with regularly spaced nuclei, moderate amounts of cytoplasm. Diff-Quik® 400×. (B) Sheet of neoplastic squamous cells with dense cytoplasmic borders and fine intracellular bridges, vesicular nuclei, and prominent, sometimes multiple, nucleoli. Papanicolaou 1000×.

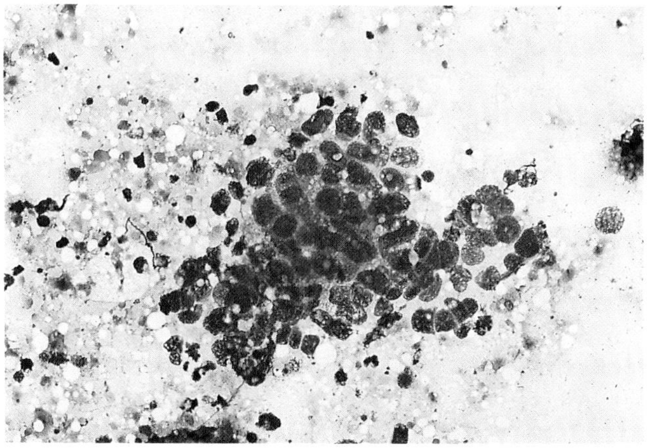

FIGURE 5.12 Sebaceous carcinoma. Undifferentiated loose cluster of malignant cells surrounded by necrosis. Note the microvesicular pattern of the cytoplasm, which is relatively clear where the cells are not crowded. This is a nonspecific feature but suggests a sebaceous carcinoma in the right clinical setting. Diff-Quik® 400×.

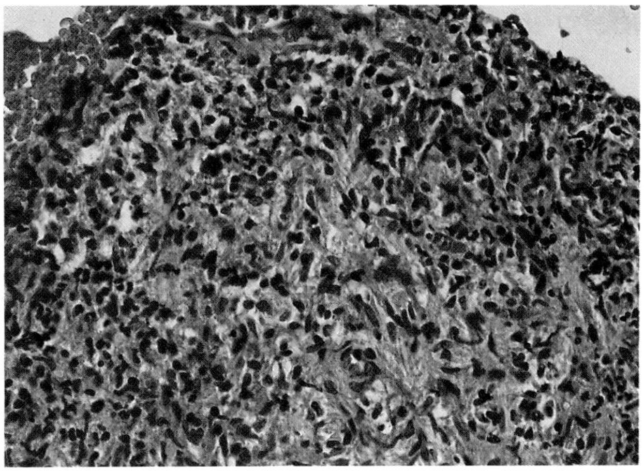

FIGURE 5.13 Kaposi's sarcoma. Cell block fragment with slit-like vascular spaces, fibroplasia, and some inflammation. The aspiration smears were nonspecific, demonstrating a few spindle cells and fat. The cell block is diagnostic only in the right clinical setting. Hematoxylin and eosin 400×.

this tumor is the neoplastic sebaceous cell.[29,30] Its distinction from the more frequent sebaceous cyst is based on nuclear features and mitotic rate. Smears show abundant lipid debris (Figure 5.12). One potential source for error in the classification of this tumor is its similarity to either metastatic breast carcinoma or renal cell carcinoma. Oil Red O stains of air-dried smears can suggest the presence of lipid.[29] PAS ± diastase can be used to identify glycogen. Estrogen/progesterone receptors may be useful in documenting breast carcinoma and are not entirely specific.

SEBACEOUS CARCINOMA—CYTOLOGIC FEATURES

Abundant material

Sebaceous cells
- **–Large cells in cohesive clusters**
- **–Abundant vacuolated (foamy) cytoplasm**
- **–Vesicular nuclei**
- **–Granular chromatin**
- **–Prominent nucleoli**

Mitoses

Necrotic debris
- **–Lipid and granular**

Vascular Neoplasms

As one would expect, the hallmark of vascular tumors is blood! It is very difficult to diagnose or subclassify these lesions based on cytology alone due to excessive blood and the limited number of cells obtained during FNAB. The major entities encountered as dermal masses include hemangioma, pyogenic granuloma, Kaposi's sarcoma, and angiosarcoma. Specific clues for differentiating among them are limited.[31–33] FNAB of pyogenic granuloma often results in loose fragments that show features of repair, including mitoses and capillary vessels surrounded by inflammatory cells. Aspirates of hemangiomas are scantily cellular with bland, spindle cells that have fragile cytoplasm. Neoplastic endothelial cells in aspirates from Kaposi's sarcoma (Figure 5.13) and angiosarcoma (Figure 5.14) are usually more plentiful with larger, more hyperchromatic nuclei. FNAB is perhaps most useful in the diagnosis of Kaposi's sarcoma in patients with cervical adenopathy.[31]

Malignant Melanoma

Most would agree that histologic examination of tissues is necessary for the initial diagnosis of melanocytic lesions, especially malignant melanoma (MM). However, if recurrence is suspected, diagnosis by FNAB is extremely accurate.[34–37] Both the cytologic and histologic features of malignant melanoma can mimic different lesions including anaplastic carcinoma, malignant lymphoma, and plasmacytoma, among others. Although on an individual basis there are no pathognomonic cytologic criteria, an accurate diagnosis of malignant melanoma can be made using a constellation of features. Woyke et al.[36] described four malignant cell types: epithelial cell, spindle cell, giant cell, and small-round cell. There is usually one predominant cell type, but other types can be present in variable amounts. The most common mixture is epithelial and spindle cell pattern. Although the association of melanin pigment with atypical cells is a strong clue to the diagnosis of MM, it is not consistently identified in smears even with the aid of electron microscopy and immunocytochemistry applied to the aspirate sample. The numerous cytologic features that can be seen with MM are listed below. Strong indicators for MM include highly cellular smears and smears with discohesive atypical cells that have intranuclear cytoplasmic inclusions (Figures. 5.15 and 5.16).

MALIGNANT MELANOMA—CYTOLOGIC FEATURES

High cellularity

Discohesive cells
- **–Epithelial, spindle, giant, small-round**

Cytoplasm
- **–Moderate to abundant**
- **–Pigment variable**
- **–Powder to cobalt blue (Diff-Quik®)**
- **–Golden brown (Papanicolaou)**

Nuclei
- **–Large**
- **–Fine to coarse chromatin**
- **–Binucleation (mirror-image cells)**
- **–Intranuclear cytoplasmic inclusions**

Nucleoli
- **–Variable number (1–3)**
- **–Often prominent**

Mitoses
- **–Atypical**

Pigment-laden macrophages

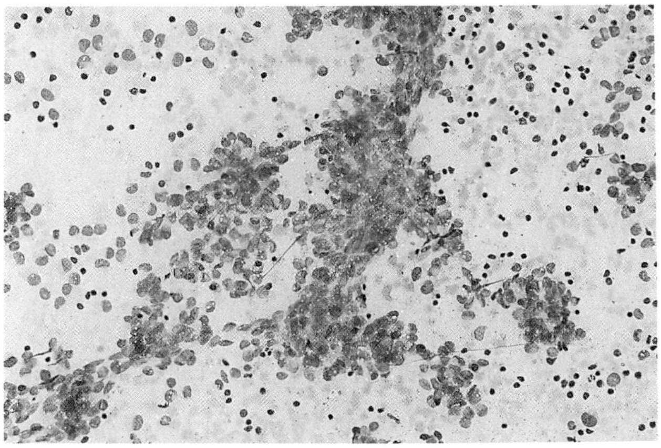
A

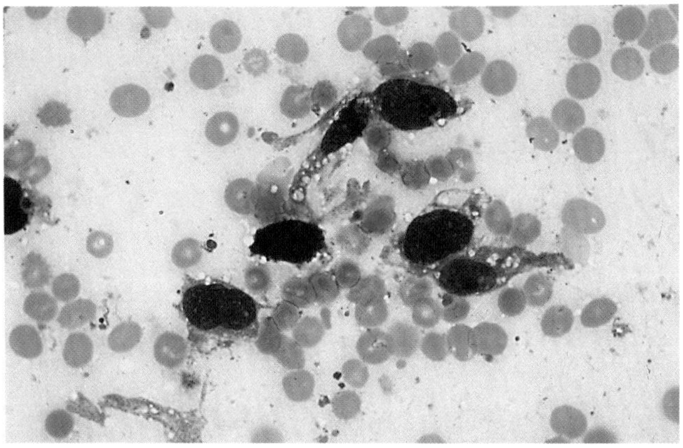
B

FIGURE 5.14 (A) Angiosarcoma. Cellular aspirate with tumor cells that have oval-shaped nuclei and irregular nuclear edges. Note the pattern of clustering and branching in some foci along a string of elongated cells. The pattern suggests a papillary tumor but without fibrovascular cores. The cell arrangement suggests the tufts of proliferating endothelial cells within small vascular spaces that is the pattern of angiosarcomas or cellular hemangioendotheliomas. Diff-Quik® 250×. (B) Angiosarcoma. Neoplastic endothelial cells with enlarged, hyperchromatic oval nuclei and fragile, elongated cytoplasmic processes in a background of blood. Diff-Quik® 1000×.

Primary Cutaneous Lymphoma

Cutaneous lymphoma may present as firm, multiple distinct nodules, elevated lesions, or plaques that range from pink to blue to brown. Aspiration cytology is often characteristic, with many discohesive, atypical lymphocytes present (Figure 5.17). Although benign lymphocytic infiltrations occur (pseudolymphoma), a monomorphic population of relatively immature lymphocytes on aspiration cytology should be thoroughly evaluated using immunocytochemistry and flow cytometry if adequate material is available. If insufficient cells are present for these ancillary studies, then a biopsy should be recommended. In contrast to cutaneous lymphoma, pseudolymphoma has small, mature lymphocytes with interspersed immunoblasts and stimulated lymphocytes.

Mycosis fungoides (MF) is another lymphoproliferative disorder that may be sampled by FNAB. Under the best of circumstances, MF, especially in its early stage, is difficult to diagnose. The presence of large convoluted (cerebriform) lymphocytes is suggestive. Identification of these cells as T lymphocytes is conclusive for lymphoproliferative processes such as MF or cutaneous peripheral T-cell lymphoma.

MALIGNANT LYMPHOMA—CYTOLOGIC FEATURES

High cellularity

Discohesive, monomorphic cells
- **–Thin rim of basophilic cytoplasm**
- **–Round nucleus**
  - **–Irregular membrane**
  - **–Folds and convolutions**
- **–Nucleoli**

Lymphoglandular bodies

Limited necrosis

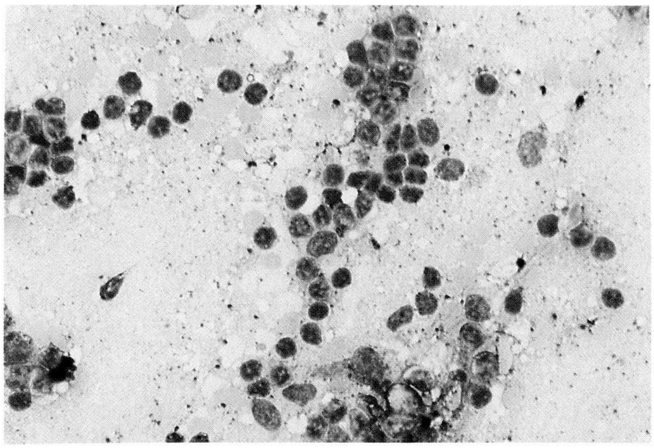

A

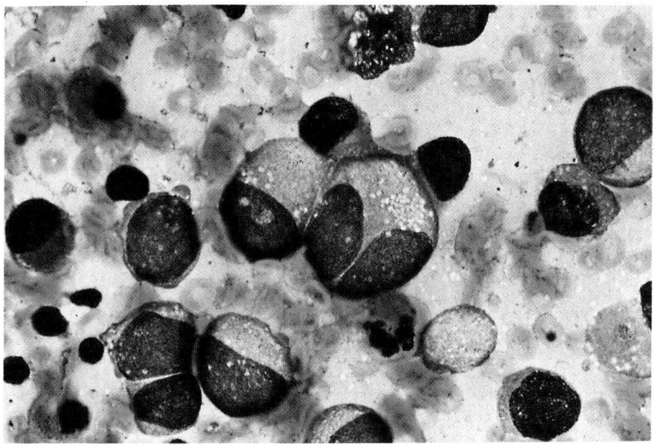

B

FIGURE 5.15 (A) Malignant melanoma. Cellular aspirate with tumor cells in small sheets with some nuclear molding. Nuclei have coarse chromatin pattern but in this example lack prominent nucleoli. Granules of black pigment can be seen in some of the cells and scattered in the background. Diff-Quik® 400×. (B) Malignant melanoma. Discohesive, pleomorphic cells with abundant, often vacuolated, cytoplasm. Binucleation (mirror-image nuclei) and pigment-laden macrophages are often present. Diff-Quik 1000×.

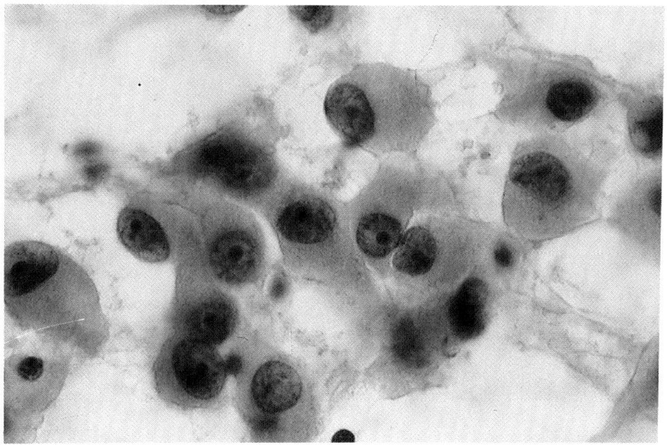

FIGURE 5.16 Malignant melanoma of parotid. Single malignant cells with eccentric position of the nucleus, prominent nucleoli. No pigment is present. Papanicolaou 1000×.

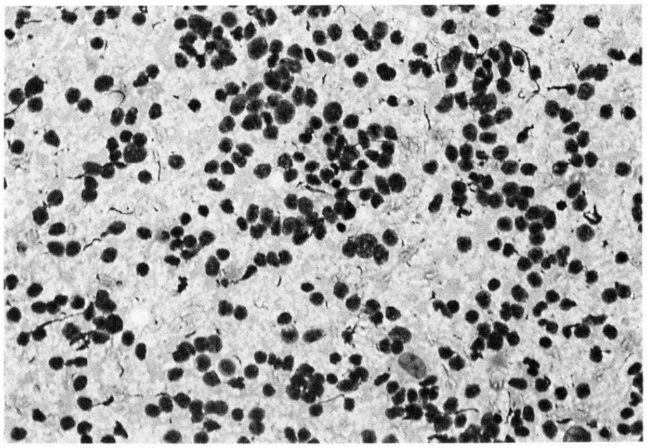

FIGURE 5.17 Primary cutaneous-mucosal lymphoma. Highly cellular smear with diffuse monotonous pattern of poorly differentiated cells. Small, round gray-staining structures in the background (lymphoglandular bodies) indicate this is lymphoid tissue. Note small clumping of the lymphoid cells, a smear pattern found in poorly differentiated lymphocytic lymphoma. This case proved to be of B-cell type by immunohistochemistry performed on cytospin preparations of the aspirate. Diff-Quik® 400×.

Benign lymphoproliferative disorders such as pseudolymphoma cutis do occur as skin nodules and as such may be sampled by FNAB.[38] In contrast to malignant lymphomas, the cytomorphology of this lesion is polymorphic with small and large lymphocytes, plasma cells, tingible body macrophages, and eosinophils. Based solely on cytomorphology, Hodgkin's disease may be a consideration. However, Reed-Sternberg cells and their variants will not be identified.

PSEUDOLYMPHOMA—CYTOLOGIC FEATURES

High cellularity

Discohesive cells

Heterogeneous population

Deep lesions

Nonneoplastic proliferations

Relatively few nonneoplastic processes that form mass lesions occur in the deep dermis. Unfortunately, when they do present there they are very difficult to categorize by cytomorphology alone. Chief among these problematic lesions are the fibrohistiocytic proliferations, which include granulation tissue, granulomatous inflammatory responses, and nodular fasciitis. All may arise due to acute or chronic trauma to the dermis or subcutis. Their primary cytologic features are compared in Table 5.4.

TABLE 5.4 Fibroblastic Proliferations—Cytologic Features

Cytologic Criteria	*Granulation Tissue*	*Granulomatous Inflammation*	*Fasciitis Nodular*
Cellularity	High	Variable	Moderate-High
Background	Inflammation(±) Blood	MNGC*	Inflammation(++) Blood
Predominant cell type	Fibroblast	Histiocyte (epithelioid)	Fibroblast
Pattern	Loose arrays Blood vessels Organized	Granulomas	Whorled Blood vessels Tissue culture
Cytoplasm	++−+++ Bipolar processes	++ Distinct borders	++−+++ Bipolar processes
Nuclei	Medium-large Pale, oval	Large Round, smooth	Medium to large Oval, plump
Nucleoli	Prominent	Present	Prominent
Mitoses	Yes, atypical	Rare	Yes, atypical

*MNGC, multinucleated giant cells

Granulation Tissue

Granulation tissue, predominantly a fibroblastic proliferation, can appear quite worrisome on FNAB cytology. Loose aggregates of plump fibroblasts associated with capillaries and small blood vessels are present with variable amounts of inflammation in a bloody background. Numerous mitoses, some atypical, in addition to large fibroblasts with large nuclei and prominent nucleoli, have resulted in false-positive diagnoses. Clues to this diagnosis are based on the pattern of spindle cell proliferation. Granulation tissue is often aspirated as large fragments of loosely arranged fibroblasts that are intimately associated with blood vessels such that they appear to be radiating out from the vessels. Numerous, scattered macrophages are identified in and around these fragments (Figures. 5.18 and 5.19). Overall, the cells composing these fragments appear organized into a coherent pattern of mesenchymal repair.

GRANULATION TISSUE—CYTOLOGIC FEATURES

Plump fibroblasts and histiocytes
- **–Loose, haphazard arrangement—often storiform**
- **–Large nuclei**
- **–Prominent nucleoli**

Capillaries and small vessels

Acute inflammatory cells in bloody background

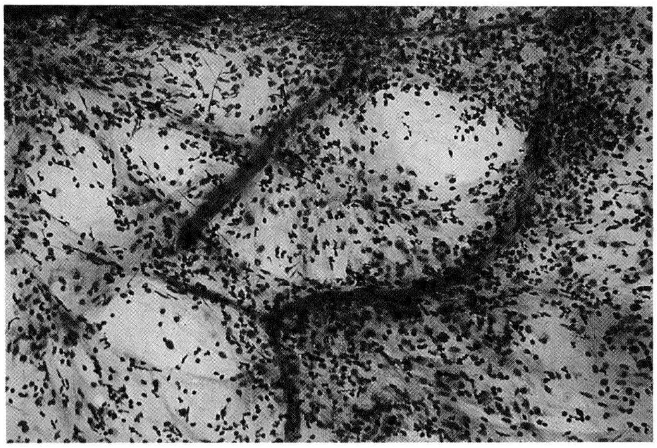

FIGURE 5.18 Granulation tissue. Highly cellular smear composed of loose aggregations of plump spindle cells, histiocytes, and inflammatory cells haphazardly traversed by capillary blood vessels. Diff-Quik® 200×.

Granulomatous Inflammation

Granulomatous processes in the skin and underlying soft tissues may be the result of infection or neoplasia. However, trauma or reaction to a foreign body is the more common etiology. Nodules within or adjacent to scars are frequently aspirated to ascertain whether or not a tumor has recurred. Suture granulomas and traumatic neuromas are the most frequent culprits for scar nodules.

Light microscopy is usually sufficient for the diagnosis of granulomatous inflammation; however, the etiology of the inflammation may not be obvious. While multinucleated giant cells with recognizable engulfed suture material are a clue to the diagnosis of suture granuloma, this entity may yield only loosely aggregated epithelioid histiocytes (Figure 5.20). This diagnosis is

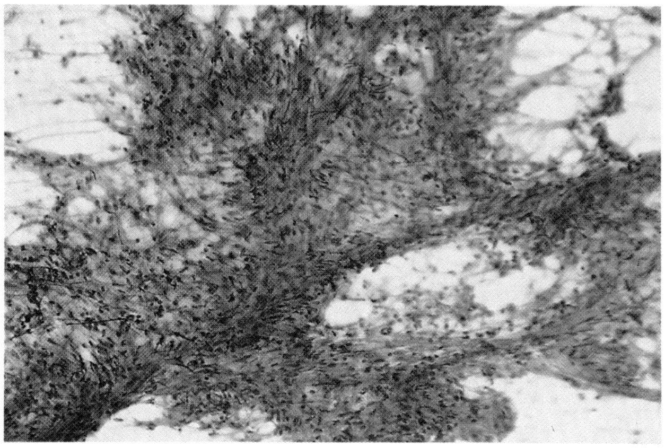

FIGURE 5.19 Granulation tissue. Arborizing capillary vessels comprise the infrastructure of this loose fragment of granulation tissue. Papanicolaou 150×.

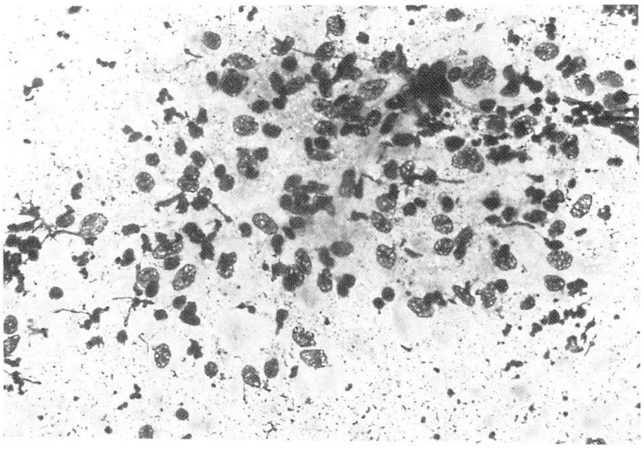

FIGURE 5.20 Suture granuloma. Loose collection of plump spindle-shaped cells with some variation in nuclear size and shape. There is an intimate mixture of inflammatory cells. The overall pattern is that of a loosely formed granuloma. Diff-Quik® 400×.

then made based on the history or presence of a previous surgical incision and the absence of cytologic features of infection. Epithelioid histiocytes arranged loosely (Figure 5.21) or as compact clusters (Figure 5.22) represent granulomas that are aspirated intact. Careful examination with polarization of smears is recommended to rule out foreign material, namely, talc, starch, or suture material. Special stains for fungi, acid-fast microorganisms, and other microorganisms should be employed if an infectious etiology is likely or if the granulomas are loosely aggregating or necrosis is present. The presence of numerous plump histiocytes without obvious granuloma formation in conjunction with inflammation may result in this lesion being confused with granulation tissue.

GRANULOMATOUS INFLAMMATION—CYTOLOGIC FEATURES

Moderate to high cellularity

Scattered plump histiocytes

Epithelioid histiocytes arranged as granulomas

Multinucleated giant cells
- **–Foreign body type**
- **–Langhan's type**

Scattered acute inflammatory cells

Background varies from clean to necrotic

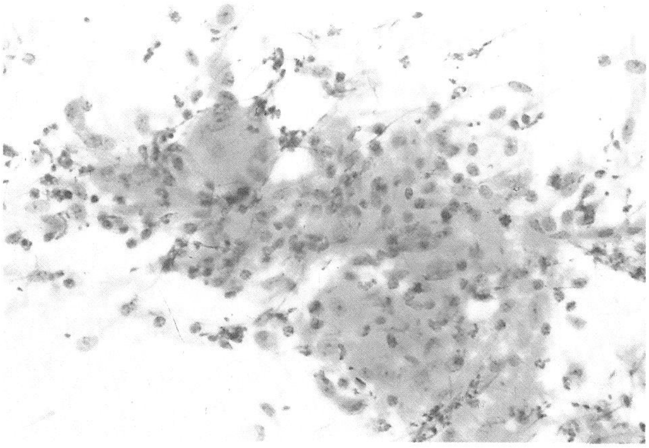

FIGURE 5.21 Granuloma, foreign body type. Granulation tissue-like pattern with suggestion of capillary running through the granuloma (flattened line of spindle cells originating at the right edge of the illustration). Multinucleated giant cell is also present at the upper margin of the granuloma. Papanicolaou 400×.

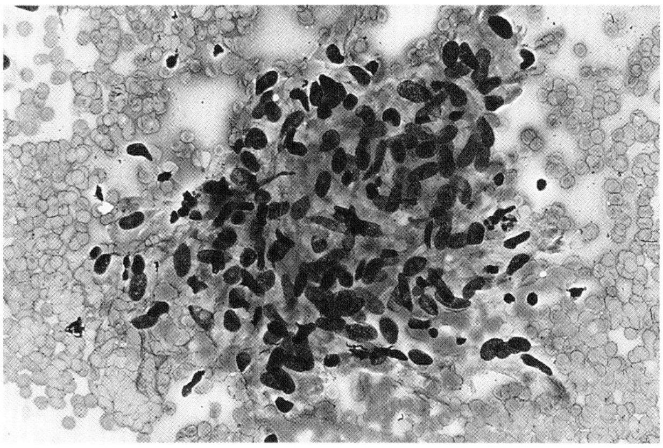

FIGURE 5.22 Compact granuloma. Dense collection of epithelioid histiocytes with "footprint" nuclei. Diff-Quik® 400×.

Nodular Fasciitis

Another entity within the category of benign, fibrohistiocytic proliferations is nodular fasciitis (NF). NF is usually perceived clinically as a subcutaneous nodule rapidly growing over the course of days to a few weeks. It is relatively firm to palpation. Often, examination of the more superficial lesions reveals their attachment to the superficial fascia. These tumors have indistinct borders. Typically occurring on the forearm, arm, and shoulder, NF can also occur on the head and neck. Smears from NF show moderate to high cellularity and numerous mitoses, some of which are atypical. Interlacing bundles of plump, spindle-shaped fibroblasts with relatively large pale nuclei and prominent nucleoli may be interspersed in an edematous or myomatous background. Scattered inflammatory cells should be present (Figure 5.23).[39–41] The smear pattern is reminiscent of fibroblasts growing in tissue culture (Figure 5.24). The aspiration cytology of NF and granulation tissue are often similar in appearance. Among the overlapping cytologic criteria are the fibroblast—the predominant cell type in both lesions—and the inflammatory background.

NODULAR FASCIITIS—CYTOLOGIC FEATURES

High cellularity

Fibroblast proliferation
- **–Haphazard arrangement—tissue culture effect**
- **–Spindle-shaped cells**
- **–Large nuclei**
- **–Prominent nucleoli**

Mitoses, often atypical

Small blood vessels and acute inflammatory cells scattered throughout

Edema or myxomatous background

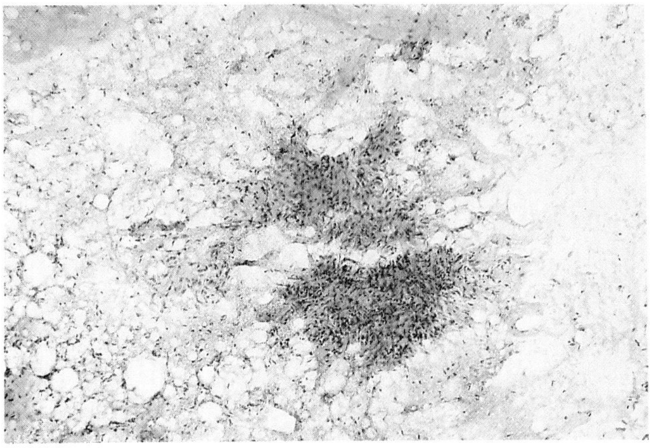

A

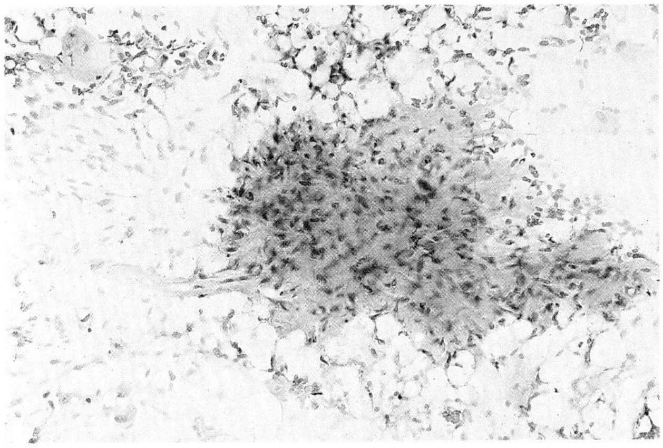

B

FIGURE 5.23 (A) Nodular fasciitis. Dense cellular fragment of spindle cells embedded in a metachromatic stroma. Individual spindle cell nuclei are seen adjacent to the fragment and at its edges. Diff-Quik® 200×. (B) Nodular fasciitis. Higher magnification showing bland, oval spindle cells haphazardly arranged in a loose stromal matrix. Papanicolaou 400×.

NEOPLASTIC PROLIFERATIONS—BENIGN

While the entire gamut of soft-tissue tumors, both benign and malignant, may occur in the head and neck, the reader is directed to monographs and papers in which the FNAB cytology of these tumors is described in detail. A few examples of the more common soft-tissue lesions that involve the head and neck and are often small and benign are included here along with some examples of soft-tissue sarcomas, which may be relatively site specific.

Traumatic Neuromas

Traumatic neuromas are usually located adjacent to scars and are not infrequently encountered in patients during long-term follow-up. FNAB of traumatic neuromas is usually quite painful and the patient will often react instinctively to this pain. Because of the patient's response and the nature of this lesion, few if any cells are obtained; however, the clinical presentation and effect of FNAB are often enough to render a diagnosis. This lesion should be in the differential diagnosis anytime FNAB of a mass adjacent to a scar is considered (Figure 5.25).

TRAUMATIC NEUROMA—CYTOLOGIC FEATURES

Scant cellularity

Spindle cells
- **–Elongate, twisted, or crescentic nuclei**
- **–Inconspicuous nucleoli**

Clean background

****Patient experiences extreme discomfort during procedure**

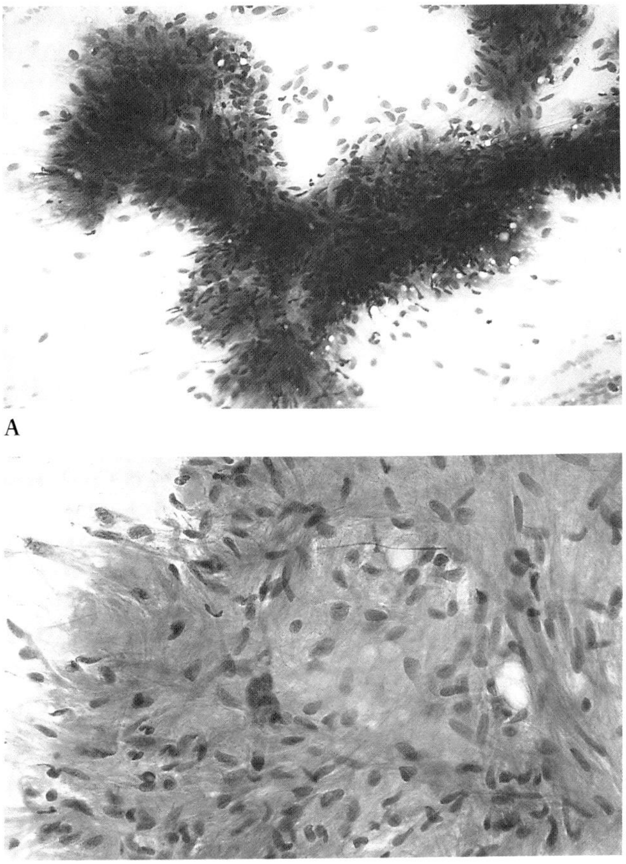

A

B

FIGURE 5.24 (A) Nodular fasciitis. Moderately cellular smear dominated by cohesive sheets of spindle-shaped cells and similar single cells coursing through fat. Note streaming pattern to the spindle-shaped cells reminiscent of fibroblasts growing in tissue culture. Papanicolaou 250×. (B) Nodular fasciitis. Higher magnification of sheet of fibroblastic cells. Nuclei are uniform and without features of malignancy. Papanicolaou 400×.

Dermatofibroma

Dermatofibroma (DF)—also known as benign fibrous histiocytoma and sclerosing hemangioma—is another fibrohistiocytic lesion that can occur as single or multiple small- to medium-sized dermal nodules. These firm, slow growing nodules are usually found on the trunk and extremities, yet they can occur on the head and neck. The overlying skin may be discolored pink to brown; the latter coloration is due to the deposition of melanin pigment and/or hemosiderin. As in NF and granulation tissue, DF is composed of fibroblasts, histiocytes, collagen, and blood vessels in a storiform, radial, or whorled arrangement. The storiform pattern with associated metachromatic stroma is often striking. Arranged as interlacing fascicles, the fibrohistiocytic cells are fusiform with bipolar cytoplasmic processes or polygonal cells with abundant cytoplasm. Nucleoli and mitoses are inconspicuous. In early phases, Touton giant cells may be present (Figures 5.26 and 5.27).

DERMATOFIBROMA—CYTOLOGIC FEATURES

Moderate to high cellularity

Storiform, radial, or whorled fragments

Fibrohistiocytic cells
- **–Fusiform/spindle**
  - **–Bipolar cytoplasmic processes**
- **–Plump, oval**
- **–Inconspicuous nucleoli**

Histiocytes
- **–Engulfed hemosiderin/melanin pigment**
- **–Touton (multinucleated) giant cells**

Blood vessels and collagen fragments

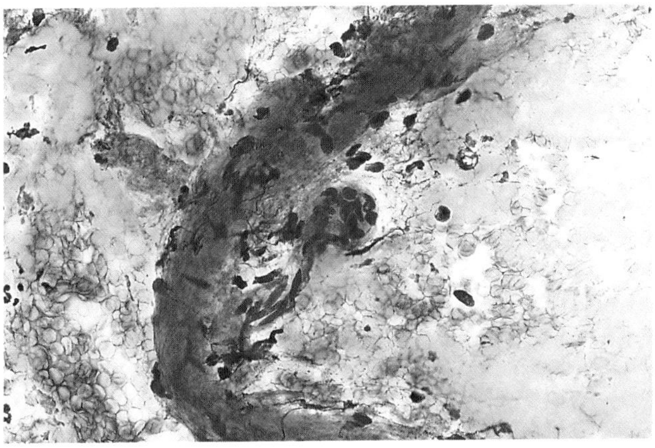

FIGURE 5.25 Neuroma. Strip of metachromatic stroma with some spindle cells embedded within it and a small circular cluster of more plump oval cells forming a Verocay-like body. The very elongated appearance of the nuclei common to nerve sheath tumors is not readily apparent in this illustration. Diff-Quik® 400×.

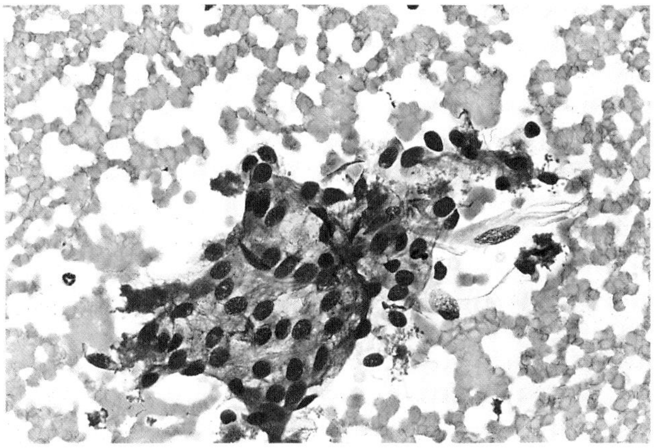

FIGURE 5.26 Dermatofibroma. Cluster of compact uniform spindle cells. Nuclei are uniform and oval to elongated and evenly spaced. Nuclear chromatin is uniform. Such cells are usually fibroblasts but the pattern is nonspecific and can be seen with scar tissue, fibromas, desmoids, fasciitis, and even smooth muscle cells with special stains. Diff-Quik® 400×.

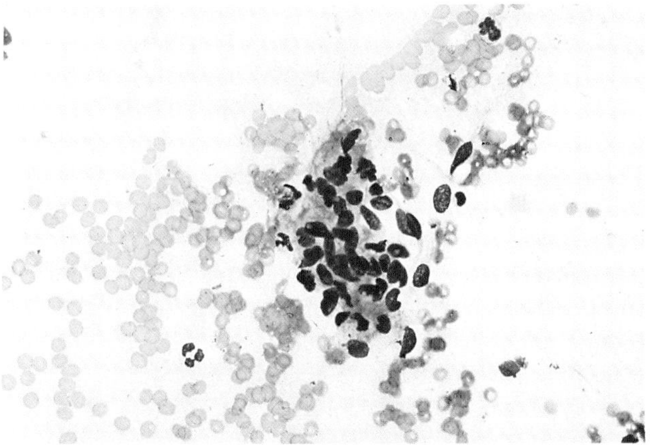

FIGURE 5.27 Dermatofibroma. Aggregate of spindle cells with somewhat irregular configuration of nuclei. The pattern is reminiscent of the storiform arrangement of the fibroblastic cells seen in dermatofibromas and dermatofibrosarcoma protuberans. Overall cellularity and clinical features determine the most likely diagnosis. Diff-Quik® 400×.

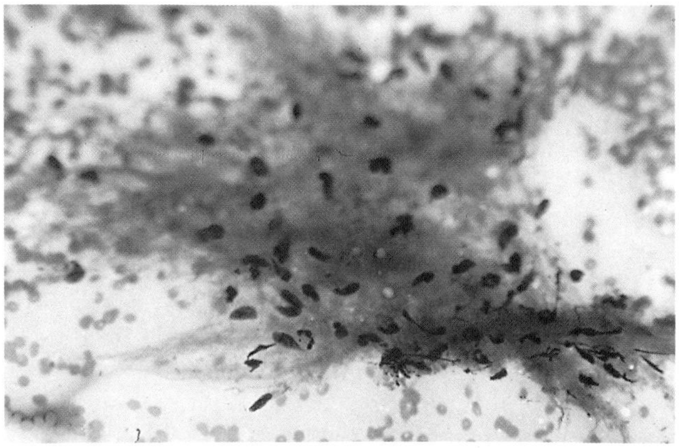

A

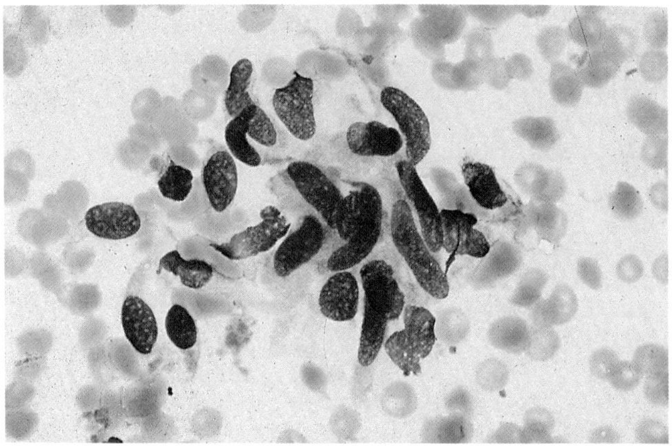

B

FIGURE 5.28 (A) Fibromatosis. Fragment of monomorphic spindle cells embedded in metachromatic stroma. Diff-Quik® 400×. (B) Fibromatosis. Loose array of spindle cells with delicate cytoplasmic processes and bland nuclear features. Diff-Quik® 1000×.

Fibromatosis

Another fibrous proliferation that occurs in the head and neck region, particularly in infants and children, is fibromatosis. When the clinical presentation is a well-circumscribed, palpable mass involving the sternocleidomastoid, often with accompanying head tilt or neck torsion (torticollis or "wry neck"), these lesions are rarely aspirated. However, if the presentation is not characteristic, FNAB is often used to rule out more significant processes that can occur as a lateral neck mass: rhabdomyosarcoma, neuroblastoma, lymphoma, developmental cysts, or hemangiomas.[42–45] Typically, aspiration smears are scant to moderately cellular and composed of a monomorphic population of loosely cohesive or single spindle cells. These cells have bland, oval to tapered nuclei, fragile cytoplasmic processes, and absent or inconspicuous nucleoli. Degenerating skeletal muscle fibers, often appearing as multinucleate cells, may be present in the background (Figure 5.28).

FIBROMATOSIS—CYTOLOGIC FEATURES

Scant to low cellularity

Monomorphic population of spindle cells
- **Oval to elongate spindle cells**
- **Unipolar and bipolar, delicate cytoplasmic processes**
- **Smooth contoured, elongate/fusiform nuclei**
- **Bland chromatin**
- **Absent or small, inconspicuous nucleoli**

Degenerating myofibers

Granular Cell Tumor (Myoblastoma)

Granular cell tumors (GCT) are well-demarcated neoplasms that can occur in almost any location, including the head and neck. Even though they are found in the subcutis, they can be palpated as hard nodules, a feature that is more typical of malignancy. FNAB of GCT are cellular with a monomorphic population of large polygonal cells. The hallmark of the tumor cells is the abundant granular cytoplasm that is rather fragile (Figure 5.29). The granularity is due to the presence of large numbers of lysosomes packing the cytoplasm. These neoplasms are benign and present no further problems when completely excised. They are most often histogenetically related to nerve sheath tumors and S-100 protein will stain the tumor cells in aspiration biopsy for confirmation.

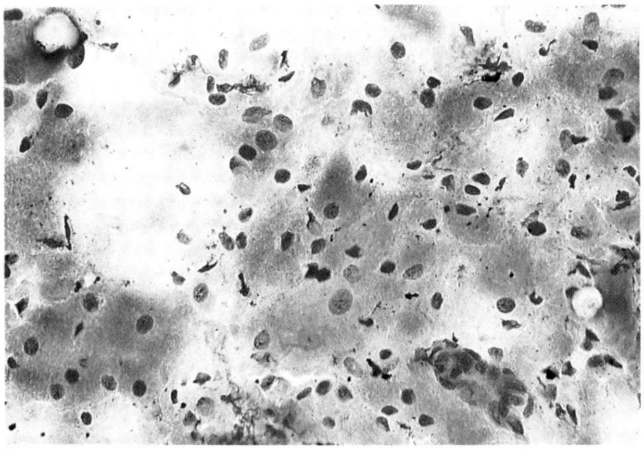

A

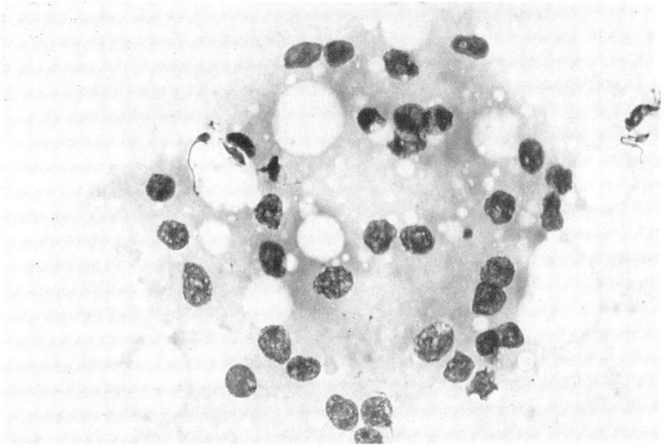

B

FIGURE 5.29 (A) Granular cell tumor. Sheets and individual cells with round, evenly spaced nuclei and abundant cytoplasm scattered in a clean background. Diff-Quik® 400×. (B) Granular cell tumor. Monomorphic cells have abundant cytoplasm that is lightly metachromatic. Striking granularity is not evident but can be enhanced with PAS stains. The nuclear chromatin is netlike and there are small nucleoli. Diff-Quik® 600×.

GRANULAR CELL TUMOR—CYTOLOGIC FEATURES

Moderate cellularity

Discohesive, monomorphic cell
- **Fragile, granular cytoplasm**
- **Round-oval, eccentric nuclei**

Background debris
- **Disrupted cytoplasm**

Immunocytochemistry
- **S-100 positivity**

Lipoma

Although more common on the trunk or extremities, lipomas can be found in the head and neck region. These tumors are usually very soft and fluctuant upon palpation. FNAB usually recovers sufficient material to diagnose these tumors. The key to successful diagnosis is to make sure the material adheres to the slides following smearing. This is especially a problem with alcohol-fixed slides. Adipose tissue can be recognized grossly because it beads up on the glass slide after smearing. Immediate fixation causes the fat globules to wash off when the slide is immersed in ethanol. Heating the bottom of the slide with a lighter or hot lamp results in more adherence with little or no damage. Adipose tissue is more likely to be retained on air-dried slides. Even the amount of adipose tissue retained on air-dried slides can be increased by fixing the slide in alcohol but removing it quickly and allowing the surface to dry completely before proceeding with the final steps of the Diff-Quik® stain. The cytomorphology is what one would expect from a fatty tumor—fat! A good preparation will reveal packets of adipose tissue surrounded by blood vessels and capillaries. Variants of lipomas exist; a good rule of thumb is to excise any fatty tumor that shows cytologic atypia.

There are a number of variants of benign lipomatous tumors. All are quite infrequent and tend to be small and subcutaneous in location. Angiolipoma has a mixture of blood vessels and fat, as the name implies, and is seen chiefly in children and young adults. The aspirate will be bloody and usually not specifically diagnostic. Myolipoma contains fat and smooth muscle. The muscle will appear as spindle cells in the aspirate mixed with fat but may not be recognized as being of smooth muscle origin. This tumor has no predilection for the head or neck. The spindle cell lipoma occurs chiefly in adults, particularly on the posterior neck and shoulder. The aspirate will be dominated by spindle cells, fibroblasts, and the fat may not be recognized (Figure 5.30). The differential diagnosis would include low-grade fibrosarcoma and nodular fasciitis. This variant of lipoma may also be

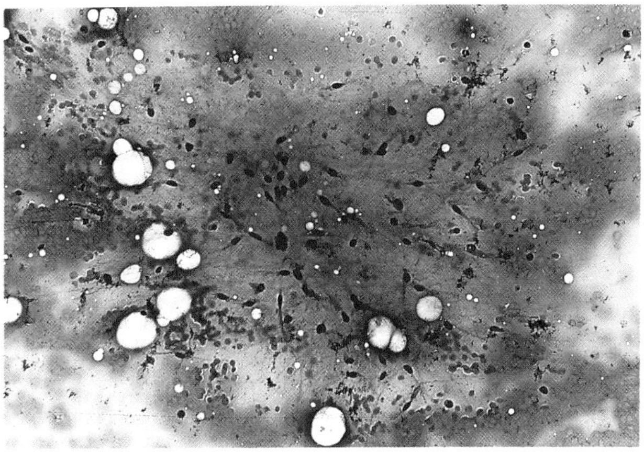

FIGURE 5.30 Spindle cell lipoma. Moderately cellular smear dominated by metachromatic myxoid stroma. Evenly dispersed stellate spindle cells without a capillary pattern. Differential diagnosis includes myxoma or myxomatous change in other soft-tissue tumors. Diff-Quik® 250×.

myxoid but lacks the branching capillary pattern of myxoid liposarcoma and typically is not a large or deeply lying tumor.[46]

Other variants include chondroid lipoma, myelolipoma, angiomyolipoma, intramuscular lipoma, neural fibrolipoma, hibernoma, and pleomorphic lipoma. This latter tumor is lumped in some reports with atypical lipoma to be described subsequently. Pleomorphic (atypical lipoma) has a predilection for the head and neck.[46]

LIPOMA—CYTOLOGIC FEATURES

Variable cellularity

Adipocytes
- **–Low nuclear to cytoplasmic ratio**
- **–Cytoplasmic vacuole**
- **–Small oval nuclei**
- **–Displaced to one side**

Interspersed blood vessels

Blood

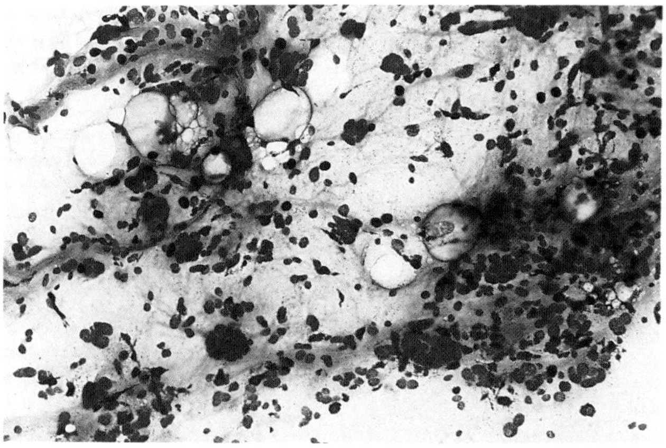

FIGURE 5.31 Atypical lipoma. Moderately cellular aspirate with abundant metachromatic stroma, spindle cells, and clusters of cells with multiple nuclei. These clusters of multinucleated cells may look epithelial. In a background of metachromatic stroma with spindle cells, the pattern simulates benign mixed tumor of salivary glands. Diff-Quik® 250×.

Atypical Lipoma

The term *atypical lipoma* has been used to describe tumors with some biologic activity that are not clearly sarcomas of adipose tissue. Location and size play a significant role in the diagnosis of atypical lipoma. Liposarcomas of the head and neck represent about 5.5 percent of this group of malignancies. Atypical lipomas are now included in the liposarcoma group because in deep locations such as the retroperitoneum they have some tendency to recur, but they do not metastasize.[46] Thus the patient is spared excessively radical surgery. The currently preferred term is *atypical lipomatous tumor*.[47] The tumors of this area tend to be small and superficial when clinically diagnosed and aspirated.[48,49]

The aspirates from atypical lipomatous tumors are moderately cellular. At low power they have some pleomorphism with relatively abundant metachromatic stroma. There is evidence of cell clumping that gives an initial suggestion of glandular structures in a spindle and myxoid background favoring a diagnosis of benign mixed tumor of salivary gland (Figure 5.31). Looking more closely at the tumor cells, multinucleated giant cells can be found. The nuclei of these cells are arranged in a rosette or circular fashion like a bouquet of flowers (Figure 5.32). Portions of the stroma and cytoplasm surrounding these cells suggest a basket, hence the term *floret* giant cells or basket of flowers. When looking at histologic sections of this tumor, the development of the aspiration pattern is evident in the myxoid stroma with the scattered floret giant cells. Despite the abundance of stroma, the branching capillary pattern of myxoid liposarcoma is lacking.

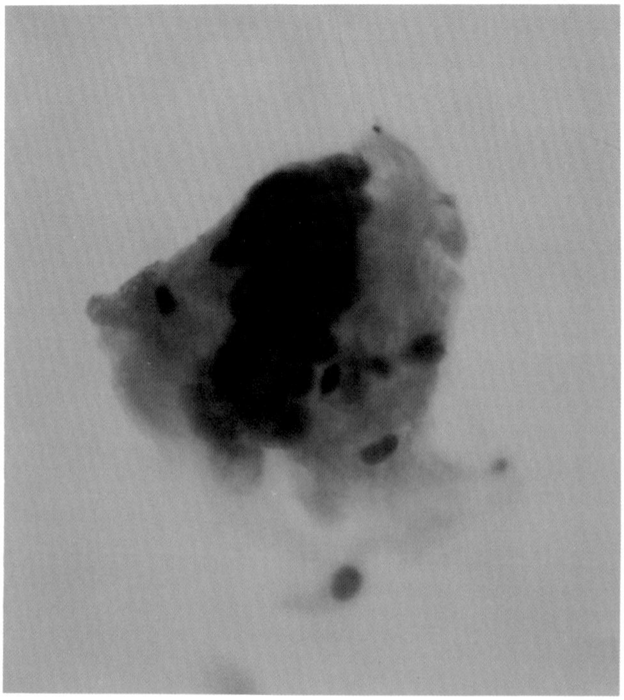

FIGURE 5.32 Atypical lipoma. The multinucleated cell with wisps of cytoplasm extending from one side of the cell with the nuclei clustered through the middle of the cell, the so-called floret or basket of flowers type giant cell. Papanicolaou 600×.

ATYPICAL LIPOMATOUS TUMOR—CYTOLOGIC FEATURES

Moderate cellularity

Floret giant cells
- **–Multiple nuclei arranged in rosette or clustered**
- **–Low nuclear to cytoplasmic ratio**
- **–Cytoplasm and stroma surrounding these cells form a "basket"**
- **–Small oval nuclei**

Myxoid stroma without branching capillary pattern

Blood

NEOPLASTIC PROLIFERATIONS—MALIGNANT

The malignant soft-tissue tumors that might be encountered on aspiration biopsy of the head and neck area are quite rare. Rhabdomyosarcoma is the most common and is usually seen in children and is located near or within the orbit (see Chapter 6). Because soft-tissue sarcomas in the head and neck are readily noticeable, they usually present with a smaller mass than would typically be found with a soft-tissue sarcoma of an extremity. These neoplasms may present in areas typically containing lymph nodes, or they may simulate a primary thyroid or salivary gland neoplasm.

Dermatofibrosarcoma Protuberans

Dermatofibrosarcoma protuberans (DFSP) is an uncommon mass in the dermis or subcutis that may be sampled by FNAB. DFSP is a slow growing nodular neoplasm of the underlying dermis that may protrude outward, resulting in a large, sometimes ulcerated tumor easily accessible to FNAB. While the majority of DFSP cases occur on the trunk or extremities, they can also be found on the scalp. Until recently,[50] there were limited attempts at primary diagnosis of this entity.[51] DFSP, as is the case in other spindle cell proliferations, has no one distinctive feature that allows definitive diagnosis. Incorporation of all available clinical, radiologic, and cytologic data can result in successful diagnosis in most cases. Like dermatofibroma, fragments with storiform architecture are often obtained during FNAB of DFSP. These fragments are metachromatic on Romanowsky-stained preparations. The presence of entrapped fibroadipose tissue, the metachromatic stromal fragments with a delicate, inconspicuous network of capillaries, and absent inflammatory cells are the most important features for cytodiagnosis (Figures 5.33 and 5.34). Osteoclastic giant cells may rarely be present and blood vessels may also be frequent in some smears of this neoplasm leading to an aspirate largely composed of blood.

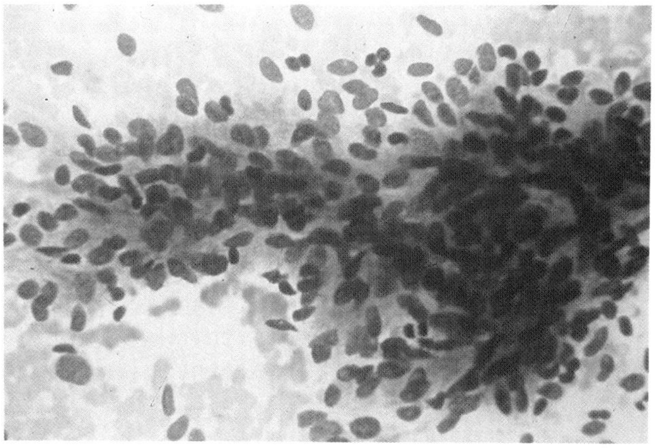

FIGURE 5.33 Dermatofibrosarcoma protuberans. Fragment of plump, oval spindle cells embedded in a dense, magenta stroma. Diff-Quik® 400×.

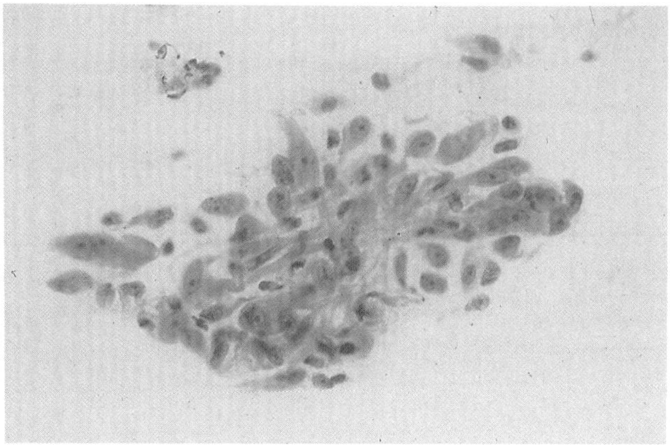

FIGURE 5.34 Dermatofibrosarcoma protuberans. Storiform fragment of oval spindle cells with small nucleoli, uniform nuclei, and cytoplasmic processes. Papanicolaou 400×.

DERMATOFIBROSARCOMA PROTUBERANS—CYTOLOGIC FEATURES

Moderate cellularity

Stromal fragments
- **–Metachromatic (magenta-Diff-Quik®)**
- **–Fibrillar matrix**
- **–Variably cellular**
- **–Storiform pattern**

Discohesive cells
- **–Plump, oval, and spindle**
- **–Moderately fine granular cytoplasm**
- **–Bipolar cytoplasmic processes**
- **–Variably sized, round nuclei**
- **–Homogeneous chromatin**
- **–Nucleoli/chromocenters**

Osteoclast giant cells, rare

Entrapped adipose tissue

Infrequent mitoses

Atypical Fibroxanthoma

This tumor typically arises in adults with actinic damaged skin. It is often ulcerated but may present initially as a subcutaneous nodule.[46] When ulcerated, it is much more likely to be biopsied by excision than aspirated. It may recur as a subcutaneous nodule and thus FNA could be useful in proving the presence of a recurrent tumor. Histologically, atypical fibroxanthoma has the same morphology as malignant fibrous histiocytoma. The aspiration pattern reflects this fact, being both cellular and pleomorphic. The tumor cells are pleomorphic with a large range in size and shape. There are single cells and small irregular sheets. Heterogeneity is the hallmark of aspiration smears from both atypical fibroxanthoma and malignant fibrous histiocytoma. Unlike some malignant fibrous histiocytomas, myxoid stroma and necrosis are rarely present.

The differential diagnosis includes principally spindle cell forms of cutaneous squamous cell carcinoma and malignant melanoma. The aspiration pattern may be dominated by spindle cells but is usually less pleomorphic in both spindle cell squamous carcinoma and malignant melanoma. The latter tumor's desmoplastic variant may have low cellularity and appear in the aspiration smear identical to fibromatoses, low-grade fibrosarcomas, or nodular fasciitis. Clinical features are important in favoring one diagnosis versus another in this group of cases; immunohistochemistry to identify markers of epithelial cells (cytokeratin) or malignant melanoma cells (S-100 protein and HMB-45) are quite useful.

ATYPICAL FIBROXANTHOMA—CYTOLOGIC FEATURES

High cellularity

Marked pleomorphism of neoplastic cells
- **–Broad range of cell size, predominantly large**
- **–Sheets and individual bizarre cells**

Individual Cells
- **–Moderate to abundant cytoplasm**
- **–Marked variation in nuclear size and shape**
- **–Clumped irregular chromatin**
- **–Some nuclei with prominent irregular nucleoli**
- **–Multinucleated giant cells, osteoclastic type and/or tumor type**

Fibrosarcoma

Fibrosarcoma is least common in the head and neck—10 percent of cases—compared to other body sites, extremities, and trunk. It presents as a slowly growing nodular mass and unless it becomes quite large from neglect the skin remains intact. This tumor was frequently overdiagnosed histologically in earlier reported series but with more recent comprehensive reviews, the description of new types of soft-tissue sarcomas, and refinements in histologic diagnosis, this sarcoma is much less frequently diagnosed than malignant fibrous histiocytoma, leiomyosarcoma, liposarcoma, synovial sarcoma, or sarcomas of muscle origin arising in soft tissue. Fibrosarcoma is usually a tumor of adults (age range 30 to 55 years), but it can occur congenitally and in infants and children. It rarely occurs in the area of the head and neck.[46]

Cytologically, FNA smears will demonstrate single cells and fascicles of spindle-shaped tumor cells with elongated and often pointed nuclei. Cellularity will parallel the degree of differentiation. Well-differentiated fibrosarcoma, which is proportionally rich in collagen, will yield relatively few and often scattered spindle-shaped tumor cells (Figure 5.35), while poorly differentiated fibrosarcoma usually provides at least moderately cellular smears with more plump-appearing, elongated tumor cells that also have more oval-shaped nuclei (Figure 5.36). The stroma, which is usually collagenous but may occasionally be myxoid, will appear metachromatic in air-dried, Romanowsky-stained preparations, thus providing a background within which to view the individual tumor cells and see a pattern similar to the histology of this tumor.

The differential diagnosis includes any spindle cell tumor but, in particular, in the head and neck, nodular fasciitis and fibromatoses. The smears of fibrosarcoma are monotonous in their appearance with little or no evidence of inflammation in contrast to the aspiration smear pattern of nodular fasciitis. Fibromatosis is heavily collagenized and yields only few or no cells to FNA. As in histologic sections, the few

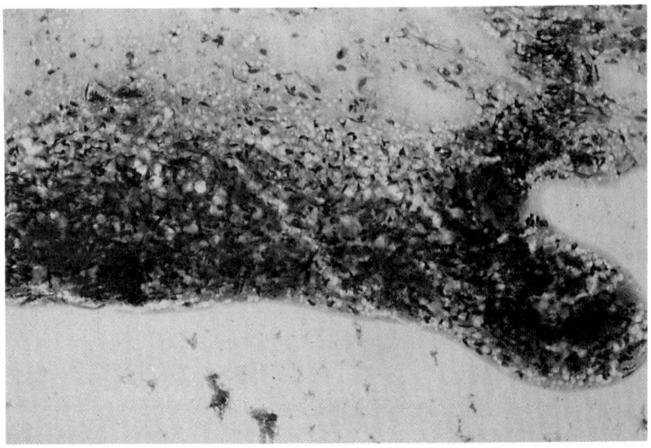

FIGURE 5.35. Well-differentiated fibrosarcoma. Sheafs of spindle-shaped cells with pointed elongated nuclei. Cells are arranged in parallel fasicles with abundant cytoplasm and metachromatic stroma. Diff-Quik® 250×.

fibroblasts that may be found on the smears from fibromatoses are thin and very elongate. Peripheral nerve-sheath tumors and smooth muscle tumors are also in the differential diagnosis. Smears from a nerve-sheath tumor will have very elongate and twisted nuclei, and, even in smears, there may be sheets of cells with evidence of palisading of the nuclei. Aspiration of a nerve-sheath tumor is often excessively painful for the patient. Smooth muscle tumors have predominantly blunt-ended nuclei in aspiration biopsy smears as they do in histologic sections, but this is a subtle feature and one that is not substantially different if the fibrosarcoma is poorly differentiated. Immunohistochemical studies performed directly on smears or on cytospins of the aspirate may aid in the differential diagnosis of these spindle cell lesions, if adequate samples can be obtained. Making some of the passes using a thin needle of the Franseen type may procure slender microcores that can be processed as a cell block, thus providing more definitive histologic features in some cases as well as material useful for immunohistochemical staining.

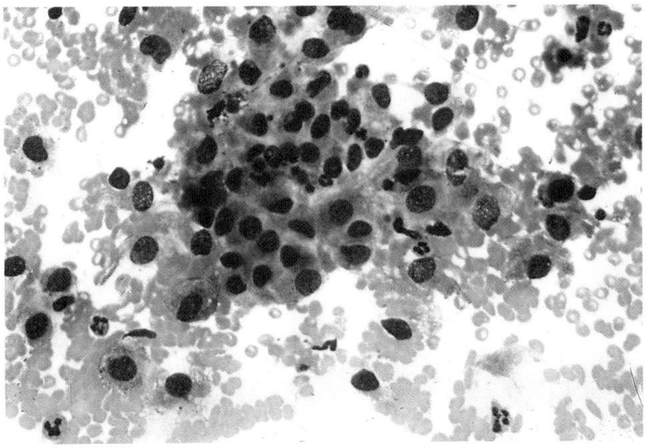

FIGURE 5.36. High-grade fibrosarcoma. Cellular aspirate dominated by spindle cells with plump oval nuclei. Nuclear chromatin is granular. Giant nuclei are not seen and cytoplasm is present at both ends of the cell, features not seen in aspirates from rhabdomyosarcomas of the head and neck. Diff-Quik® 400×.

FIBROSARCOMA—CYTOLOGIC FEATURES

Cellularity
- **High in poorly differentiated forms**
- **Modest in moderately differentiated forms**
- **Sparse to nonexistent in well-differentiated desmoid types**

Individual cells
- **Spindle-shaped, elongated typical fibroblasts (moderately differentiated)**
- **Plump, short, obviously malignant cells (poorly differentiated forms)**
- **Thin tapering in well-differentiated forms**
- **Pleomorphism is minimal**
- **Multinucleated giant cells absent**
- **Thin elongated nuclei (well-differentiated forms) becoming plump with loss of differentiation**

Stroma and cytoplasm
- **Myxoid metachromatic stroma essentially absent**
- **Cytoplasm metachromatic (well and moderately differentiated)**

Rhabdomyosarcoma

Rhabdomyosarcoma is the most common of the soft-tissue sarcomas in children and is nearly as prevalent in both adolescents and young adults. The prevalence of this tumor was high in adults in the past, but it is now known that most of those tumors were sarcomas of other types, often malignant fibrous histiocytoma. Today, rhabdomyosarcoma is rare in adults over 45 years of age. There are several histologic subtypes: embryonal, botryoid, alveolar, and pleomorphic. Rhabdomyosarcoma is the most common sarcoma of the head and neck (43 percent of the cases) with the orbit and nasal cavity dominating (19.5 and 13.1 percent, respectively). In general, the tumor is rapidly growing, so that within the orbit there is displacement of the glove and diplopia and blurred vision (see Chapter 6). In the nasopharynx, the tumor may be easily confused at first with enlarged adenoids; within the mastoid, middle ear, and ear canal, problems in hearing and a suspicion of inflammation may for a time obscure the diagnosis.[46]

A mass in any of these areas may be sampled by FNA. In a recent report of 17 cases of rhabdomyosarcoma diagnosed by fine needle aspiration biopsy, 5 occurred in the area of the head and neck. The smears were highly cellular with a predominantly undifferentiated small-round-cell pattern (Figure 5.37). There was a mixture of single cells and cohesive cell clusters. The individual cells had a high nuclear to cytoplasmic ratio. Comparison with aspiration smears of other small-round-cell tumors revealed two features that pointed predominantly toward a diagnosis of rhabdomyosarcoma—intracytoplasmic vacuoles and bi- or multinucleation (Figure 5.38).[52] Of interest was the finding of a tigroid background to the smear in 3 of the 17 cases, a feature usually seen in aspiration smears from metastatic seminoma.

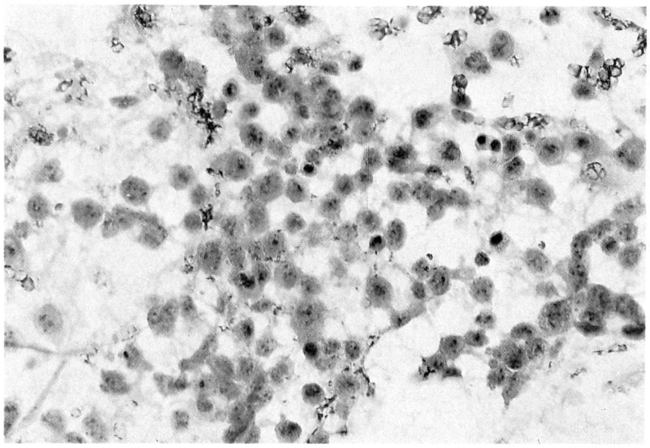

FIGURE 5.37 Rhabdomyosarcoma. Cellular aspirate with predominance of small undifferentiated round cells. Small cytoplasmic tags can be seen at the edge of some cells. Cells are in very loose clusters with many single cells. Nuclear chromatin is coarsely granular with irregular nuclear membranes. There are scattered, very small necrotic cells. The pattern is very nonspecific, indicating only an undifferentiated small-round-cell tumor. Papanicolaou 400×.

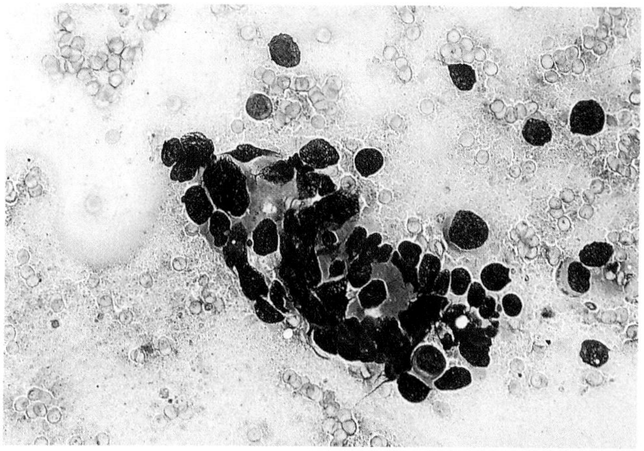

FIGURE 5.38 Rhabdomyosarcoma. Both small undifferentiated cells are present with some enlarged individual nuclei. This is a characteristic feature of rhabdomyosarcoma in the differential diagnosis of other small-round-cell tumors. There is some striped (tigroid) background that can be seen in the upper right of the figure. This is a feature found in some aspiration smears of a small number of rhabdomyosarcomas. Diff-Quik® 400×.

RHABDOMYOSARCOMA—CYTOLOGIC FEATURES

Cellularity
- **High**
- **Small undifferentiated anaplastic cells**
- **Single cells and clusters**
- **Multinucleated cells**

Individual cells
- **High nuclear to cytoplasmic ratio**
- **Finely granular chromatin**
- **Visible nucleoli**
- **Peripheral cytoplasmic vacuoles**
- **Dense cytoplasmic tags on some cells**

Background
- **Tigroid in a few cases**
- **Metachromasia, little or none**

Liposarcoma

Only 5.6 percent of all of the cases of liposarcomas occur in the head and neck. They are seen predominantly in the fifth and sixth decade of life and are quite rare in children. Clinically, they are slowly growing masses. The common histologic types are myxoid and round cell. There are transitional tumors of both these types. The myxoid variety has spindle-shaped cells that are rather uniform, separated by a branching capillary pattern, so-called "chicken-wire" pattern, that is the histologic hallmark of this tumor. The round-cell type of liposarcomas are highly cellular with few large lipoblasts, a cell type also relatively sparse in the myxoid variety. The third variety is the well-differentiated liposarcoma, which looks very much like mature fat in many areas except that there is a subtle increase in cellularity and atypia of individual adipocytes. There are some additional histologic variations on these three patterns.[46]

Cytologically, aspirates from liposarcoma are moderately cellular when of the myxoid variety, highly cellular if of round-cell type, and of relatively low cellularity when well differentiated. The smears of the myxoid type have an abundance of metachromatic stroma with evenly spaced and uniform spindle-shaped cells and rare lipoblasts. In scanning the smear microscopically, the branching capillary pattern that is typical histologically for myxoid liposarcoma usually becomes evident (Figure 5.39). This smear pattern is most important in the diagnosis as the individual spindle shaped cells do not have frankly malignant features.

The round-cell variety has high-cellularity smears with small, uniform but clearly malignant cells. These tumor cells have a high nuclear to cytoplasmic ratio, irregularly distributed clumped chromatin, and prominent nucleoli. The aspiration pattern mimics a poorly differentiated carcinoma that, in the head and neck, could easily lead to a mistaken diagnosis because liposarcomas are so uncommon in this area. There is a peculiar metachromatic background of fragmented material, presumably cytoplasm, that is a clue to the diagnosis because this is not seen with poorly differentiated carcinomas (Figure 5.40).

Well-differentiated liposarcoma looks predominantly like mature fat. This tumor is not likely to be encountered in the head and neck, particularly in contrast to pleomorphic or so-called "atypical lipoma." The

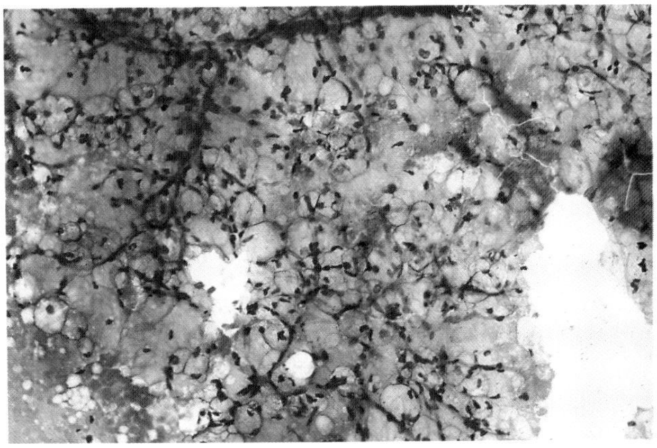

FIGURE 5.39 Myxoid liposarcoma. Moderately cellular aspirate with metachromatic stroma containing relatively small, uniform spindle cells. There is little variation in nuclear size. Note branching capillary pattern throughout the aspirated fragment, a major clue to the diagnosis of myxoid liposarcoma. Diff-Quik® 250×.

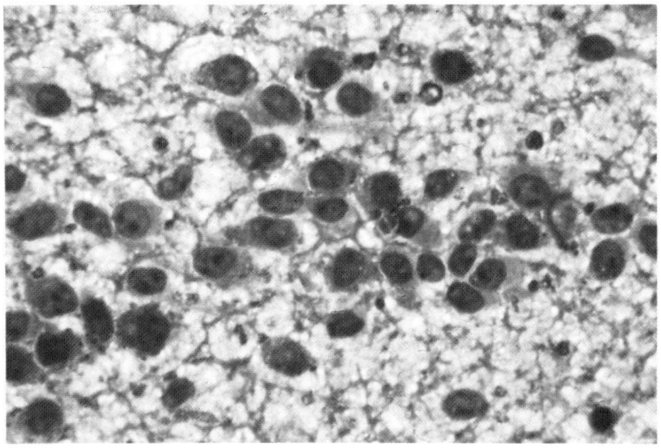

FIGURE 5.40 Round-cell liposarcoma. Cellular aspirate with round to oval undifferentiated tumor cells. Lipoblasts are few in these tumors and not easily seen on aspiration smears. Note the reticulated background that is metachromatic. This seems to be a feature of round-cell liposarcomas. Diff-Quik® 400×.

smears of well-differentiated liposarcoma will be of low cellularity with some cells having a more prominent nucleus than would be expected with mature adipose tissue. Given this feature and the observation that a lesion has been slowly but consistently increasing in size, at least the possibility of well-differentiated liposarcoma has to be raised in reporting the aspiration biopsy (Figure 5.41).

LIPOSARCOMA—CYTOLOGIC FEATURES

Cellularity
- **Moderate, myxoid type**
- **High, round-cell type**
- **Low, well-differentiated, lipoma-like type**

Individual cells
- **Spindle and uniform, myxoid type**
- **Round and uniform with prominent nucleoli, granular chromatin, round-cell type**
- **Mature fat with some increase in nuclear size and variation in nuclear shape, well differentiated, lipoma-like**
- **Scattered vacuolated lipoblasts, rare in round-cell type, uncommon in myxoid type, relatively common in well-differentiated type**

Stroma and background
- **Myxoid metachromatic with branching capillary pattern, myxoid type.**
- **Granular metachromatic "background," round-cell type**
- **Mature fat with minimal metachromasia, predominantly cytoplasmic, lipomalike**

Synovial Sarcoma

Synovial sarcoma of the head and neck accounted for 9 percent of all cases reported by Enzinger and Weiss in the third edition of their textbook on soft tissue sarcomas. Half of these cases were of internal structures, equally divided between the larynx and pharynx. This sarcoma is seen in adolescents and young adults with 90 percent of the cases in Enzinger and Weiss's series under 50 years of age.[46]

The tumor has three histologic patterns: biphasic—composed of both spindle cell and epithelial areas, monophasic spindle-cell type, and monophasic epithelial type. The monophasic epithelial type is quite rare and difficult to differentiate from carcinoma.[46]

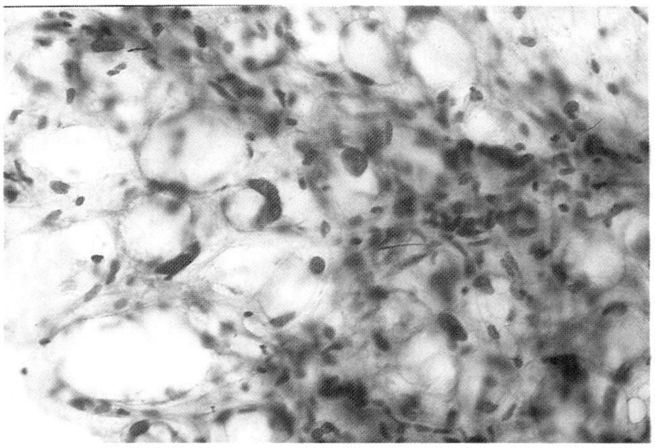

FIGURE 5.41 Differentiated liposarcoma. Cellular aspirate composed of discrete adipocytes with enlarged, eccentrically placed hyperchromatic nuclei. Endothelial cells comprising a fine vascular network are seen traversing the cellular cluster. Papanicolaou 1000×.

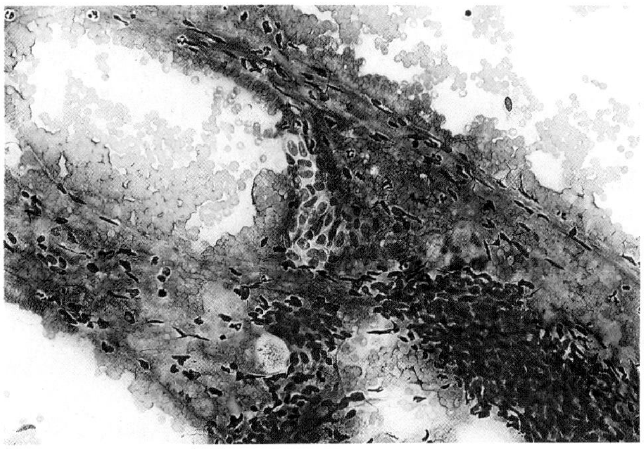

FIGURE 5.42 Synovial sarcoma. Moderately cellular aspirate with a compact sheet of spindle cells and small cluster of more epithelial-appearing cells with more abundant cytoplasm in the center of the illustration. Moderate amounts of metachromatic stroma concentrated to some extent at the periphery of the cell groupings. Diff-Quik® 250×.

The cytologic features reflect predominantly the spindle cell, poorly differentiated, fibrosarcomatous pattern of this tumor.[53,54] The smears are cellular with plump elongated cells appearing in clusters and also as single cells. There is some metachromatic stroma that is chiefly seen at the periphery of the cell groupings (Figure 5.42). The suggestion of the epithelial component is the tighter clusters of cells with a hint at gland formation and these same cells having slightly more abundant cytoplasm (Figure 5.43). This biphasic pattern is not readily apparent on smears in most cases but can be found more easily in cell block material or may be discerned from immunostaining spindle-cell areas for cytokeratin. The monophasic spindle-cell variety will have the same cytologic pattern as poorly differentiated fibrosarcoma, while the monophasic epithelial type will appear as a poorly differentiated carcinoma, making for a very difficult specific cytologic diagnosis in an aspirate from a mass in the head and neck.

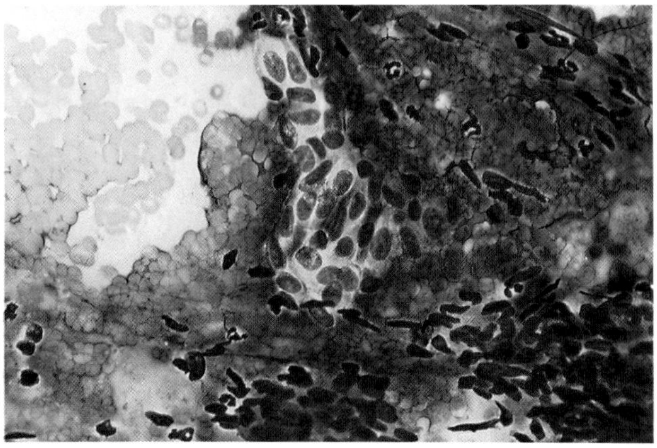

FIGURE 5.43 Synovial sarcoma. Higher magnification of the juxtaposition of the epithelial-appearing cell cluster adjacent to the spindle-cell compact sheet. This is the cytologic pattern of the typical biphasic synovial sarcoma. Diff-Quik® 400×.

SYNOVIAL SARCOMA—CYTOLOGIC FEATURES

Cellularity
- **–High**
- **–Sheets and single, plump but elongated cells**
- **–Small tighter clusters of cells indicate biphasic pattern**

Individual cells
- **–Plump and spindle shaped**
- **–Moderately high nuclear to cytoplasmic ratio**
- **–Uniform but undifferentiated-appearing nuclei**
- **–Nucleoli inconspicuous**

Stroma
- **–Small amounts of metachromatic stroma applied tightly to edges of cell clusters**

IMMUNOLOGIC AND CYTOGENETIC MARKERS

In addition to traditional methods of histologic grading and clinical staging, an increasing number of monoclonal antibodies have been used to refine the diagnosis of soft-tissue sarcomas and to estimate prognosis.[55] At the molecular level, there are not a remarkable number of genetic markers that appear to be relatively specific for certain types of soft-tissue sarcomas. These are summarized in Table 5.5.

In many cases, FNA can provide an adequate sample for both immunohistochemistry and identification of some chromosome alterations by fluorescent *in situ* hybridization (FISH) techniques. These studies may allow a more precise diagnosis when cytomorphology is not that specific. Advantage is gained in treatment planning and the use of adjuvant therapy where indicated.

ACCURACY

Limited information is available regarding the diagnostic accuracy of FNAB of primary skin and subcutaneous masses. The primary reason for this is the lack of a significant volume of cases for any particular entity at any one institution or that any one individual has had the opportunity to diagnose. Certainly FNAB is very accurate in the diagnosis of recurrent or metastatic malignancies, especially if cytologic and/or histologic material of the primary tumor is available

TABLE 5.5 Genetic Alterations Associated with Soft-Tissue Sarcomas

Histologic Diagnosis	*Genetic Alteration*
Rhabdomyosarcoma	Expression of the MYOD1 muscle-specific gene
Alveolar	t(2;13) (q37;q14) and variant t(1;13) (p36;q12)
solid form	t(2;13)f
Embryonal	+11 (trisomy); deletion of 11p15, loss of heterozygosity
Synovial sarcoma	t(X;18) (p11.2q11.2) and variants involving 18q11.2
Osteosarcoma	13q14 (loss of the retinoblastoma tumor suppressor gene)
MFH	Characterized by abnormalities at diverse sites including 1q11, 3p12, 11p11, and 19p13
Liposarcoma	t(12;16) (q13;p11)
Myxoid liposarcoma and solitary lipomas	Rearrangements of chromosome 12 with chromosome 16 and other autosomes
Malignant peripheral nerve-sheath tumors	17p13 in the region of the p53 tumor suppressor gene, also 17q11 in the vicinity of the neuro-fibromatosis 1 gene
Ewing's sarcoma/PNET	t(11;22) (q24;q11.1-12) indistinguishable patterns protooncogenes, c-myc N-myc, c myb, c-mil/raf-1, c-fes, c-sis
Clear-cell sarcoma	+8 (trisomy), t(22)
Epithelioid sarcoma	+2
Chondrosarcoma, myxoid	t(2,13);t(9;22)(q31;q12.2)
Fibrosarcoma	+8, +11, +17 (trisomies)
Leiomyosarcoma	t(12;14); others
Alveolar soft-part sarcoma	+12 (trisomy); del(17)
Fibromatosis (desmoid)	del(5)(q13-q31); some Gardner's syndrome
Dermatofibrosarcoma	+8
Hemangiopericytoma	t(12;19)t(13;22)

for examination. This includes malignant melanomas, lymphomas, and carcinomas. Accuracy in the diagnosis of spindle cell and fibrohistiocytic proliferations and adenexal tumors is variable. Accuracy of diagnosis for these lesions depends equally on the availability of all relevant clinical information and the experience of the cytopathologist. Many cytopathologists are reluctant to categorize these processes much beyond benign, malignant, or inconclusive.

PITFALLS AND COMPLICATIONS

Pitfalls in the diagnosis of primary cutaneous entities are numerous and have for the most part already been discussed. Problems are likely to be encountered when the pathologist succumbs to the *too little syndrome:*

Too little clinical information
Too little material
Too little familiarity with FNAB criteria

The antidote is painful. The pathologist must insist on being provided with adequate clinical data and a good aspiration biopsy that is well prepared and stained; he or she must not be cajoled or bullied into rendering a diagnosis that he/she is uncomfortable with due to lack of experience or knowledge.

Another problem is that many of the cytologic features of these lesions overlap to the extent that the differential diagnoses are many and are difficult to elim-

TABLE 5.6 Differential Diagnosis of Basaloid Lesions Encountered in Fine Needle Aspiration Biopsy

Basal cell carcinoma	Merkel-cell carcinoma
Basosquamous carcinoma	Squamous cell carcinoma
Eccrine spiradenoma	Other appendageal neoplasms
Metastatic carcinoid	Metastatic small-cell carcinoma
Malignant melanoma	Malignant lymphoma

inate. Basaloid cells are particularly problematic; the differential diagnosis is listed in Table 5.6.

As Table 5.6 indicates, it is possible to encounter many different neoplasms during FNAB of skin nodules. While some can be eliminated based on history and physical examination, others may need ancillary techniques, electron microscopy, flow cytometry, and/or immunochemistry to differentiate them further.

Complications

There are no serious complications that occur due to FNAB of the skin or subcutaneous region. Transient discomfort and limited bleeding, at most a small hematoma, are the only problems encountered. The latter is treated with pressure to the puncture site and a small pressure bandage (a 2 × 2 gauze pad held in place by an adhesive bandage). No infection has ever been documented as a result of FNAB.

REFERENCES

1. Brownstein MH, Helwig EB. Patterns of cutaneous metastases. *Arch Dermatol* 1972;105:862–868.

2. Brownstein MH, Helwig EB. Spread of tumors to the skin. *Arch Dermatol* 1973;107:80–83.

3. Dvorak AM, Monahan RA. Metastatic adenocarcinoma of unknown primary site. *Arch Pathol Lab Med* 1982;106:21–24.

4. Pak HY, Forster BA, Yokata SB. The significance of cutaneous metastasis from visceral tumors diagnosed by fine-needle aspiration biopsy. *Diagn Cytopathol* 1987;3:24–29.

5. Reyes CV, Jensen J, Eng AM. Fine needle aspiration cytology of cutaneous metastases. *Acta Cytol* 1993;37:142–148.

6. Linsk JA, Fransen S. *Clinical aspiration cytology.* Philadelphia: J.B. Lippincott Co., 1983, pp. 281–296.

7. Ramzy I. *Clinical cytopathology and aspiration biopsy: Fundamental principles and practice.* Norwalk, CT: Appelton and Lange, 1990.

8. Bibbo M. *Comprehensive cytopathology.* Philadelphia: W.B. Saunders Co., 1991.

9. Koss LG, Woyke S, Olszewski W. *Aspiration biopsy: Cytologic interpretation and histologic bases.* New York: Igaku-Shoin, 1992, pp. 409–458.

10. Layfield LJ, Glasgow BJ. Aspiration biopsy cytology of primary cutaneous tumors. *Acta Cytol* 1993;37:679–688.

11. Ramzy I, Rone R, Schantz HD. Squamous cells in needle aspirates of subcutaneous lesions: A diagnostic problem. *Am J Clin Pathol* 1986;85:319–324.

12. Woyke S, Olszewski W, Eichelkraut A. Pilomatrixoma: A pitfall in the aspiration cytology of skin tumors. *Acta Cytol* 1982;26:189–194.

13. Bhalotra R, Jayaram G. Fine-needle aspiration cytology of pilomatrixoma: A case report. *Diagn Cytopathol* 1990;6:280–283.

14. Gomez-Aracil V, Azua J, San Pedro C, Romero J. Fine-needle aspiration cytologic findings in four cases of pilomatrixoma (calcifying epithelioma of Malherbe). *Acta Cytol* 1990;34:842–846.

15. Unger P, Watson C, Phelps RG, Dangue P, Bernard P. Fine needle aspiration cytology of pilomatrixoma (calcifying epithelioma of Malherbe): A case report. *Acta Cytol* 1990;34:847–850.

16. Ortiz J, Macias CG, Abad M, Flores T, Paz JI, Bullon A. Pilomatrixoma: A description of two cases diagnosed by fine-needle aspiration. *Diagn Cytopathol* 1995;12:155–157.

17. Masood S, Hardy NM. Fine needle aspiration cytology of chondroid syringoma: Report of a case. *Acta Cytol* 1988;32:482–484.

18. Gottschalk-Sabag S, Glick T. Chondroid syringoma diagnosed by fine-needle aspiration: A case report. *Diagn Cytopathol* 1994;10:152–155.

19. Srinivasan R, Rajwanshi A, Padmanabhan V, Dey P. Fine needle aspiration cytology of chondroid syringoma and syringocystadenoma papilliferum: A report of two cases. *Acta Cytol* 1993;37:535–538.

20. Varsa EW, Jordan SW. Fine needle aspiration cytology of malignant spiradenoma arising in congenital eccrine spiradenoma. *Acta Cytol* 1990;34:275–277.

21. Malberger E, Tillinger R, Lichtig C. Diagnosis of basal cell carcinoma with aspiration cytology. *Acta Cytol* 1984;28:301–304.

22. Haddad MG, Silverman JF. Fine-needle aspiration cytology of metastatic basal cell carcinoma of the skin to the lung. *Diagn Cytopathol* 1994;10:15–19.

23. Szpak CA, Bossen EH, Linder J, Johnston WW. Cytomorphology of primary small-cell (Merkel-cell) carcinoma of the skin in fine needle aspirates. *Acta Cytol* 1984;28:290–296.

24. Mellblom L, Akerman M, Carlen B. Aspiration cytology of neuroendocrine (Merkel-cell) carcinoma of the skin. *Acta Cytol* 1984;28:297–300.

25. Kawamoto EH, Geisinger KR, Leonard DD, Pol RS. The cytologic appearance of Merkel-cell carcinoma in fine needle aspirates. *Acta Cytol* 1984;28:650.

26. Domgala W, Lubinski J, Lasota J, Giryn I, Weber I, Osborn M. Neuroendocrine (Merkel-cell) carcinomas of the skin: Cytology, intermediate filament typing and ultrastructure of tumor cells in fine-needle aspirates. *Acta Cytol* 1987;31:267–275.

27. Skoog L, Schmitt FC, Tani E. Neuroendocrine (Merkel-cell) carcinoma of the skin: Immunocytochemical and cytomorphologic analysis on fine-needle aspirates. *Diagn Cytopathol* 1990;6:53–57.

28. Al-Kaisi NK. Fine-needle aspiration cytology of metastatic Merkel-cell carcinoma. *Diagn Cytopathol* 1991;7:184–188.

29. Hood IC, Qizilbash AH, Salama SS, Young JEM, Archibald SD. Needle aspiration cytology of sebaceous carcinoma. *Acta Cytol* 1984;28:305–312.

30. Gal R, Prialnic M, Savir H, Kessler E. Aspiration cytology of metastatic sebaceous carcinoma. *Acta Cytol* 1986;30:91–92.

31. Hales M, Bottles K, Miller T, Ljung BM. Diagnosis of Kaposi's sarcoma by fine-needle aspiration biopsy. *Am J Clin Pathol* 1987;88:20–25.

32. Gagliano EF. Fine needle aspiration of Kaposi's sarcoma in lymph nodes—A case report. *Acta Cytol* 1987;31:25–28.

33. Perez-Guillermo M, Perez JS, Rojo BG, Gil AH. Fine needle aspiration cytology of cutaneous vascular tumors. *Cytopathology* 1992; 3:231–244.

34. Yamada T, Itou U, Watanabe Y, Ohashi S. Cytologic diagnosis of malignant melanoma. *Acta Cytol* 1972;16:70–76.

35. Hajdu SI, Savine A. Cytologic diagnosis of malignant melanoma. *Acta Cytol* 1973;17:320–327.

36. Woyke S, Domagala W, Czerniak B, Strokowska M. Fine needle aspiration cytology of malignant melanoma of the skin. *Acta Cytol* 1980; 24:529–538.

37. Nance KV, Park HK, Silverman JF. Fine needle aspiration cytology of desmoplastic malignant melanoma: A case report. *Acta Cytol* 1991;35: 765–769.

38. Kumar PV, Roozitalab MH, Hambarsoomian B, Sotoodeh M. Fine needle aspiration cytologic findings in pseudolymphoma cutis. *Acta Cytol* 1991;35: 337–340.

39. Dahl I, Akerman M. Nodular fasciitis: A cytological and histological study of 13 cases. *Acta Cytol* 1981;25:215–223.

40. Azua J, Arraiza A, Delgado B, Romeo C. Nodular fasciitis initially diagnosed by aspiration cytology. *Acta Cytol* 1985;29:562–565.

41. Powers CN, Berardo MD, Frable WJ. Fine-needle aspiration biopsy: Pitfalls in the diagnosis of spindle cell lesions. *Diagn Cytopathol* 1994; 10:232–241.

42. Gonzales J, Ljung BM, Guerry T, Schoenrock LD. Congenital torticollis: Evaluation by fine-needle aspiration biopsy. *Laryngoscope* 1989;99:651–654.

43. Wakely PE, Price WG, Frable WJ. Sternomastoid tumor of infancy (Fibromatosis colli): Diagnosis by aspiration cytology. *Mod Pathol* 1989;2:378–381.

44. Zaharopoulos P, Wong JY. Fine-needle aspiration cytology in fibromatoses. *Diagn Cytopathol* 1992; 8:73–78.

45. Raab SS, Silverman JF, McLeod DL, Benning TL, Geisinger KR. Fine needle aspiration biopsy of fibromatoses. *Acta Cytol* 1993;37:323–328.

46. Enzinger FM, Weiss SW. *Soft tissue tumors*, 3rd ed. St. Louis: Mosby-Yearbook, 1993, pp. 269–282, 352–355, 390–423, 431–450, 539–545, 757–762.

47. Evans HL. Liposarcomas and atypical lipomatous tumors: A study of 66 cases followed for a minimum of 10 years. *Surg Pathol* 1988;1:41.

48. Walaas L, Kindblom L-G. Lipomatous tumors: A correlative cytologic and histologic study of 27 tumors examined by fine needle aspiration cytology. *Hum Pathol* 1985;16:6–18.

49. Akerman M, Rhydholm A. Aspiration cytology of lipomatous tumors. A ten-year experience at an orthopedic oncology center. *Diagn Cytopathol* 1987; 3:295–302.

50. Powers CN, Hurt MA, Frable WJ. Fine-needle aspiration biopsy: Dermatofibrosarcoma protuberans. *Diagn Cytopathol* 1993;9:145–150.

51. Perry MD, Furlong JW, Johnston WW. Fine-needle aspiration cytology of metastatic dermatofibrosarcoma protuberans. *Acta Cytol* 1986;30: 507–512.

52. de Almeida M, Stastny JF, Wakely PE Jr., Frable WJ. Fine-needle aspiration biopsy of childhood rhabdomyosarcoma: Reevaluation of the cytologic criteria for diagnosis. *Diagn Cytopathol* 1994;11: 231–236.

53. Koivuniemi A, Nickels J. Synovial sarcoma diagnosed by fine needle aspiration biopsy: A case report. *Acta Cytol* 1978;22:515–518.

54. Aisner SC, Seidman JD, Burke KC. Aspiration cytology of biphasic and monophasic synovial sarcoma. A report of two cases. *Acta Cytol* 1993;37:413–417.

55. Frable WJ. Pathologic classification of soft tissue sarcomas. *Sem Surg Oncol* 1994;10:332–339.

CHAPTER

6

Miscellaneous Lesions of the Head and Neck

Although we have subdivided the head and neck into several discrete chapters: lymph nodes, salivary gland, thyroid, and skin and soft tissue, there are still diverse entities that can be encountered on FNAB in this region. The concept of FNAB as a diagnostic tool of the otolaryngologist, head, and neck surgeon is not new. In the 1970s, FNAB was often discussed in the surgical literature.[1–3] Currently, a significant percentage of FNABs in this region are performed to rapidly confirm the clinical impression of squamous cell carcinoma, either as an initial diagnosis, metastasis, or recurrence.[4–9] Another group of lesions commonly encountered are cysts, the result of either embryonal remnants or inflammatory conditions. Obviously the surgical management of malignant, benign, and inflammatory lesions is sufficiently different that this rapid, outpatient (clinic) procedure has been extensively utilized by these specialists. These lesions are, for the most part, straightforward diagnoses with the collaboration of pathologist and surgeon. However, there are numerous, relatively uncommon conditions encountered often enough that a specific diagnosis is difficult for the pathologist with limited FNAB experience. The literature is replete with single case reports and small series of these unusual lesions such that some cytologic criteria for them are being or have been developed.

TECHNIQUE

While there is no specific technique recommended for FNAB of masses in the head and neck, positioning of the patient is very important. An examining chair, similar to those used by the dentist or otolaryngologist, provides the best support with a secure head/neck rest. When FNAB of masses in the scalp or face is performed, it is important to have the patient's head stabilized. It is quite natural for the patient to move away from the needle as it approaches a mass located in any of these areas. A posterior and/or lateral head rest provides a level of reassurance to the patient and support for the clinician. Masses located in the anterior neck may be more apparent and easier to stabilize if the patient rotates his or her head in the contralateral direction. Similarly, masses in the posterior neck may be more accessible if the head is tilted forward.

The presence of a mass near the major vessels (external jugular vein or carotid artery) should not dissuade the clinician from performing FNAB. The most common fear is that penetration of the vessel by the needle will cause excessive bleeding or frank hemorrhage. In fact, the use of fine needles results in relatively little damage even if the penetration is through the vessel. If this does occur, it is usually signaled by rapid blood flow into the syringe, which can be quite startling if an artery has been punctured. First and most important, DON'T PANIC! This can result in improper withdrawal of the needle, resulting in a tear. The needle should be withdrawn in a controlled fashion and firm pressure applied to the puncture site. If a major blood vessel is punctured, it should be treated just as a venipuncture or as arterial blood gas sampling—pressure should be applied for 5 to 10 minutes, as indicated. It should be remembered that arterial blood is sampled for blood gas studies via needle puncture, usually without complications.

Aspiration of masses within the oral cavity can present difficult but not insurmountable problems. Because visualization of the mass or lesion can be quite helpful in placement of the needle, a strong light source, either from a head lamp, mirror, or flexible light source (freestanding or attached to the examining chair) is necessary. It is essential to keep both hands free to perform the FNAB. In addition, patients tire quickly if they are required to keep their mouths open for any length of time. Bite blocks or the less sophisticated gauze packing rolled around a tongue depressor should be placed appropriately to give the patient relief from the exertion of keeping the mouth open while the procedure is underway. Bite blocks should be positioned to avoid obstructing the view of the mass and to allow a clear path for the needle. Topical (spray) anesthetic may be used to provide limited local anesthesia. Although the gauge of the needle remains small, 23 to 25 gauge, 7.7 to 12.8 centimeter (3 to 5 inches) needles will be required to reach lesions in the posterior pharynx. Often, two fingers of the left hand can be inserted into the mouth to guide and reinforce the longer and more flexible needle while the right hand controls the aspiration gun.

An alternative approach is to use the Franseen needle guide with 20-centimeter needle, if the lesion can be palpated through the mouth. The needle guide, originally designed for prostate aspiration, is secured in place over the finger and palm of the gloved examining hand with a second glove. The palpating finger locates the lesion and pushes against it firmly. Once the examining finger has secured the point for aspiration, the needle is advanced through the guide and into the mass. An assistant will usually be necessary to initiate the placement of the needle into the guide and the attachment of the aspirating syringe to the needle after the aspirator has advanced the needle into the mass. A bite block is also necessary and a chair with head rest so that the patient cannot move away as the needle enters the mass. Topical anesthesia is recommended for this procedure, which is best utilized for lesions at the base of the tongue and adjacent areas in the oral cavity. It is important to remember that the target for biopsy should be palpable within the oral cavity to effectively biopsy it in this manner.[10]

Clinical signs and symptoms arising from masses in the pharynx and nasopharynx result in their identification by CT or magnetic resonance imaging (MRI) with confirmation by endoscopic aspiration and biopsy. A bulge in the pharyngeal wall produced by a mass may be the only evidence of tumor. Aspiration may prove difficult to perform in the conventional fashion. The introduction of flexible endoscopes has allowed physicians to visualize and sample these masses via flexible needles in a manner similar to techniques employed in bronchoscopic and mediastinal aspiration biopsies.[11] This is usually an outpatient procedure and the patient may only require mild sedation and topical anesthesia.

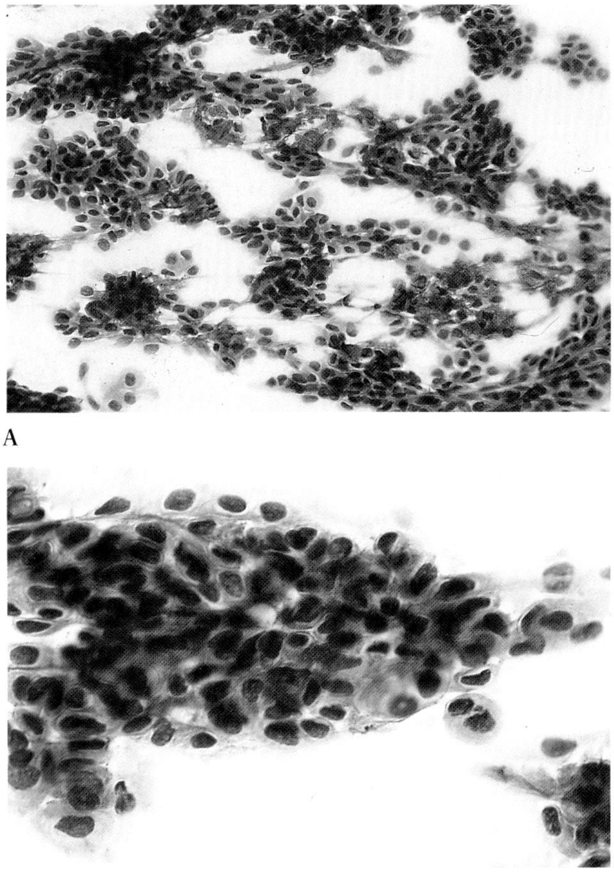

A

B

FIGURE 6.1 (A) Acrospiroma. Cellular smear composed of cohesive irregular sheets of ovoid cells with bland nuclei and amphophilic cytoplasm. Papanicolaou 200×. (B) Higher power of single sheet demonstrating a suggestion of squamous features that can be seen with some skin adenexal tumors cytologically and histologically. Papanicolaou 400×.

MASSES OF THE HEAD

Scalp and Face

The majority of lesions that can occur as facial and scalp masses have been discussed in Chapter 5. Masses frequently identified in this region include epidermoid cysts and primary skin carcinomas; squamous cell, basal cell, and Merkel-cell carcinomas, and cutaneous appendage tumors. An example of an aspirate from an acrospiroma is illustrated in Figure 6.1.

Dermal and subcutaneous lesions such as Kaposi's sarcoma, dermatofibrosarcoma protuberans, and not uncommonly, metastatic carcinoma may also be encountered. An example of an unusual case is illustrated in Figure 6.2. The aspirate was from a 5.0-millimeter nodule recently noted in the scalp of a 12-year-old patient. The patient had been treated by radiation therapy at the age of 2 for medulloblastoma of the cerebellum. This had been successful, but the patient developed a pelvic mass at the age of 11 that on removal proved to be a leiomyosarcoma arising in the right ovary. The scalp lesion was metastatic leiomyosarcoma, clinically the only apparent metastasis 1 year after removal of the ovarian tumor.

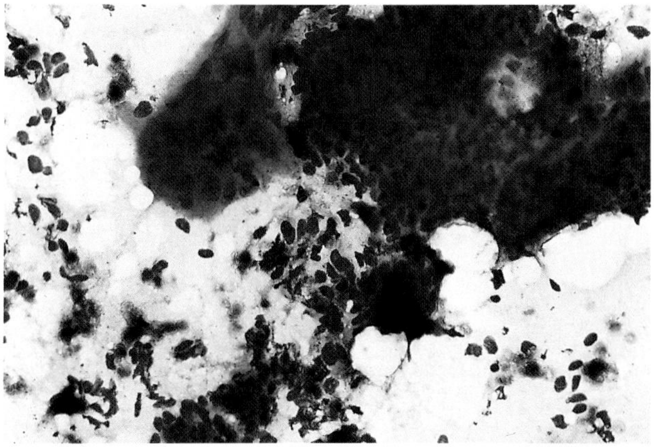

FIGURE 6.2 Metastatic hemangiopericytoma. Tight and loose clusters of spindle-shaped, plump cells. The variable pattern suggests a skin adenexal tumor. Comparison to the original ovarian hemangiopericytoma revealed a good match between the cytologic features and the histology. Diff-Quik® 400×.

Skull and Jaw

Masses of the head are not limited to the skin and soft tissues but may also occur in the bones of the skull and jaw. Lesions of the bones of the head and neck are predominantly tumors; they require skill in aspiration to obtain adequate material for diagnosis, clinical experience with this type of case, and some expertise in evaluating bone radiographs. It is important to be able to translate conventional histopathology to the cytologic smear. Bone tumors are particularly challenging under the best of circumstances, and accurate diagnosis by FNAB requires collaboration with clinician and radiologist and correlation with the cytologic features. This section is intended as an overview of lesions that may be encountered, albeit infrequently in the skull and jaw.

The procedure for FNAB of bone lesions is not appreciably different from standard aspiration technique. Masses arising in the bony cortex are often destructive and offer little resistance to the fine needle as it penetrates the periosteum. Other bone tumors may have a soft-tissue component that can be sampled using traditional 3.8-centimeter (1.5 inch) or 7.7-centimeter (3-inch) 22- to 25-gauge needles. Difficulty arises in attempts to sample an intramedullary lesion that requires penetration of the intact cortical bone. Approaches may vary depending on the physician's experience and training. Needles such as a Jamshidi or Illinois may be used to extract a core of cortical bone directly above the mass followed by direct aspiration using the same type of needle or the insertion of a fine needle through the tract created by the large-bore needle. This has the benefit of being a rapid, outpatient procedure that requires only local anesthesia. A second choice for problem cases may be an intraoperative aspiration biopsy under general anesthesia. In these instances, an orthopedic surgeon drills through the cortical bone and then inserts the fine needle and performs the aspiration.

Giant-Cell Tumor of Bone

Although more commonly identified in the epiphysis or metaphysis of the bones of the extremities, giant-cell tumor of bone may rarely be encountered in the facial bones, particularly the jaw. In the flat bones of the craniofacial region, giant-cell tumor is seen as a complication of Paget's disease. True giant-cell tumor of the jaw, not associated with Paget's disease, is quite rare.[12] The chief difficulty in diagnosis is distinguishing this neoplasm from other giant-cell lesions such as hyperparathyroidism (brown tumor) and reparative granulomas that are much more frequent in this region. Ramzy suggests the use of the description "benign giant cell containing proliferative lesion."[13] Cytomorphology should be correlated with radiology (osteolytic or blastic, multicentricity) and clinical data (metabolic state of the patient, history of trauma, Paget's disease) to arrive at a more specific diagnosis.[14–16] Giant-cell tumor, a friable and highly vascular tumor, produces a radiolytic lesion that is easily identified and aspirated. This neoplasm is a biphasic tumor composed of multinucleated (osteoclast-type) giant cells and a stromal component composed of spindle cells (Figure 6.3). The ratio of stromal cells to giant cells varies from case to case. Aspirates are often bloody but there is usually little difficulty obtaining adequate material with one or two aspirations. One clue to the diagnosis of giant-cell tumor is the recognition that the nuclei of both the spindle cells and giant cells are morphologically similar, suggesting a coalescence of the stromal cells into giant cells (Figure 6.4). Giant cells are not specific for giant-cell tumor because they

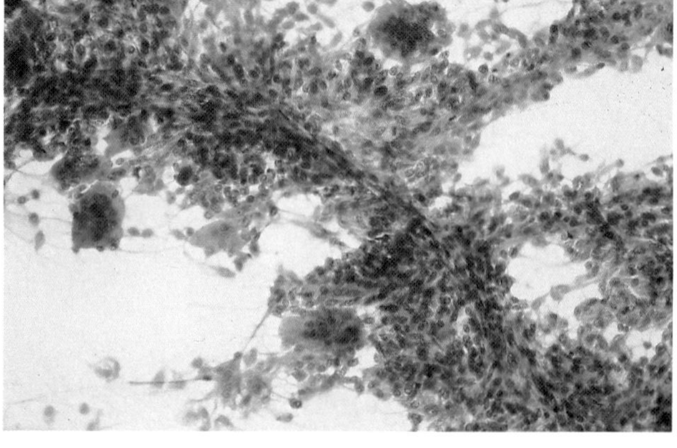

FIGURE 6.3 Giant-cell tumor. Cellular smear with cohesive fragments of spindle cells and scattered multinucleated giant cells. In this limited field, the even distribution of the giant cells suggests giant-cell tumor rather than a reactive process. Papanicolaou 200×.

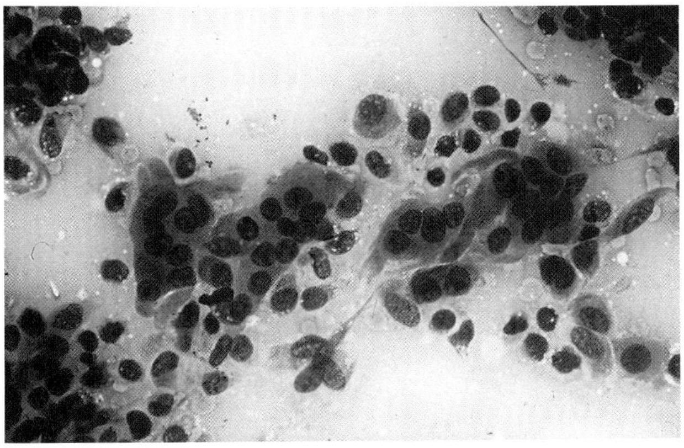

FIGURE 6.4 Giant-cell tumor. The nuclei of the spindle cells are identical to those of the giant cells suggesting the latter are formed by a coalescence of spindle cells. Diff-Quik® 400×.

are often associated with other lesions, for example, giant cell reparative granuloma of the jaw. Their presence is a reaction to the disease process (inflammatory response) rather than a component of it.[12]

Giant-cell tumors are usually benign tumors, but a small percentage can metastasize. While increased cellularity and mitotic activity and cytologic atypia are suggestive of malignancy, these features may not be present in other malignant giant-cell tumors. Measurement of DNA ploidy has not been found to be of value in predicting the behavior of giant-cell tumor of bone.[17]

GIANT-CELL TUMOR OF BONE

Bloody background

Bimorphic population
- **–Spindle "stromal" cells**
  - **–Sheets, fragments, or less often dispersed**
  - **–Spindle, plump, oval**
  - **–Moderate cytoplasm—bipolar cytoplasmic processes**
  - **–Oval nuclei with finely granular chromatin**
  - **–Membrane may be indented**
  - **–Chromocenters and/or small nucleoli**

Multinucleated (osteoclastic) giant cells
- **–Enmeshed in stromal fragments or single and dispersed**
- **–Abundant dense cytoplasm**
- **–Few to numerous nuclei, membrane may be indented**
- **–Finely granular chromatin**
- **–Nucleolus**

****Nuclei of both cell types are similar in appearance**

Plasmacytoma

Multiple myeloma, a systemic disease, is often diagnosed by a combination of serum or urine studies (protein electrophoresis) that identify a dysproteinemia/urea with subsequent monoclonal spike and bone marrow aspiration and biopsy of iliac crest that retrieves a sample of marrow containing the neoplastic plasma cells. With the exception of multiple myeloma lesions of the skull or a clinical presentation involving soft tissue, FNAB is rarely used to diagnose this condition. However, it is very useful for identifying the variant of multiple myeloma—plasmacytoma or plasma cell tumor (PCT). PCT, usually a solitary lesion, most commonly presents in the head and neck region as a soft-tissue mass but may occur as a solitary bone lesion, usually within the jaw.[12,18–20] As in the giant-cell tumor of bone, this lesion is osteolytic and easily penetrated by a fine needle. The discohesive nature of this tumor assures adequate recovery of cells. The cytomorphology of multiple myeloma

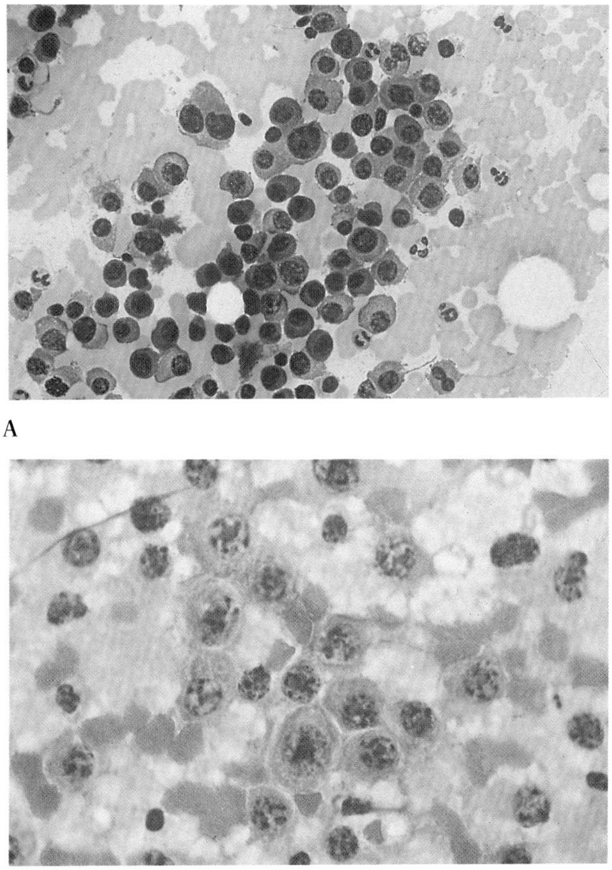

A

B

FIGURE 6.5 (A) Plasma cell tumor. Numerous, discohesive plasma cells of varying size. Note the variation in nuclear size, occasional double-nucleated tumor cells, and consistent eccentric position of the nucleus with adjacent perinuclear clear area. Diff-Quik® 200×. (B) Neoplastic plasma cells with prominent central nucleoli and "clock face" chromatin pattern. Papanicolaou 400×.

and PCT is identical—that is, numerous neoplastic plasma cells are present and show varying degrees of differentiation (Figure 6.5). A few other tumors will closely mimic PCTs: melanoma, immunoblastic lymphomas, and undifferentiated carcinomas. Inflammatory conditions with abundant, reactive plasma cells are seldom mistaken for a PCT. The correlation of radiologic and clinical findings and, if necessary, immunocytochemical analysis will solidify the diagnosis.[21,22]

PLASMA CELL TUMOR

Bloody background

Monomorphic population
- **–Neoplastic plasma cells**
  - **–Varying degrees of differentiation (normal-appearing plasma cells to extreme atypia)**
  - **–Abundant basophilic cytoplasm**
  - **–Prominent perinuclear hof (Golgi body)**
  - **–Mono- or binucleated**
  - **–Nucleus with coarse chromatin ("clock face pattern")**
  - **–Large, prominent nucleoli**
- **Mitoses**

Osteosarcoma

Osteosarcoma, with the exception of myeloma, is the most common primary tumor of bone, though it occurs relatively infrequently in the bones of the head and neck. Most osteosarcomas are high-grade malignancies and by definition produce at least some osteoid. In the head and neck, the jaw is the most common site. Patients present with pain and loose teeth. Osteosarcoma of the craniofacial bones is seen in patients usually over the age of 25 years; in much older individuals, it is most likely to be associated with an underlying process involving the skull or jaws, such as Paget's disease. Radiographically, osteosarcomas are bone-destructive tumors that produce a lytic, sclerotic, or mixed lytic and sclerotic appearance.[23] Because of the destruction of the bone cortex by the time of presentation, aspiration biopsy is relatively simple.[24–27]

Cytologically, the smears are cellular and full of single, plump tumor cells with an oval to slightly spindle shape (Figure 6.6). The tumor cells are large and the nuclei vary in size and have prominent nucleoli. A few multinucleated giant cells may be present. Small fragments or rather abundant metachromatic stroma may be identified on air-dried smears stained with one of the Romanowsky stains. The tumor cells may appear trapped haphazardly within the metachromatic material, which is osteoid, mimicking the histologic pattern of this tumor (Figure 6.7). Osteosarcoma arising in Paget's disease of the skull appears highly anaplastic both in tissue and on aspiration smears.

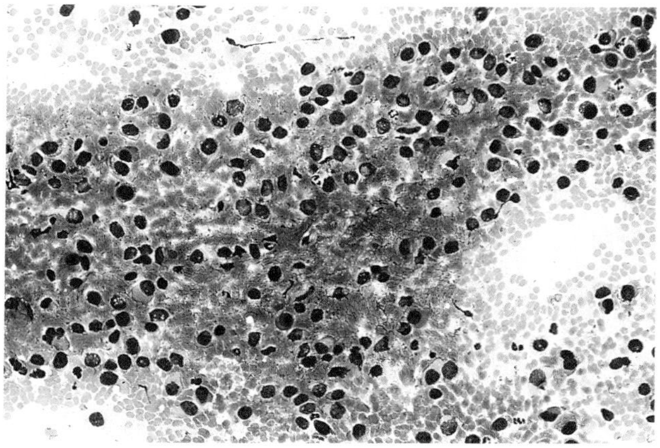

FIGURE 6.6 Osteosarcoma. Cellular smear with scattered discohesive cells and fragment of metachromatic osteoid. Matrix in the smears of osteosarcoma may be prominent or quite limited. Diff-Quik® 250×.

OSTEOSARCOMA

Cellularity, high

Pleomorphic population of plump, oval to spindle-shaped tumor cells
- **–Large nuclei**
- **–Coarse chromatin**
- **–Prominent nucleoli**
- **–Scattered binucleated tumor cells**
- **–Few multinucleated osteoclasts**
- **–Mitoses**

Metachromatic stroma, abundant to scant
- **–Tumor cells juxtaposed to stroma (osteoid)**

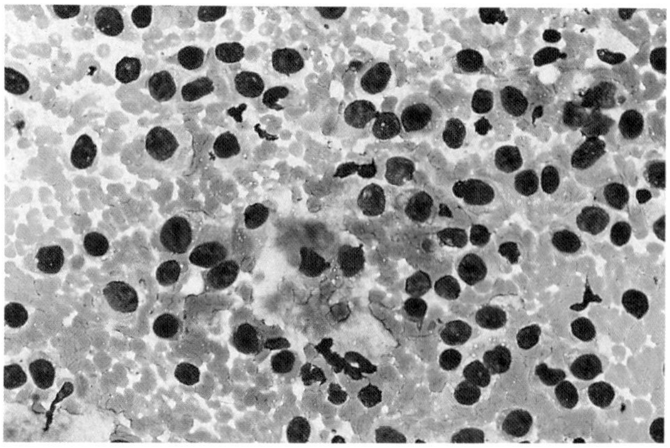

FIGURE 6.7 Osteosarcoma. Plump, oval cells with large nuclei and prominent nucleoli. Osteoid stains as a metachromatic, amorphous material on Romanowsky stains. Two tumor cells in the center of the field appear to be embedded within the stroma, simulating the histologic pattern of malignant osteoid. Diff-Quik® 400×.

Chondrosarcoma

With the exception of myeloma, chrondrosarcoma is the second most common malignant neoplasm of bone, but it is a very uncommon primary in the jaw or craniofacial bones.[23] With relationship to the bone, this tumor occurs centrally within the medullary canal, peripherally—extending both outward from the bony cortex and invading the medullary canal, or juxtacortical. There are several histologic subtypes: mesenchymal, dedifferentiated, and clear cell. Primary chondrosarcoma is a neoplasm of later onset, occurring from the fifth to seventh decade, unless it results as a malignant growth from chondroma or osteochrondroma, when it occurs earlier.[12]

Aspirates of chondrosarcoma are affected by differentiation of the tumor. Those forming differentiated cartilage will have dominance of metachromatic stroma in nodules entrapping isolated chondrocytes. The latter may have double nuclei and appear as cells embedded in the metachromatic matrix within lacunar spaces, simulating the histologic pattern of cartilage (Figure 6.8). Less-differentiated forms retain much of the metachromatic stroma but have increased numbers of cytologically malignant cartilage cells. They exhibit nuclear variation and abnormalities in chromatin distribution (Figure 6.9). Some areas of the smear may have a spindle cell, fibrosarcomatous pattern. The dedifferentiated forms and mesenchymal types have smears that are highly cellular and frankly malignant but may lack any other identifying features of origin from cartilage. Unlike other tumors of bone, dedifferentiated chrondrosarcoma may demonstrate positive immunostaining for S-100 protein, cytokeratin, and epithelial membrane antigen (EMA).

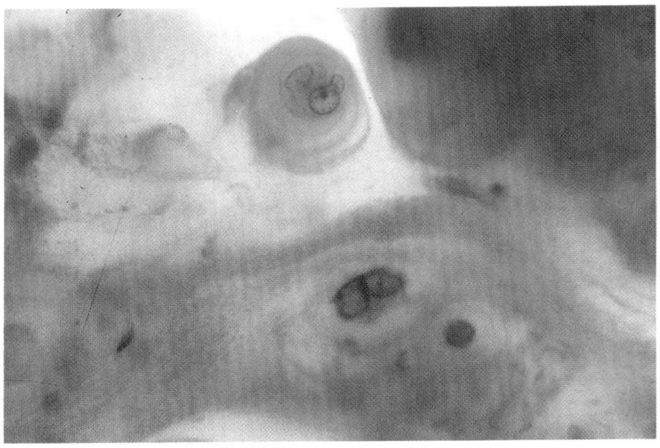

FIGURE 6.8 Well-differentiated chondrosarcoma. Rounded cells in lacunar spaces, outlined by a thick cytoplasmic and stromal interface. Two cells in this field are binucleate chondrocytes, a cytologic and histologic feature of well-differentiated chrondrosarcoma. Papanicolaou 1000×.

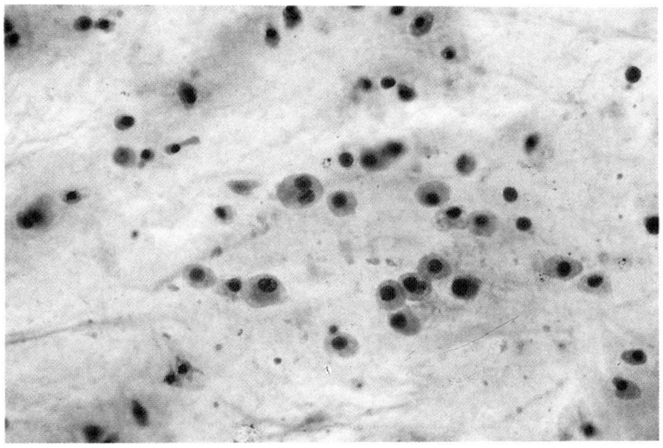

FIGURE 6.9 Dedifferentiated chrondrosarcoma. Smear with increased cellularity and round plasmacytoid-like cells and nonspecific appearance of background stroma. A few smaller spindle-shaped cells are also present. Papanicolaou 400×.

CHONDROSARCOMA

Cellularity
- **Moderate, dominated by stroma, well-differentiated examples**
- **High, less evident stroma, dedifferentiated**

Chondrocytes
- **Differentiated lacunar cells, a few multinucleated in differentiated forms**
- **Pleomorphic tumor cells with malignant nuclear features in dedifferentiated forms**

Stroma
- **Abundant metachromatic with fibrillar pattern surrounding individual chondrocytes in differentiated forms. Resembles normal cartilage closely.**
- **Less, but recognizable, metachromatic stroma that suggests a cartilagenous neoplasm surrounds both individual and groups of cells.**
- **Simulates metastatic epithelial tumor**

Oral Cavity and Pharynx

The majority of paroral FNABs are for the diagnosis of neoplasms of the oral mucosa, tonsils, or posterior pharynx. Tumors occurring in the minor salivary gland are less often encountered.[28–31] The two most frequently occurring tumors of this region are the benign mixed tumor (pleomorphic adenoma) and squamous cell carcinoma. These neoplasms have been discussed in Chapters 2 and 5. Inflammatory processes, either infectious (tuberculosis, actinomycosis, blastomycosis) or radiation-induced injury, are also frequently identified.[31,32] Drainage of abscesses or hematomas, while

TABLE 6.1 Dental Lesions Identified by Fine-Needle Aspiration Biopsy

Adenomatoid odontogenic tumor
Ameloblastoma
Cementifying fibroma
Cementoma
Odontoma
Odontogenic cysts
radicular
developmental
keratocyst
glandular

performed with a fine needle, are not done for the purpose of diagnosis and are therefore not considered in this chapter.

A specialized area of FNAB includes "dental" lesions of the oral cavity and jaw (Table 6.1). A knowledge of embryonal and developmental anatomy is absolutely necessary for accurate diagnosis of most of these processes. The institutions most likely to provide definitive diagnoses of these conditions using FNAB are medical centers with a high-volume dental clinic and oral pathologists familiar with FNAB. The histologic patterns encountered with these entities are quite variable. Illustrated in Figure 6.10 is an example of ameloblastic carcinoma, recurrent in the jaw. There are overlapping and nonspecific cytologic patterns, particularly for those neoplasms that have no or limited epithelium.

In particular, FNAB of odontogenic cysts is often nonspecific: inflammation with histiocytes and either squamous, columnar, or cuboidal epithelium resulting in a generic diagnosis of "benign cysts with epithelial lining."[30] An experienced oral pathologist may be able to further classify these cysts (Table 6.1). Non-specific inflammatory lesions are often encountered and result in an equally nonspecific diagnosis. Generally these aspirates reveal inflammatory cells admixed with epithelial cells, scattered histiocytes, and cellular debris. Fibroblasts may also be encountered if the process is resolving and forming granulation tissue or scar. Multinucleated giant cells may be encountered sporadically in these conditions; however, the presence of Langhans-type giant cells should initiate a search for an infectious etiology such as tuberculosis.

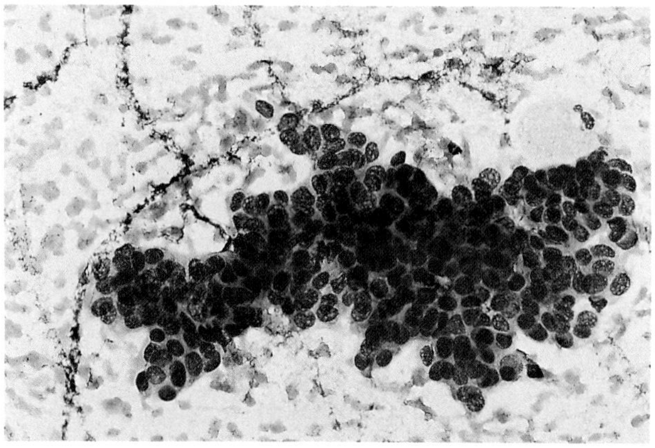

FIGURE 6.10 Ameloblastic carcinoma. Islands and trabecular pattern of epithelial cells in a very limited, metachromatic stromal background. Stellate reticulum is absent in this tumor. The basic cytologic pattern is that of a well-differentiated adenocarcinoma. Location of the neoplasm and comparison with prior histology establish the correct diagnosis. Diff-Quik® 400×.

NASAL CAVITY, SINUSES, AND NASOPHARYNX

Nasopharyngeal Carcinoma

Although direct aspiration biopsy of the nasopharynx is not frequent, the diagnosis of nasopharyngeal carcinoma (NPC) by FNAB is not uncommon. Initial diagnosis of this undifferentiated carcinoma, often referred to as lymphoepithelioma, is more commonly made from aspiration of metastasis to cervical lymph nodes.[33,34] There are two recognizable histologic patterns of NPC based on the distribution of lymphoid elements: Schmincke's and Regaud's. In the former pattern, lymphocytes are dispersed among tumor cells while in the latter they surround aggregates of the carcinoma. FNAB smears of NPC are usually very cellular with the tumor cells scattered singly and in clusters. The distribution of lymphoid elements, mostly mature lymphocytes, will give an indication of the overall histologic pattern. The individual neoplastic cells are large with scant cytoplasm, large nuclei, and prominent nucleoli

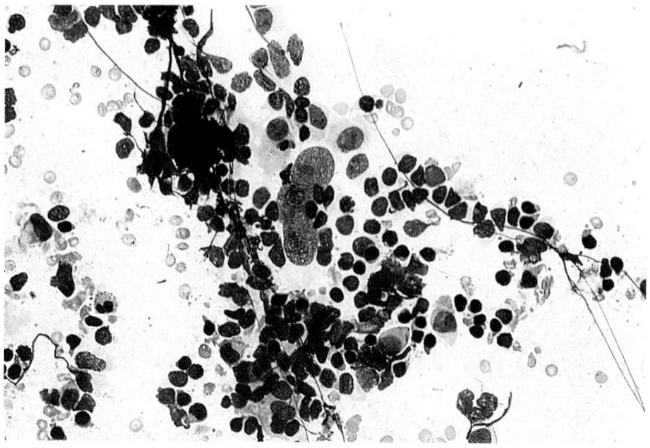

FIGURE 6.11 Nasopharyngeal carcinoma. Pleomorphic epithelial cells surrounded by small mature lymphocytes. The tumor cells are represented by large naked nuclei in this field. DiffQuik® 400×.

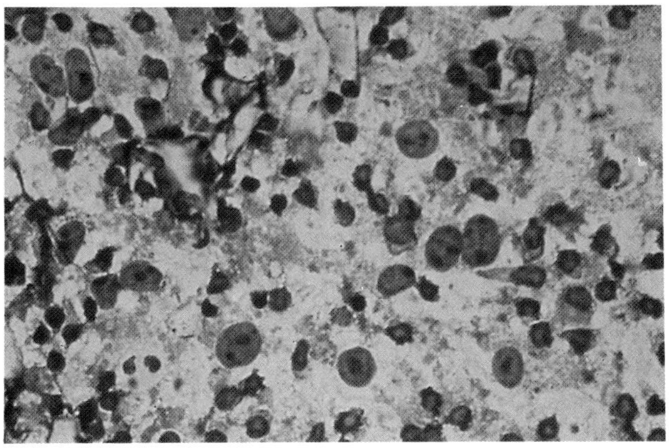

FIGURE 6.12 Nasopharyngeal carcinoma. Numerous degenerating epithelioid cells in a background of lymphocytes and necrosis. The tumor cells are large naked nuclei with very prominent nucleoli. Fragments of cell cytoplasm simulate lymphoglandular bodies and the presence of large single cells may suggest a diagnosis of large-cell lymphoma. Diff-Quik® 400×.

(Figure 6.11). Mitotic figures may sometimes be identified. Problems in recognition may occur when the tumor cells are few in number and the lymphoid population is dominant. Necrosis and a granulomatous reaction may also occur, thus obscuring the true diagnosis (Figure 6.12).[35] Immunostains on aspiration smears of cytospins may be helpful when the diagnosis is suspected, but tumor cells are not easily identified.

When using cytokeratin in this situation, some caution is necessary because dendritic reticulum cells, normal inhabitants of lymph nodes, will stain positively with cytokeratin, resembling epithelial cells.[36]

NASOPHARYNGEAL CARCINOMA

High cellularity

Biphasic population
- **–Large epithelial cells**
  - **–High nuclear to cytoplasmic ratio**
  - **–Minimal cytoplasm**
  - **–Prominent nucleoli**
  - **–Occasional mitoses**
- **–Lymphocytes**
  - **–Intermingling with tumor cells (Schmincke)**
  - **–Surrounding clusters of tumor cells (Regaud)**

Malignant Lymphoma

Malignant lymphoma may arise in the lymphoid tissue that is present throughout the nasopharynx. Because lymphomas are frequently monomorphic and lack cohesion, aspirates are very cellular, providing material not only for cytomorphology but for immunophenotyping as well. The cytologic criteria necessary for a diagnosis of lymphoma are reviewed in detail in Chapter 4.

Olfactory Neuroblastoma

A small, round, blue cell tumor of childhood, olfactory neuroblastoma (esthesioneuroblastoma) occurs frequently in the orbital and nasal cavity but is seen usually in young adults rather than children. Like neuroblastomas that occur elsewhere, these tumors are quickly recognized in aspiration smears as small-round-cell undifferentiated neoplasms (Figure 6.13). Further characterization as a neuroblastoma occurs when rosettes containing delicate, eosinophilic fibrillar material, or "neuropil," are identified. Dispersed single cells with elongated nuclei and DNA artifact can be seen in variable amounts in the background.[37,38] Distortion of these fragile cells is most likely due to vigorous smear preparation. As an adult disease, the differential diagnosis includes lymphoma and metastatic small-cell carcinoma from the lung. Immunostains for leukocyte common antigen will help in differentiating malignant lymphoma, but neuroendocrine markers are less helpful as there is wide variation in the number of small-cell carcinomas of the lung that will stain for neuron-specific enolase or chromogranin.[39]

OLFACTORY NEUROBLASTOMA

High cellularity

Dispersed small blue cells
- **–Minimal cytoplasm**
- **–Round nuclei (salt and pepper chromatin)**
- **–Nucleoli**

Rosette formation

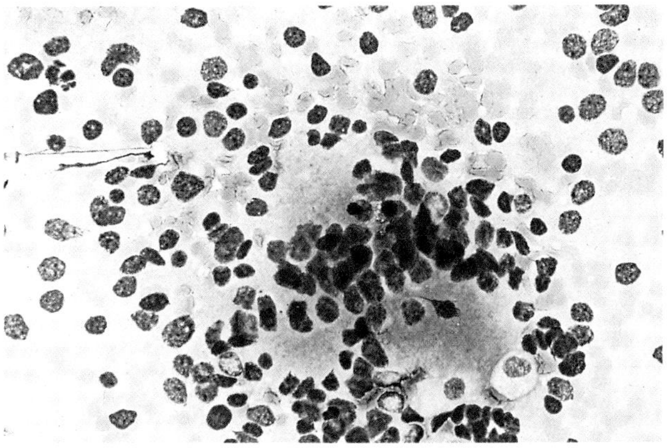

FIGURE 6.13 Olfactory neuroblastoma. Undifferentiated round cells with wispy red cytoplasm representing "neuropil." Clustering of tumor cells in the center of the illustration suggests a rosette. The primary diagnosis is small-round-cell tumor that is differentiated more specifically after the application of special stains. Diff-Quik® 400×.

Diagnostic Accuracy, Problems, and Pitfalls

The accuracy of FNAB in the diagnosis of oral and pharyngeal lesions is dependent upon (1) the skill of the aspirator and (2) the experience of the interpreter. These are familiar but extremely important phrases. In the studies specifically targeting this region, accuracy ranged from 88% to 100%.[1,28,31] The higher rates reflect stringent criteria for obtaining an adequate sample. Those FNABs that were paucicellular as well as those that were acellular or blood only were not included. Unfortunately, this can be a very high number of samples if the procedure is not done consistently by experienced physicians. False-positive diagnoses were rare (1 case) and false-negative diagnoses were due to inadequate sampling in those studies that attempted diagnosis on aspirates of low cellularity. Castelli et al. indicate that FNAB of the oral cavity is less sensitive and less specific than FNAB of superficial lesions.[29] This probably reflects the reluctance of many to perform aspiration in this region and the reluctance, due to lack of expertise in oral pathology, to render specific diagnoses on FNAB performed by clinicians. This does not appear to be a problem in those institutions that have oral pathology services or a high volume of cases such that pathologists gain the necessary experience in dealing with the many and variable conditions in this area. As suggested above, diagnostic difficulty is usually encountered when the pathologist tries to render a diagnosis on scant material or on aspirates that are obscured by blood or inflammation.

ORBIT AND EYELID

FNAB of the orbit and to a lesser extent the eyelid requires both technical expertise and thorough knowledge of the anatomy of these two areas. It should not be attempted without having considerable experience with fine needle aspiration biopsy generally. Although the anatomy of the orbit is complex, orbital aspirations are not technically difficult if a palpable mass is present. However, they may be disconcerting to the uninitiated, and as such require the aspirator to be secure and confident in his/her ability. Typically, oculoplastic surgeons, orbital surgeons, and cytopathologists have the experience to perform these aspirations with minimal complications and maximum diagnostic efficacy. In the past, cytopathology was limited to the interpretation of direct conjunctival smears with a minimal focus on FNAB.[40] However, several groups have vigorously pursued the utility of FNAB in the diagnosis of orbital lesions. Recently, a textbook dedicated to FNAB of the orbit has been published.[41] The two major indications for FNAB of the orbit are the diagnosis of an unresectible malignancy, thus eliminating the need for an incisional biopsy, and confirmation of orbital metastases.[42–48]

Technique

Standard aspiration technique is used for FNAB of eyelid and orbital tissues. Knowledge of the anatomy is crucial for accurate placement of the needle. FNAB with or without aspiration has been performed successfully on superficial, extraocular masses.[49] While 22-gauge needles have been used in the past, currently smaller needles 25, 27, and 30 gauge are preferred (Figure 6.14). Only slight discomfort is experienced; therefore, local anesthesia is not recommended. Both CT and ultrasound (B-scan) image guidance have been used for localization of intraconal and retrobulbar masses.[48,50–52] CT guidance offers precise targeting of deeply situated tumors while ultrasound appears more useful in masses located in the mid- and anterior orbit.

Lesions

A detailed cytologic description of the numerous conditions found in the orbit and periorbital region is beyond the scope of this text. However, many of the processes mentioned in this chapter are described elsewhere in this book, especially in Chapters 4 and 5.

Palpable masses of both upper and lower eyelids are easily and adequately sampled by FNAB using either

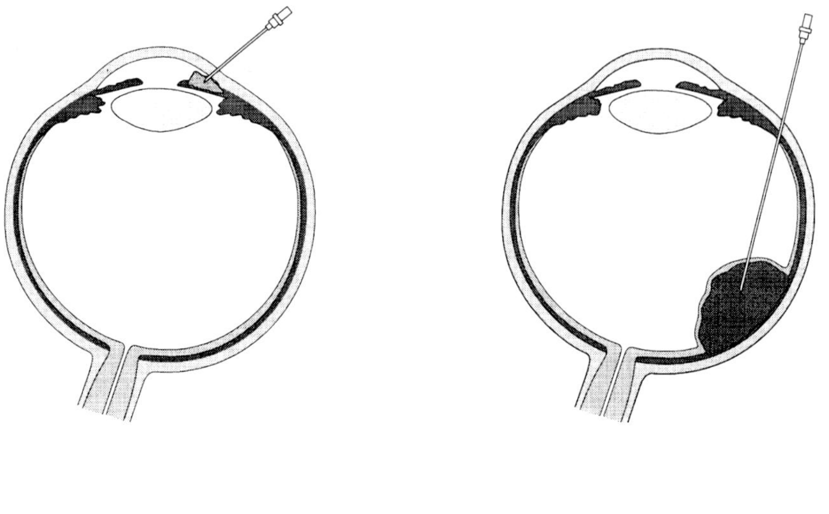

FIGURE 6.14 Indirect FNAB of intraocular lesions. (A) Sampling of mass within the anterior chamber by needle biopsy may be performed with or without aspiration. (B) FNAB of posterior intraocular masses requires longer needles, often with radiologic (ultrasonography) guidance.

aspiration or nonaspiration technique. The most common neoplasms that occur in this region are squamous and basal cell carcinomas followed less frequently by malignant melanoma and sebaceous carcinoma. The cytologic features of these malignancies are described elsewhere (Chapter 5). Most pathologists are familiar with the cytologic features of these tumors such that FNAB represents a rapid and accurate technique that can be followed by definitive treatment, usually wide local excision.[53]

Other regions that can harbor palpable masses include eyebrow, lacrimal gland, orbital roof and floor, and inner and outer canthus. A variety of benign and malignant processes can be found in these areas: dermoid cyst, inflammation, abscess, squamous papilloma, meningioma, eosinophilic granuloma, adenoid cystic carcinoma, adenocarcinoma, plasmacytoma, rhabdomyosarcoma.[47,49] An abscess due to mucormycosis is illustrated in Figure 6.15. Diagnosis of this condition can be a medical emergency because of the destructive nature of the organisms and their ability to invade blood vessels. An example of adenoid cystic carcinoma of the lacrimal gland invading the orbit is seen in Figure 6.16. This neoplasm grows slowly but invades bone soft tissue and perineural spaces, making it quite difficult to resect with a negative surgical margin. An example of a meningioma is seen in Figure 6.17. The whorled pattern is distinctive but the resemblance to squamous cell carcinoma can make the specific diagnosis difficult. Another example of rhabdomyosarcoma of the alveolar type involving the orbit is depicted in Figure 6.18. Other than the pleomorphic pattern of rhabdomyosarcoma, the alveolar and embryonal types look essentially identical in FNAB smears.

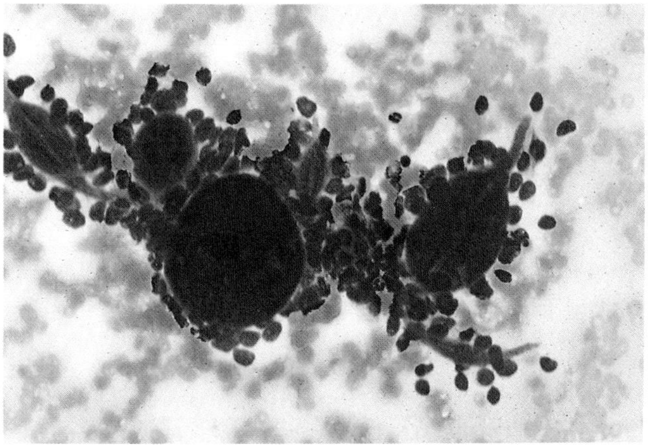

FIGURE 6.16 Adenoid cystic carcinoma arising in the lacrimal gland. Metachromatic hyaline globules surrounded by small, uniform basaloid cells are a key feature in the diagnosis of this neoplasm. Diff-Quik® 200×.

Accuracy

Diagnostic accuracy is primarily dependent upon the experience of the aspirator as well as the cytopathologist. As with FNAB of other body sites, close cooperation among ophthalmologist, radiologist, and cytopathologist will ensure the best results. This is reflected in the literature: the majority of reports with reasonably high accuracy rates (80% to over 92%) are the result of this collaboration.[45–47,49,53,54] Indeed, in the 1986 study by Zajdela et al., not only were the authors able to establish a diagnosis of malignancy in 95 percent of their cases, but they also accurately classified 87 percent of these malignancies.[49] However, one study in particular disputed this level of diagnostic accuracy,

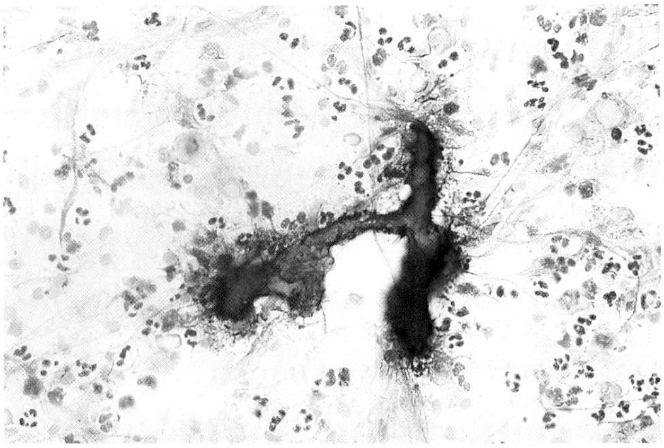

FIGURE 6.15 Mucormycosis involving the orbit. Thick, irregular fragments of nonseptate hyphae in a background of acute inflammatory cells and blood. Organisms may be few in number and difficult to detect without a careful search of the smears. In contrast, a much larger number of organisms may be found with special stains such as Gomori methamine silver that are performed on smears from the same aspirate. Diff-Quik® 400×.

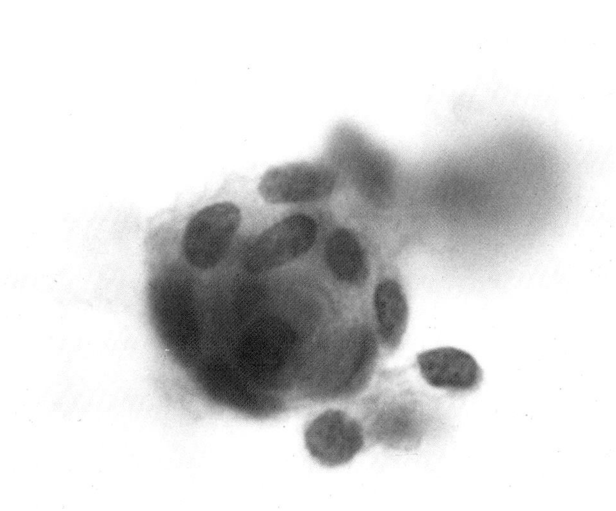

FIGURE 6.17 Meningioma appearing in the orbit. Small spindle cells with abundant cytoplasm wrap around each other creating whorls. The vague laminar appearance of the cytoplasm in the center of this cell cluster suggests early formation of a psammoma body. Papanicolaou 1000×.

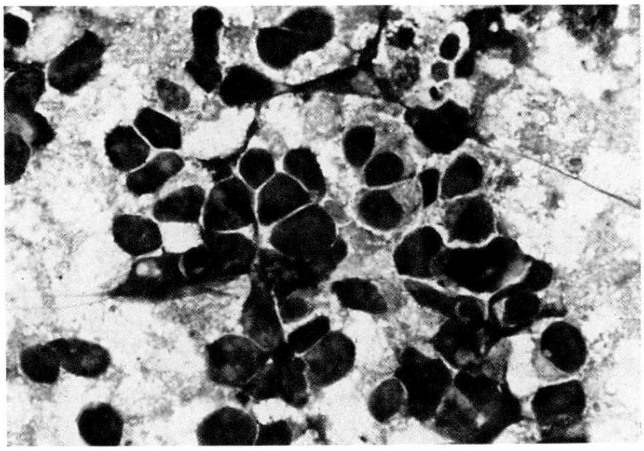

FIGURE 6.18 Alveolar rhabdomyosarcoma of the orbit. Cellular smears with discohesive small cells with oval irregular nuclei and scant cytoplasm. Muscle differentiation may not always be present in these lesions. Detection of a few much larger nuclei or multiple nuclei found in rhabdomyosarcomas aid cytologically in the differential diagnosis among other small-round-cell tumors. Diff-Quik® 400×.

suggesting that it may be much lower—in the range of 47 percent.[55] In this study, Krohel et al. performed FNAB of orbital masses using direct visualization concurrent with or immediately following open surgical biopsy. Of FNAB on 34 patients, 11 (32 percent) yielded minimal or nondiagnostic material; 7 patients (21 percent) resulted in an inaccurate or misleading diagnosis by cytopathologists blinded to the histopathologic results. This prompted Krohel et al. to recommend FNAB only for patients with strongly suspected metastatic tumors or for those patients with secondary neoplasms, such as sinus tumors, that have been previously biopsied. It should be noted that approximately 50 percent of the lesions sampled in this study would not routinely lend themselves to FNAB.[46]

Problems and Pitfalls

Arguably, the lack of experience due to limited exposure to orbital aspiration specimens may be the greatest threat to diagnostic accuracy.[56] One specific pitfall that may result in false-positive diagnoses is the failure to recognize normal glandular tissue in aspirate material.[57] In their 1984 study, Dekker et al. discussed the possibility that the presence of glandular epithelial inclusions may be the result of inadvertent sampling of the lacrimal gland rather than a neoplasm. FNABs of inflammatory lesions and lymphoproliferative processes are also difficult to accurately diagnose; this is also true of orbital biopsies. Fortunately the treatment for lymphomas and benign lymphoid hyperplasia is similar—radiation therapy. The judicious use of ancillary techniques such as immunocytochemistry is very helpful in this situation. Electron microscopy is another ancillary technique that is quite useful, especially in distinguishing small-round-cell tumors such as neuroblastoma, retinoblastoma, and rhabdomyosarcoma and occasionally in distinguishing eosinophilic granuloma from lymphoma.

Another pitfall is a recurrent theme—the attempt to render specific diagnoses on limited material. Careful selection of appropriate lesions and accurate clinical evaluation as well as adequate sampling will eliminate the tendency to overdiagnose. In addition, several lesions of the orbit and periorbital tissue are fibrous or mesenchymal and therefore difficult to aspirate. Examples of these include meningioma, hemangioma, glioma, fibrous histiocytoma, neurofibroma, and neurilemmoma.[46]

Complications

Needle Tract Seeding

There has always been and will probably continue to be speculation and concern over needle tract seeding (NTS) resulting from FNAB of any body site, including the orbit. Experimental studies, designed to evaluate the risk of tumor dissemination, do indicate that tumor cells may be deposited along the needle tract following aspiration biopsy.[58–62] However, these experimental models are not ideal and the data obtained from these studies fail to correlate with clinical, *in vivo*, observations. Certainly the number of uncontrolled variables increases in the clinical setting. Tumor implantation has been attributed to various factors, including inexperienced operators, the use of large diameter cutting needles and core biopsy needles, a high number of passes, and the absence of normal parenchyma overlying the neoplasm.[63] Presumably, the biologic characteristics of the tumor cells, namely, growth potential, cohesiveness, and the number of cells seeded, play an important role.[64] Engzell et al. have speculated that the number of tumor cells deposited in the needle tract may be too small to maintain viability, especially in the face of a vigorous host response.[58] Both Glasgow et al.[61] and Karioglu et al.[60] identified tumor cells in needle tracts following FNAB on eyes that had been anucleated for diagnosis of melanoma and retinoblastoma, respectively. Both studies used small-gauge needles, 30 gauge and 25 gauge. Quantitative analysis revealed that the number of tumor cells in the tracts was less than that associated with viable tumor growth. This may explain the absence of documented NTS in patients who have had orbital FNAB. Another possibility is the use of indirect FNAB, that is, the use of tumor-free tissue (sclera and conjunctiva) and fluids (vitreous and aqueous humor) to cleanse the needle of tumor cells.[61,65] However, the direct route (transocular or scleral) has not been implicated in NTS in the clinical setting.

Hemorrhage

The majority of studies report no significant morbidity using FNAB with and without radiologic guidance.[47,50–52,56,66,67] There are a few reports of complications that include orbital or conjunctival hemorrhage, motility disturbance, ptosis, blindness, and death.[44,45,68] With the exception of hemorrhage, these complications are extremely rare. Serious consequences, especially those reported by Liu,[68] were related to faulty technique. Several variables may contribute to orbital hemorrhage: technique, location of the mass, patients with increased intraocular pressure, and lack of apparent close clinical monitoring after FNAB. Hemorrhage is more likely to occur if aspiration is used rather than the needle-only technique, if the mass is deep, requiring additional needle passes, and if there is inadequate compression of the globe following FNAB. It is important to note that successful performance and diagnosis of orbital FNAB, similar to FNAB elsewhere, is highly dependent on experience.

MASSES OF THE NECK

It is often difficult to discuss FNAB of the head and neck as a region because it contains so many distinct areas such as salivary gland, oral cavity, thyroid, and so forth. Even considered separately, the neck contains numerous structures, any one of which can develop an inflammatory, infectious, or neoplastic process. The most common mass in the neck to be sampled by FNAB is the enlarged, palpable lymph node, discussed in Chapter 4.

Cysts

Another common neck mass is the cyst. FNAB is often used to confirm the clinical and/or radiologic impression of a cystic lesion. When palpated, these masses can be fluctuant, giving slightly under pressure, or they can be very tense and firm with a distinct curvature felt during examination. The origins of cysts are diverse. Some commonly encountered cysts include branchial cleft cyst and thyroglossal duct cyst (embryologic), abscess (infectious), retention cysts and cystic degeneration of thyroid and salivary gland lesions (degeneration), and lymphangiomas (neoplastic). When the amount of fluid obtained during FNAB exceeds 1 milliliter and/or there is decompression of the mass during aspiration, a cyst has been sampled. The fluid obtained may be clear, turbid, viscous, yellow, or even bloody. The amount of fluid obtained should be recorded and then sent for analysis. The type of analysis selected will be based in part on the clinical data and location of the cyst. For example, crystal-clear fluid obtained from a mass in the midanterior neck may be a

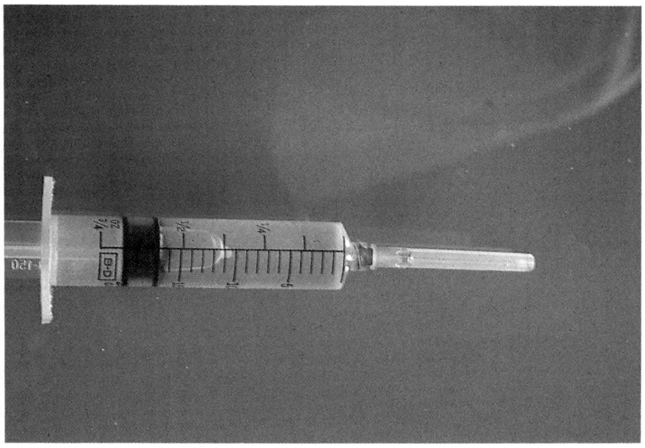

FIGURE 6.19 Parathyroid cyst. Syringe with clear fluid. Cyst did not recur and did not need to be excised. Parathormone level in the fluid was markedly elevated.

parathyroid cyst (Figure 6.19). Cellularity is minimal or absent. If necessary, the fluid may be sent for parathormone analysis rather than microscopy. However, there is no other type of cyst of the neck that has water-clear fluid on aspiration.[69] When thick, creamy material is obtained or if the immediate interpretation indicates neutrophils and debris, then the material should be apportioned with some sent (in a sterile fashion) to microbiology for culture. Blood or blood-tinged fluid should be examined closely for viable cells because this finding may indicate a neoplastic condition.

Branchial Cleft Cyst

These congenital, squamous-lined cysts are most common in the lateral neck, often partially obscured by the sternocleidomastoid muscle. As a result of their location and their predominant cytologic feature, namely, squamous cells and debris, the primary differential diagnosis is squamous cell carcinoma. A clue to the benign nature of this cyst is the presence of mature and

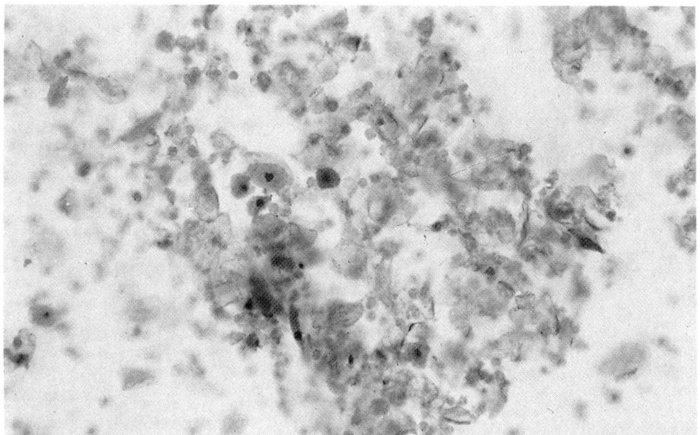

FIGURE 6.20 Branchial cleft cyst. Moderately cellular smear composed of scattered mature squamous cells and granular debris. Papanicolaou 200×.

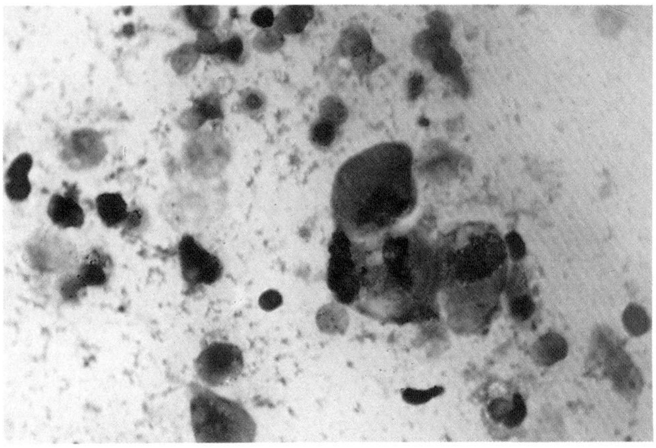

FIGURE 6.21 Branchial cleft cyst. Squamous cells with moderate nuclear atypia. Severe atypia or atypia in the absence of inflammation may require surgical biopsy to exclude squamous cell carcinoma. Differentiating degenerative atypia of a squamous-lined cyst from a necrotic metastatic squamous cell carcinoma can be quite difficult in some cases. Diff-Quik® 400×.

anucleate squamous cells, features quite similar to epidermal inclusion cysts (Figure 6.20). Although most FNABs of branchial cleft cysts consist of squamous cells, germinal center fragments and lymphocytes can be seen if the stromal layer of the cyst is sampled. When acutely inflamed, the resultant squamous atypia can be severe enough to warrant excisional biopsy to confirm the absence of squamous cell carcinoma in patients predisposed to this cancer (Figure 6.21).

BRANCHIAL CLEFT CYST

Mature and anucleate ghost squamous cells

Cellular debris/proteinaceous material

Lymphocytes and occasional germinal centers

****Squamous atypia pronounced if acutely inflamed cyst**

Thyroglossal Duct Cyst

Like branchial cleft cysts, the thyroglossal duct cysts are congenital anomalies most often located in the anterior neck (midline) often at the level of the hyoid bone. FNAB usually recovers varying amounts of cyst fluid with scant cellularity. While thyroid elements may be present, more often rare columnar or squamous cells and scattered inflammatory cells are observed in a dense proteinaceous background. Cholesterol crystals may be plentiful (Figure 6.22). Rarely papillary carcinoma has been documented to occur within these cysts.[70]

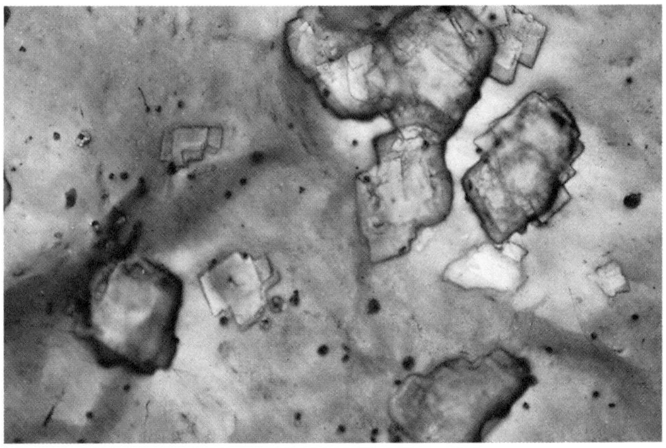

FIGURE 6.22 Thyroglossal duct cyst. Abundant proteinaceous debris, cholesterol crystals, and scattered lymphocytes are often the predominant pattern in these cysts. Diff-Quik® 200×.

THYROGLOSSAL DUCT CYST

Cyst Fluid
- **–Proteinaceous**
- **–Cholesterol crystals**

Scattered squamous or columnar cells

Acute and/or chronic inflammatory cells

Occasional thyroid elements

Lymphoepithelial Cysts

Lymphoepithelial cysts are described in Chapter 2. The incidence of these cysts has increased with the epidemic of infection with the human immunodeficiency virus (HIV) and may be an early as well as late manifestation of HIV infection and subsequent destruction of the immune system.

Infectious Processes

A wide variety of infectious agents responsible for cervical lymphadenopathy and skin and subcutaneous nodules have been diagnosed by FNAB. The increased incidence of immunocompromised patients due to HIV infection, chemo- and radiation therapy, and organ transplantation has also resulted in an increase in routine and unusual infections. The cytologic criteria necessary for the diagnosis of infectious agents are well established, many of which were developed from FNAB material of lymph nodes and other masses in the head and neck region, where FNAB is used routinely in the workup and diagnosis of lymphadenopathy.[32,71–82]

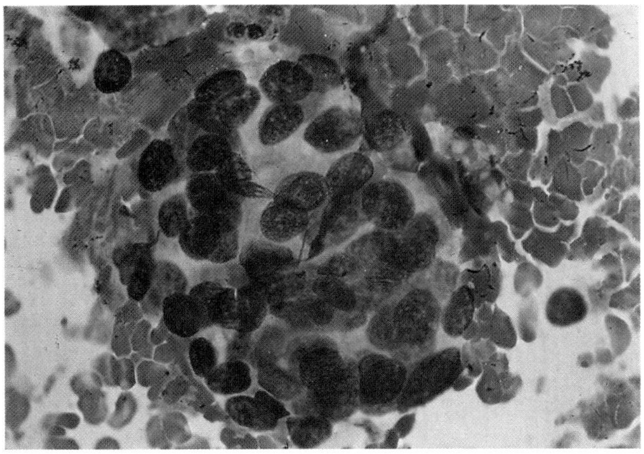

FIGURE 6.23 Carotid body tumor. Cells with uniform, bland oval nuclei arranged in "organoid" or ball-like clusters in a background of blood. Diff-Quik® 600×.

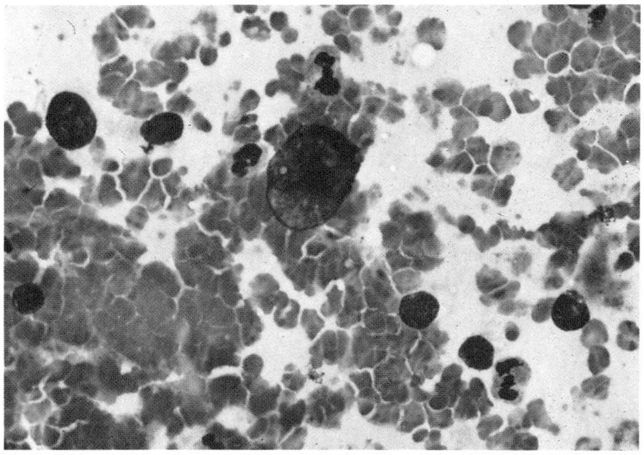

FIGURE 6.24 Carotid body tumor. Scattered cells with giant nuclei, often stripped of cytoplasm. Marked variation in nuclear size is common in the paragangliomas. Diff-Quik® 400×.

Carotid Body Tumor

Paragangliomas, so-called carotid body tumors, are infrequently encountered in FNAB of the neck. They are usually located at the carotid bifurcation and may be adherent to it. As a result, many physicians are reluctant to sample the mass. In addition, the mass is often pulsatile and vigorous palpation can result in a syncopal reaction, especially in older individuals. Carotid body tumors, similar to the thyroid and other endocrine organs, have a rich vascular supply; however, the possibility of extensive hemorrhage is virtually eliminated with the use of fine needles. Perforation of the adjacent carotid is a possibility if the aspirator is inexperienced. Complications have occurred in the past but more recently have not seemed to be a problem with skill and use of very fine needles.[83,84] Direct pressure over the puncture site for several minutes, similar to the procedure used for arterial blood gas punctures, is adequate to control any bleeding.

Cytologically, aspiration of carotid body tumors presents a population of monomorphic cells that are often in clusters or a ball-like arrangement (Figure 6.23). Stripped nuclei of variable sizes may be seen in either a clean background or with blood. A few very large giant nuclei are present that are usually stripped of cytoplasm (Figure 6.24). Because the aspiration morphology of endocrine organs is similar, follicular carcinoma of the thyroid metastatic to the lateral neck, or other carcinomas, particularly non-small cell types from the lung, are also a consideration. It is quite rare for either one of those malignancies to have the free giant nuclei as part of the smear pattern.

CAROTID BODY TUMOR

Cellularity high

Monomorphic cell population
- **–Oval or polygonal medium sized cells**
- **–Rosettes or organoid pattern**
- **–Moderate, slightly granular cytoplasm**
- **–Red (neuroendocrine) granules on Diff-Quik®**
- **–Smooth, round but variably sized nuclei**
- **–Conspicuous nucleoli**
- **–Stripped small or giant nuclei in the background**

***Necrosis and high mitotic rate suggest malignant carotid body tumor**

Ectopic Thyroid

The presence of thyroid tissue outside of the thyroid gland proper is not unusual. The most commonly aspirated sites for ectopic thyroid are retrosternal and anterior mediastinum. In the anterior neck, many of these masses come to the physician's attention when enlargement occurs. This enlargement is often the result of a nonneoplastic process, namely, a goiter, or due to a small amount of bleeding into a goiter. Excision of ectopic thyroid is usually for cosmetic purposes or to eliminate obstruction when the mass is large enough to make breathing or swallowing difficult. The typical aspiration smear will show abundant colloid and bland follicular cells, often in small sheets or follicles.

Cystic fluid containing cholesterol crystals and hemosiderin-laden macrophages may be present, suggesting prior hemorrhage and degeneration. It may not be clear clinically that these nodules of thyroid tissue are separate from the thyroid proper, but nodules of non-neoplastic thyroid can become separated from the thyroid and appear in the neck as an isolated mass. Most ectopic thyroid is in the midline and may appear as a mass at the base of the tongue.[85]

Extracranial Meningioma

Although rare, meningiomas have been sporadically reported to occur in various regions of the head and neck, including the cervical area, orbit, and nasal cavity.[86–90] Aspiration cytology shows small collections of whorled spindle cells with bland uniform nuclei (Figure 6.25). Nucleoli are usually inconspicuous, and occasionally, small nuclear intracytoplasmic inclusions may be seen. The cytoplasm is ill-defined and has a fibrillary quality. Psammoma bodies are rarely encountered in their entirety. Differentiation from squamous cell carcinoma may be a problem, but the cells of meningioma are quite bland. Clinical correlation, particularly with sites in the orbit or nasal cavity, is obviously important.

EXTRACRANIAL MENINGIOMA

Cellularity moderate

Background clean

Small, cohesive collections of spindle cells in whorls
- **–Uniform, oval nuclei**
- **–Bland chromatin**
- **–Inconspicuous nucleoli**
- **–Indistinct cytoplasm**

Occasional psammoma bodies

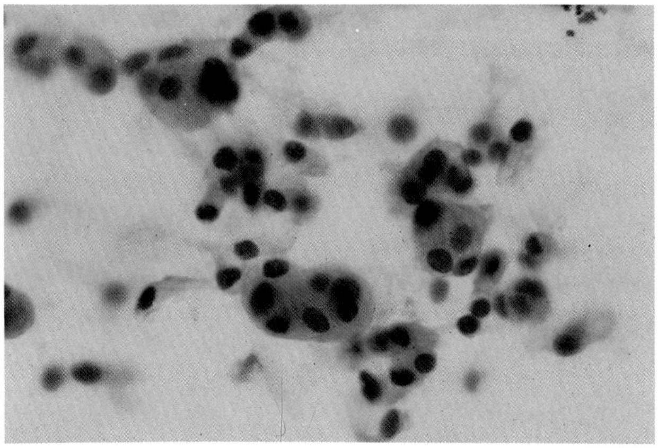

A

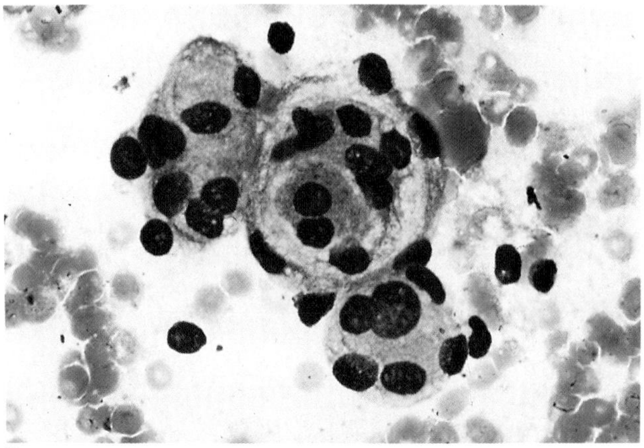

B

FIGURE 6.25 Extracranial meningioma. (A) Clusters of cells without as definitive a picture of whorls of cells as seen in the prior example of orbital meningioma (see Figure 6.17). The cells are bland, oval to slightly spindle-shaped and represent a transitional-type meningioma. Papanicolaou 600×. (B) A more definite whorling pattern is seen at higher magnification. Diff-Quik® 1000×.

Fat Necrosis

While fat necrosis is most often sampled in breast aspirations, it can be encountered in other superficial and deep locations, including the head and neck. The etiology of this process is often related to trauma and/or surgical procedures.[91] In many ways, the aspiration cytology of fat necrosis is similar to granulation tissue—the presence of histiocytes, multinucleated giant cells, and cell debris with chronic inflammation (Figure 6.26). However, fragments of adipose tissue, scattered adipocytes, and foamy-appearing histocytes whose cytoplasm is laden with small fat droplets are the predominant features (Figure 6.27). Although the yield from aspirations of normal adipose tissue is variable due to the lack of adherence to glass slides, this is usually not a problem with fat necrosis. The resolution of this process is usually fibrosis and scar formation.

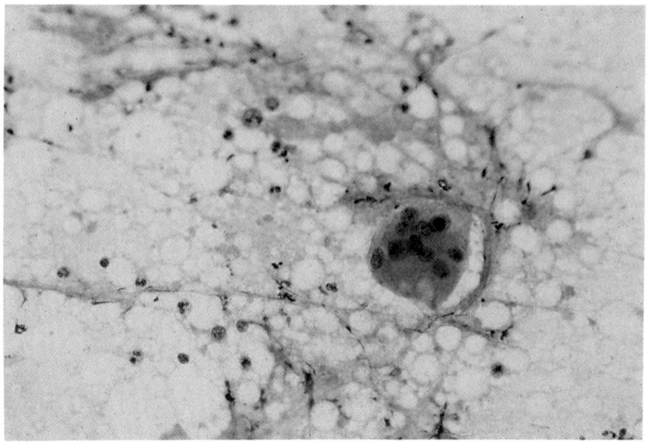

FIGURE 6.26 Fat necrosis. Multinucleated giant cell in a background of inflammation and disrupted adipose tissue. Papanicolaou 400×.

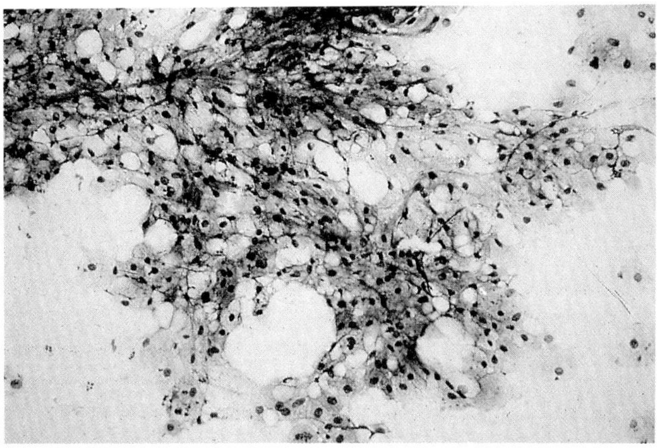

FIGURE 6.27 Fat necrosis. Small vessel traversing loosely cohesive, foamy histiocytes. Adipose tissue and individual fat vacuoles will appear as smooth, punched-out circles of varying sizes in Romanowsky stains. Increased cellularity and a somewhat myxoid appearance with the presence of a capillary blood vessel at the top of the illustration would raise the possibility of a well-differentiated liposarcoma, particularly if the aspiration smear is not considered within the clinical context of the case. Diff-Quik® 200×.

FAT NECROSIS

Cellularity variable

Background microvesicular droplets and cell debris

Loose fragments of fat and stroma

Adipocytes and foamy histiocytes

Scattered chronic inflammation (lymphocytes and plasma cells)

Radiation Effect

Although surgery is the treatment of choice for most neoplasms of the head and neck, radiation therapy is often an adjunctive modality, especially in the treatment of squamous cell carcinomas. Radiation affects the tissues of this region as it does in gynecologic and respiratory cytology. There is a progression from tumor necrosis and the subsequent inflammatory response to healing with granulation tissue and fibrosis. These phases vary in duration and severity. In the head and neck, FNAB is often the initial procedure used to evaluate masses that have arisen in previously treated areas. Its goal is to identify the presence of persistent or recurrent carcinoma; therefore, a positive finding eliminates the need for further workup. However, in the absence of a positive aspirate, the clinician has a more difficult decision—whether or not to biopsy for confirmation of the FNAB findings. In these situations, it is helpful to understand the response of normal tissue to radiation. In general, the cytologic findings should mirror the expected treatment response based upon the time interval. Once again, history is absolutely crucial to the cytopathologist when evaluating these specimens.

No matter what phase is sampled, the hallmark of radiation effect on benign cells is the preservation of a normal nuclear to cytoplasmic ratio. The remaining features associated with radiation effect (multinucleation, bizarre forms, vacuolization) are all secondary to this finding. In the early (acute) phase of treatment response, there may be considerable cell debris, acute inflammation, and scattered foreign body multinucleate giant cells. Aspirate material obtained at this time may suggest infection or abscess as well as an inflammatory process. As time progresses, normal parenchymal elements may or may not be identified, depending on the site sampled. For example, salivary gland may have atrophied, leaving small, atypical intercalated duct cells that can be misinterpreted as carcinoma, while soft tissues of the neck may be only minimally disrupted. Most reported problems with FNAB following aspiration have occurred with breast lesions.[92,23]

As the duration between treatment and aspiration biopsy increases (chronic phase), so does the likelihood that FNAB will yield granulation tissue and/or fibrosis. When granulation tissue becomes exuberant, a mass effect is often palpated. FNAB of these areas may produce abundant material but also may result in some hemorrhage due to the increased vascularity of the region. Aspiration smears typically show scattered fibroblasts and histiocytes in a loose, often myxoid, stroma. Numerous arborizing capillaries and small vessels can be seen throughout these fragments (Figure 6.28). These smears may resemble other fibroblastic proliferations such as nodular fasciitis.

Successful radiation therapy often leaves the skin and underlying tissues extremely firm, secondary to fibrosis and scar formation, making penetration of the tissues by a fine needle difficult. As expected, under these circumstances it is a problem to obtain an adequate sample. At times these smears are often the most treacherous to diagnose because of their scant cellularity and the atypia of the few cells encountered (Figure 6.29). In most cases, the differential diagnosis will be between radiation effect and squamous cell carcinoma. Clues indicating radiation effect include atypical cells with a normal nuclear to cytoplasmic ratio, bland chromatin, cytoplasmic vacuolation, and wispy cytoplasmic processes.

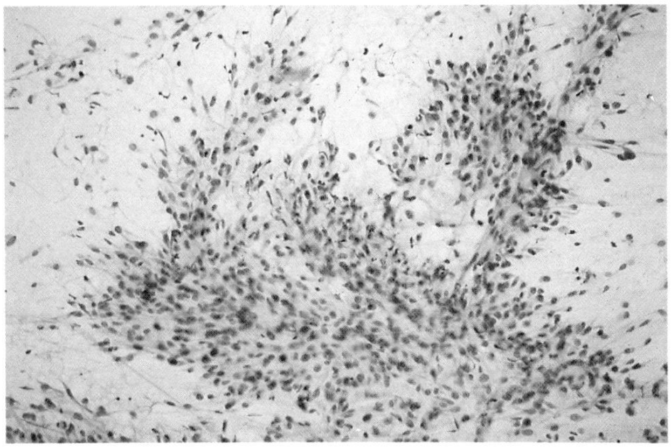

A

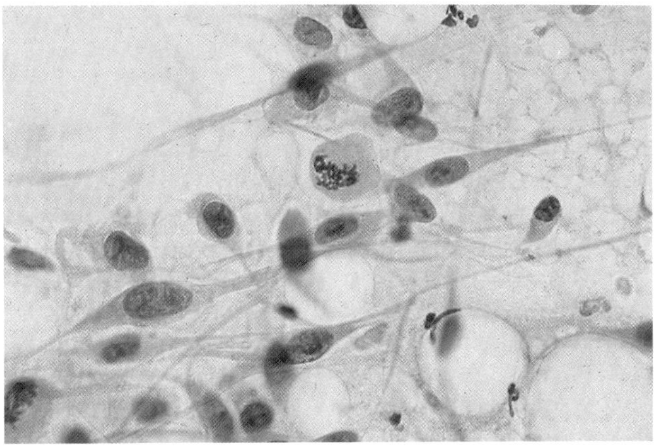

B

FIGURE 6.28 Radiation reaction, early chronic phase. (A) Spindle cells with slender bipolar cytoplasmic processes arranged along arborizing vessels. Mitoses are common in the early phases of a granulation tissue response. Papanicolaou, 400×. (B) Higher magnification demonstrates the details of the proliferating fibroblasts as the repair process evolves following radiation therapy. Note bizarre mitotic figure. Papanicolaou, 1000×.

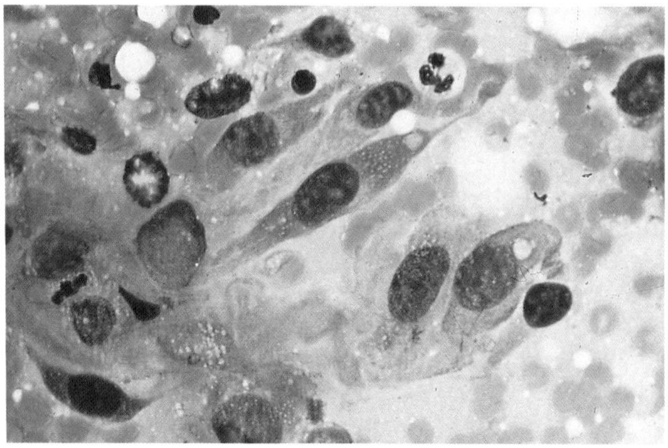

FIGURE 6.29 Radiation reaction, atypia. Fibroblasts with bipolar cytoplasmic processes, large plump nuclei, nucleoli, and clumped chromatin. Nuclear to cytoplasmic ratio is still within normal limits in these actively proliferating fibroblasts. Diff-Quik® 600×.

RADIATION EFFECT (ACUTE PHASE)

Cellularity moderate to high

Abundant acute inflammation

Scattered multinucleated giant cells

Cell debris and necrosis

Nonviable tumor cells may be present immediately posttreatment

RADIATION EFFECT (CHRONIC PHASE)

Cellularity variable
- **–Moderate (Granulation tissue)**
  - **–Loosely cohesive fragments**
  - **–Fibroblasts with atypia, plump I histiocytes**
  - **–Capillaries and small vessels, arborizing pattern**
  - **–"Dirty" background—cell debris and blood**
- **Scant (Fibrosis)**
  - **–Scattered small fragments of hyalinized collagen (usually obtained with 22-gauge rather than 23 to 27-gauge needles)**
  - **–Single, isolated atypical fibroblasts**
  - **–Relatively clean background**

REFERENCES

1. Frable WJ, Frable MA. Thin needle aspiration biopsy: The diagnosis of head and neck tumors revisited. *Cancer* 1979;43:1541–1548.
2. Russ JE, Scanlon EF, Christ MA. Aspiration cytology of head and neck masses. *Am J Surg* 1978; 136:342–347.
3. Meyers DS, Templer J, Davis WE, Balch JA. Aspiration cytology for the diagnosis of head and neck masses. *Otolaryngology* 1978;86:650–655.
4. Mondal A, Mukherjee D, Chaterjee DN, Saha AM, Mukerjee AL. Fine needle aspiration biopsy cytology in diagnosis of cervical lymphadenopathies. *J Ind Med Assoc* 1989;87:281–283.
5. Abram AC, Nabizadeh S, Feldman PS, Cantrell RW, Levine PA. Fine needle aspiration (FNA) in diagnosing recurrent squamous cell carcinoma of the head and neck: Truth or consequences? *Laryngoscope* 1993;103:1073–1075.
6. Banks ER, Frierson HF, Covell JL. Fine needle aspiration cytologic findings in metastatic basaloid squamous cell carcinoma of the head and neck. *Acta Cytol* 1992;36:126–131.
7. Oyafuso MS, Longatto FA, Ikeda MK. The role of fine-needle aspiration cytology in the diagnosis of

head and neck excluding the thyroid and salivary glands. *Tumori* 1992;78:134–136.

8. Schwartz R, Chan NH, MacFarlane JK. Fine needle aspiration cytology in the evaluation of head and neck masses. *Am J Surg* 1990;159:482–485.

9. van den Brekel MWM, Castelijins JA, Stel HV, Luth WJ, Valk J, van der Waal I, Snow GB. Occult metastatic disease: Detection with US and US-guided fine-needle aspiration cytology. *Radiology* 1991;180: 457–461.

10. Linsk AJ, Franzen S. *Clinical aspiration cytology,* 2nd ed. New York: J.B. Lippincott Co., 1989, p. 40.

11. Lubis MND. The technical procedure and the value of fine needle aspiration biopsy of the nasopharynx. *Pathology* 1993;25:35–38.

12. Fechner RE, Mills, SE. *Atlas of Tumor Pathology. Tumors of the Bones and Joints.* Washington, DC: Armed Forces Institute of Pathology, 1992, pp. 101, 112, 113, 118, 119, 174, 181–182, 218, 219.

13. Ramzy I, Aufdemorte TB, Duncan DL. Diagnosis of radio lucent lesions of the jaw by fine needle aspiration biopsy. *Acta Cytol* 1985;29:419–424.

14. Stormby N, Akerman N. Cytodiagnosis of bone lesions by means of fine needle aspiration biopsy. *Acta Cytol* 1973;17:166–172.

15. Sneige N, Ayala AG, Corrasco CH, Murray J, Raymond AK. Giant cell tumor of bone: A cytologic study of 24 cases. *Diagn Cytopathol* 1985;1:111–117.

16. Powers CN, Bull JM, Raval P, Schmidt WA. Fine-needle aspiration of a solitary pulmonary nodule following treatment of metastatic giant-cell tumor of bone. *Diagn Cytopathol* 1991;7:286–289.

17. Sanerkin NG. Malignancy, aggressiveness, and recurrence in giant cell tumor of bone. *Cancer* 1980; 46:1641–1649.

18. Das DK, Gupta SK, Sehgal S. Extramedullary plasma cell tumors: Diagnosis by fine needle aspiration cytology. *Diagn Cytopathol* 1986;2:248–251.

19. Powers CN, Wakely PE, Silverman JF, Kornstein MJ, Frable WJ. Fine needle aspiration biopsy of extramedullary plasma cell tumors. *Mod Pathol* 1990; 3:648–653.

20. Koss LG, Woyke S, Olszewski O. *Aspiration biopsy: Cytologic interpretation and histologic bases,* 2nd ed. New York: Igaku-Shoin, 1992, p. 651.

21. Geisinger KR, Buss DH, Kawamoto EH, Ahl EJ. Multiple myeloma: The diagnostic role and prognostic significance of exfoliative cytology. *Acta Cytol* 1986; 30:334–340.

22. Elson CE, Johnston WW. Cytology of plasma cell neoplasms (abstract). *Acta Cytol* 1989;33:726.

23. Dahlin DC, Unni KK. *Bone tumors. General aspects and data on 8,542 cases,* 4th ed. Springfield, IL: Charles C. Thomas, 1986, pp. 270–271.

24. Thommesen P, Frederiksen P. Fine needle aspiration biopsy of bone lesions. Clinical value. *Acta Orthop Scand* 1976;47:137–143.

25. DeSantos LA, Murray JA, Ayala AG. The value of percutaneous needle biopsy in the management of primary bone tumors. *Cancer* 1979; 43: 735–744.

26. Layfield LJ, Glasgow BJ, Anders KH, Mirra JM. Fine needle aspiration cytology of primary bone lesions. *Acta Cytol* 1987;31:177–184.

27. Ayala AG, Raymond AK, Ro JY, Carrasco CH, Fanning CV, Murray JA. Needle biopsy of primary bone lesions: M.D. Anderson experience. *Pathol Ann* 1989;24:219–251.

28. Das DK, Gulati A, Bhatt NC, Mandal AK, Khan VA, Bhambhani S. Fine needle aspiration cytology of oral and pharyngeal lesions: A study of 45 cases. *Acta Cytol* 1993;37:333–342.

29. Castelli M, Gattuso P, Reyes C, Solans EP. Fine needle aspiration biopsy of intraoral and pharyngeal lesions. *Acta Cytol* 1993;37:448–450.

30. Gunhan O, Dogan N, Celasun B, Sengun O, Onder T, Finci R. Fine needle aspiration cytology of oral cavity and jaw bone lesions: A report of 102 cases. *Acta Cytol* 1993;37:135–141.

31. Mondal A, Raychourdhuri BK. Peroral fine needle aspiration cytology of parapharyngeal lesions. *Acta Cytol* 1993;37:694–698.

32. Das DK, Bhatt NC, Khan VA, Luthra UK. Cervicofacial actinomycosis: Diagnosis by fine needle aspiration cytology. *Acta Cytol* 1989;33:278–280.

33. Chan MKM, McGuire LJ, Lee JCK. Fine needle aspiration cytodiagnosis of nasopharyngeal carcinoma in cervical lymph nodes: A study of forty cases. *Acta Cytol* 1989;33:344–350.

34. Powers CN, Raval P, Schmidt WA. Fine needle aspiration cytology of metastatic lymphoepithelioma: A case report. *Acta Cytol* 1989;33: 254-258.

35. Koss LG, Woyke S, Olszewski W. *Aspiration biopsy. Cytologic interpretation and histologic bases,* 2nd ed. New York: Igaku-Shoin, 1992, pp. 247–248.

36. Kornstein MJ, Kardos TF, Wakely PE Jr., et al. Dendritic reticulum cells and immunophenotype in fine needle aspirates of lymph nodes: Value in the subclassification of non-Hodgkin's lymphomas. *Am J Clin Pathol* 1990;94:165–169.

37. Fagan MF, Rone R. Esthesioneuroblastoma: Cytologic features with differential diagnostic considerations. *Diagn Cytopathol* 1985;1:322–326.

38. Wozniak JM, Rak J. Cytologic appearance of esthesioneuroblastoma in a fine needle aspirate. *Acta Cytol* 1988;32:377–380.

39. True LD. *Atlas of diagnostic immunohistopathology.* Philadelphia: J.B. Lippincott Co., 1990, pp. 11:16–11:17.

40. Naib ZM. Cytology of ocular lesions. *Acta Cytol* 1972;16:178–185.

41. Glasgow BJ, Foos RY. *Ocular cytopathology.* Stoneham, MA: Butterworth-Heinemann, 1992.

42. Westman-Naeser S, Naeser P. Tumors of the orbit diagnosed by fine needle biopsy. *Acta Ophthalmol* 1978;56:969–976.

43. Augsberger JJ, Shields JA, Folberg R, Lang W, O'Hara BJ, Claricci JD. Fine needle aspiration biopsy in the diagnosis of intraocular cancer: Cytologic-histologic correlations. *Ophthalmology* 1985;92:39–49.

44. Kennerdell JS, Dekker A, Johnson B, Dunois PJ. Fine needle aspiration biopsy: Its use in orbital tumors. *Arch Ophthalmol* 1979;97:1315–1317.

45. Kennerdell JS, Dekker A, Johnson BL. Orbital fine needle aspiration biopsy: The results of its use in 50 patients. *Neuro-Ophthalmology* 1980;1:117–121.

46. Kennerdell JS, Slamovits TL, Dekker, A, Johnson BL. Orbital fine-needle aspiration biopsy. *Am J Ophthalmol* 1985;99:547–551.

47. Zajdela A, Vielh P, Schlienger P, Haye C. Fine-needle cytology of 292 palpable orbital and eyelid tumors. *Am J Clin Pathol* 1990;93:100–104.

48. Dresner SC, Kennerdell JS, Dekker A. Fine needle aspiration biopsy of metastatic orbital tumors. *Survey Ophthalmol* 1983;27:397–398.

49. Zajdela A, deMaublanc MA, Schlienger P, Haye C. Cytologic diagnosis of orbital and periorbital palpable tumors using fine-needle sampling without aspiration. *Diagn Cytopathol* 1986;2:17–20.

50. Dubois PJ, Kennerdell JS, Rosenbaum AE, Dekker A, Johnson BR, Swink CA. Computed tomographic localization for fine needle aspiration biopsy of orbital tumors. *Radiology* 1979;131:149–152.

51. Spoor TC, Kennerdell JS, Dekker A, Johnson BL, Rehkopf D. Orbital fine needle aspiration biopsy with B-scan guidance. *Am J Ophthalmol* 1980;89: 274–277.

52. Czerniak B, Woyke S, Daniel B, Krzysztolik Z, Koss LG. Diagnosis of orbital tumors by aspiration biopsy guided by computerized tomography. *Cancer* 1984;54:2385–2389.

53. Arora R, Rewari R, Betheria SM. Fine-needle aspiration cytology of eyelid tumors. *Acta Cytol* 1990;34:227–239.

54. Dey P, Radhika S, Rajwanshi A, Ray R, Nijhawan R, Das A. Fine needle aspiration biopsy of orbital and eyelid lesions. *Acta Cytol* 1993;37:903–907.

55. Krohel GB, Tobin DR, Chavis RM. Inaccuracy of fine needle aspiration biopsy. *Ophthalmology* 1985;92:666–670.

56. Augsburger JJ, Shields JA. Fine needle aspiration biopsy of solid intraocular tumors: Indications, instrumentation, and techniques. *Ophthal Surg* 1984; 15:34–40.

57. Dekker A, Johnson BL, Kennerdell JS. Occurrence of benign glandular tissue in orbital aspirates: Importance of recognizing its lacrimal gland origin. *Acta Cytol* 1984;28:171–174.

58. Engzell U, Esposti PL, Rubio C, Sigurdson A, Zajicek J. Investigation on tumor spread in connection with aspiration biopsy. *Acta Radiol Ther Phys Biol* 1971;10:385–397.

59. Ryd W, Hagmar B, Eriksson O. Local tumor seeding by fine-needle aspiration biopsy. *Acta Pathol Microbiol Immunol Scand (A)* 1983; 91:17–21.

60. Karcioglu ZA, Gordon RA, Karcioglu GL. Tumor seeding in ocular fine needle aspiration biopsy. *Ophthalmology* 1985;92:1763–1767.

61. Glasgow BJ, Brown HH, Zargoza AM, Foos RY. Quantitation of tumor seeding from fine needle aspiration of ocular melanomas. *Am J Ophthalmol* 1988;105:538–546.

62. Owen ER, Kark AE. Fine-needle aspiration of tumours. *Lancet* 1989;1(8651):1384–1385.

63. Roussel F, Dalion J, Benozio M. The risk of tumoral seeding in needle biopsies. *Acta Cytol* 1989; 33:936–939.

64. Haddad FS, Somsin AA. Seeding and perineal implantation of prostatic cancer in the track of the biopsy needle: Three case reports and a review of the literature. *J Surg Oncol* 1987;35:184–191.

65. Jakobiec FA, Coleman DJ, Chattock A, Smith M. Ultrasonically guided needle biopsy and cytologic diagnosis of solid intraocular tumors. *Ophthalmology* 1979;86:1662–1678.

66. Meyer E, Malberger E, Gdal-On M, Zonis S. Fine-needle aspiration of orbital lesions. *Ann Ophthalmol* 1983;15:635–638.

67. Westman-Naeser S, Naeser P. Tumors of the orbit diagnosed by fine needle biopsy. *Acta Ophthalmol* 1978;56:969–976.

68. Liu D. Complications of fine needle aspiration biopsy of the orbit. *Ophthalmology* 1985;92: 1768–1771.

69. Lowhagen T, Tamo EM, Skoog L. Salivary glands and rare head and neck lesions. In Bibbo M. (ed.), *Comprehensive cytopathology*. Philadelphia: W.B. Saunders Co., 1991, p. 641.

70. Pitts W, Tani E, Skoog L. Papillary carcinoma in fine needle aspiration smears of a thyroglossal duct lesion. *Acta Cytol* 1988;32:599–601.

71. Silverman JF (ed.). *Guides to clinical aspiration biopsy. Infectious and inflammatory diseases and other nonneoplastic disorders*. New York: Igaku-Shoin, 1991.

72. Ashton PR. Infectious organisms in cytologic material. *Lab Med* 1983;14:227–233.

73. Bailey TM, Akhtar M, Ali MA. Fine needle aspiration biopsy in the diagnosis of tuberculosis. *Acta Cytol* 1985;29:732–736.

74. Cavett JR, McAfee R, Ramzy I. Hansen's disease (leprosy). Diagnosis by aspiration biopsy of lymph nodes. *Acta Cytol* 1986;30:189–193.

75. Covell JL, Feldman PS. Identification of infectious microorganisms. In Silverman JF (ed.), *Guides to clinical aspiration biopsy. Infectious and inflammatory*

diseases and other nonneoplastic disorders. New York: Igaku-Shoin, 1991, pp. 47–81.

76. Finfer MD, Perchick A, Burstein DE. Fine needle aspiration biopsy diagnosis of tuberculous lymphadenitis in patients with and without the acquired immunodeficiency syndrome. *Acta Cytol* 1991;35: 325–332.

77. Greaves TS, Strigle SM. The recognition of *Pneumocystis carinii* in routine Papanicolaou-stained smears. *Acta Cytol* 1985;29:714–720.

78. Gupta AK, Nayar M, Chandra M. Reliability and limitations of fine needle aspiration cytology of lymphadenopathies: An analysis of 1,261 cases. *Acta Cytol* 1991;35:777–783.

79. Johnston WW. The cytopathology of opportunistic infections of the lung and other body sites. In Weid GL, Koss LA, Reagan JW (eds.), *Compendium on diagnostic cytology*. Chicago: International Academy of Cytology, 1983, pp. 282–294.

80. Kardos TF. Lymph nodes. In Silverman JF (ed.), *Guides to clinical aspiration biopsy. Infectious and inflammatory diseases and other nonneoplastic disorders*. New York: Igaku-Shoin, 1991, pp. 105–137.

81. Metre MS, Jayaram G. Acid fast bacilli in aspiration smears from tuberculous lymph nodes: An analysis of 255 cases. *Acta Cytol* 1987; 31: 17–19.

82. Pollock PG, Koontz FP, Vina TF. Cervicofacial actinomycosis. Rapid diagnosis by fine needle aspiration. *Arch Otolaryngol* 1978;101:491–494.

83. Engzell U, Franzen J, Zajicek J. Aspiration biopsy of tumors of the neck: II, Cytologic findings in 13 cases of carotid body tumors. *Acta Cytol* 1971; 15:25–30.

84. Hood IC, Qizilbash AH, Young JEM, Archibald SD. Fine needle aspiration biopsy cytology of paragangliomas: Cytologic light microscopic and ultrastructural studies of three cases. *Acta Cytol* 1983; 27:651–657.

85. Rosai J, Carcangiu ML, DeLellis RA. *Atlas of tumor pathology. Tumors of the thyroid gland*. Washington D.C.: Armed Forces Institute of Pathology, 1992, pp. 318–320.

86. Dusenbery D, Ducatman BS, Fetter TW. Extradural spinal meningioma presenting as a neck mass. Diagnosis by aspiration cytology. *Arch Pathol Lab Med* 1987;111:483–485.

87. Gonzalez-Campora R, Otal-Salavverri C, Hevia-Vazquez A. Fine needle aspiration of recurrent ectopic meningioma. *Acta Cytol* 1989;33:85–88.

88. Solares J, Lacruz C. Fine needle aspiration cytology diagnosis of an extracranial meningioma presenting as a cervical mass. *Acta Cytol* 1987;31:502–504.

89. Rorat E, Yang W, DeLaTorre R. Fine needle aspiration cytology of parapharyngeal meningioma. *Acta Cytol* 1991;35:497–500.

90. Bose S, Kapila K, Sarkar C, Verma K. Fine-needle aspiration cytology meningiomas with unusual presentations. *Diagn Cytopathol* 1988;4:258–261.

91. Walker WP, Smith RJH, Cohen MB. Fine-needle aspiration biopsy of subcutaneous fat necrosis of the newborn. *Diagn Cytopathol* 1993;9:329–332.

92. Ku NK, Mela NJ, Fiorica JV, et al. Role of fine needle aspiration cytology after lumpectomy. *Acta Cytol* 1994;38:927–932.

93. Peterse JL, Thunnissen FBJM, van Heerde P. Fine needle aspiration cytology of radiation-induced changes in nonneoplastic breast lesions. Possible pitfalls in cytodiagnosis. *Acta Cytol* 1989;33:176–180.

Index